COAGULATION AND BLOOD TRANSFUSION

DEVELOPMENTS IN HEMATOLOGY AND IMMUNOLOGY

Volume 26

The titles published in this series are listed at the end of this volume.

Coagulation and Blood Transfusion

Proceedings of the Fifteenth Annual Symposium on Blood Transfusion, Groningen 1990, organized by the Red Cross Blood Bank Groningen-Drenthe

edited by

C.Th. SMIT SIBINGA
Red Cross Blood Bank Groningen-Drenthe, The Netherlands

P.C. DAS
Red Cross Blood Bank Groningen-Drenthe, The Netherlands

and

P.M. MANNUCCI
Haemophila and Thrombosis Centre, Milan, Italy

SPRINGER SCIENCE+BUSINESS MEDIA, B.V.

Library of Congress Cataloging-in-Publication Data

International Symposium on Blood Transfusion (15th : 1990 : Groningen, Netherlands)
Coagulation and blood transfusion : proceedings of the Fifteenth International Symposium on Blood Transfusion, Groningen, 1990 / organised by the Red Cross Blood Bank Groningen-Drenthe ; edited by C. Th. Smit Sibinga, P.C. Das, P.M. Mannucci.
p. cm. -- (Developments in hematology and immunology ; v. 26)
Includes index.
ISBN 978-1-4613-6740-6 ISBN 978-1-4615-3900-1 (eBook)
DOI 10.1007/978-1-4615-3900-1
1. Blood--Transfusion--Congresses. 2. Blood--Coagulation--Congresses. I. Smit Sibinga, C. Th. II. Das, P. C. III. Mannucci, P. M. (Pier Mannuccio) IV. Stichting Rode Kruis Bloedbank Groningen/Drente. V. Title. VI. Series: Developments in hematology and immunology ; 26.
[DNLM: 1. Blood Coagulation--congresses. 2. Blood Transfusion--congresses. W1 DE997VZK v. 26 / WH 310 I585c 1990]
RM171.I564 1990
615'.39--dc20
DNLM/DLC
for Library of Congress 91-20824

ISBN 978-1-4613-6740-6

Printed on acid-free paper

Baxter

Acknowledgement

This publication has been made possible through the support of Baxter, which is gratefully acknowledged.

CONTENTS

Moderators and speakers XI

Foreword XIII

I. Principles and fundamentals

The mechanisms of thrombin formation
H.C. Hemker 3

Structure-function relationships of human coagulation proteins
L.W. Hoyer 17

The role of calcium in coagulation and anticoagulation
M.E. Mikaelsson 29

Effect of blood collection on the hemostatic potential of coagulation proteins
R. Pflugshaupt 39

Factor VIII yields from anticoagulant exchanged Haemonetics Ultralite™ plasma
J. Speak 49

Discussion 55

II.Preservation aspects

Platelet function preservation
S. Holme 67

Platelet adhesion to the vessel wall
J.J. Sixma 83

Trends in the production and use of coagulation factor concentrates
J.K. Smith 93

Immunoaffinity purification of Factor VIII/von Willebrand factor complex
K. Koops 103

Structural and functional properties of recombinant coagulation factors
A. Pavirani 119

Discussion 125

III. LABORATORY ASPECTS

Platelet counting and function testing
B. Brozovic 137

Selection of platelet apheresis donors for alloimmunized patients by ELISA platelet crossmatch versus HLA-matching
K. Sintnicolaas 151

Clinical efficacy of platelet concentrates
J.Th.M. de Wolf 159

Principles of coagulation factor assays
A.M.H.P. van den Besselaar 165

Standardization of clotting factor assays
T.W. Barrowcliffe 175

Protein C and S in swiss blood donors
R. Pflugshaupt 187

Clinical efficacy of clotting factor concentrates: survival, recovery and hemostatic capacity
I.M. Nilsson 193

Discussion 207

IV. Clinical consequences

Principles in the treatment of bleeding
P.M. Mannucci 219

The effect of chronic exposure to clotting factor concentrates on the immune system
C.R.M. Hay 227

Liver transplantation and blood usage
R.A.F. Krom 241

The use of aprotinin in cardiopulmonary bypass and the impact on hemostasis and blood transfusion
W. van Oeveren 247

Discussion 251

Index 263

MODERATORS AND SPEAKERS

Moderators

P.M. Mannucci (chairman)	– Haemophilia and Thrombosis Centre Angelo Bianchi Bonomi Milan, I
P.C. Das	– Red Cross Blood Bank Groningen-Drenthe Groningen, NL
L.W. Hoyer	– American Red Cross The Jerome H. Holland Laboratory Rockville, MD, USA
M. Mikaelsson	– Kabi Biopharma Stockholm, S
J.J. Sixma	– Department of Haematology University Hospital Utrecht Utrecht, NL
C.Th. Smit Sibinga	– Red Cross Blood Bank Groningen-Drenthe Groningen, NL
J.Th.M. de Wolf	– Department of Internal Medicine University of Groningen Groningen, NL

Speakers

T.W. Barrowcliffe	– National Institute for Biological Standards and Control Potters Bar, UK
A.M.H.P. van den Besselaar	– RELAC, University Hospital Leiden Leiden, NL

B. Brozovic – North London Blood Transfusion Centre
London, UK

C. Hay – Royal Liverpool Hospital
Liverpool, UK

S. Holme – American Red Cross Blood Services
Tidewater Region Norfolk, VA, USA

K. Koops – Bio-Intermediair
Groningen, NL

R.A.F. Krom – Mayo Clinics
Rochester, MN, USA

T. Lindhout – Department of Biochemistry
University of Limburg
Maastricht, NL

I.M. Nilsson – Allmänna Hospital
University of Lund
Malmö, S

A. Pavirani – Transgene
Strassbourg, F

R. Pflugshaupt – Blood Transfusion Service of the
Swiss Red Cross
Bern, CH

K. Sintnicolaas – Dr. Daniël den Hoed Kliniek
Rotterdam, NL

J.K. Smith – Plasma Fractionation Laboratory
Churchill Hospital
Oxford, UK

Prepared discussants

J. Speak – Manchester Royal Infirmary
Department of Haematology
Manchester, UK

FOREWORD

With great pleasure I welcome you to the City of Groningen. In more than one way there is cause for celebration.

Today marks the third lustrum of the annual international symposium on blood transfusion, organized by the Rode Kruis Bloedbank Groningen-Drenthe. In my opinion it has been a remarkable initiative of the Bloedbank, to start organizing a scientific conference, as it did, in 1976. It meant, among others, that in case of success the initiative would grow to be an annual item on the international congress calender. It also meant that a possible third lustrum would coincide with the celebration of the 950th anniversary of the City of Groningen.

I am happy to note that the initiative has been successful: over the past fourteen years the Rode Kruis Bloedbank Groningen-Drenthe has succeeded in organizing an annual symposium on blood transfusion, with a different theme each year, and with an average attendance of 250 participants from some 26 countries world-wide. The platform created with the special formula of the symposium, for science and industry, has been well balanced and beneficial to both.

Mr. Chairman, ladies and gentlemen, I like to compliment the organizers with the success that they have attained. Allow me to mention the name of just one person, in whom I like to thank everyone who has been involved in creating the annual Bloedbank-symposia: my warm congratulations to Dr. Smit Sibinga and his staff.

I mentioned the anniversary of the City of Groningen. Throughout this festive year a large number of activities has been programmed, ranging from the ribbons that decorate two of our famous church towers, to scientific, cultural and sports events.

Many of these activities have an international character, which is not at all surprising since Groningen has a great number of international contacts. Among others and in particular in the field of education and science.

With our University, our Institutes for Higher Professional Training, and the State Agricultural College we accommodate some 35,000 students at a total of 150 branches of study. Scientific research is directed towards commercial pathways through the Zernike Science Park: an important link between training, research and the business-community, moreover it helps high-tech companies to a solid start.

The University's Transfer Point gives advise to companies with problems in the field of process-technology or organization.

And, as you know, the Rode Kruis Bloedbank Groningen-Drenthe is located in our city. I assure you that we are proud of the prominent position that the Bloedbank has internationally in professional circles. I am sure that this symposium will not be the last in the Rode Kruis Bloedbank Groningen-Drenthe tradition!

A.A.M.F. Staatsen
Mayor of the City of Groningen

I. PRINCIPLES AND FUNDAMENTALS

THE MECHANISMS OF THROMBIN FORMATION

H.C. Hemker, S. Béguin and T. Lindhout

The formation of thrombin in the blood results from a complicated series of chemical and physical interactions; its subsequent inactivation also. In vivo these opposite mechanisms (activation-inactivation) are tuned so precisely that the blood remains fluid in the vessels but any leak is promptly mended. When this equilibrium is disrupted either bleeding or thrombosis will ensue. It is readily possible at this moment to give a plausible scheme of the biochemical reactions that contribute to the formation and to the disappearance of thrombin. It is considered common knowledge that there exist two pathways that explain the mechanism of the coagulation of blood: the intrinsic pathway operative when coagulation is started by contact of blood with glass or other foreign surfaces, and the extrinsic pathway triggered by the addition of tissue thromboplastin. In both cases, calcium is essential. However, these standard schemes of blood coagulation are essentially based on in vitro experiments. They perfectly explain why blood clots in glass or under the influence of a large excess of tissue factor. These situations will not however necessarily apply in vivo. Recent research allows to obtain an idea of what reactions that are biochemically possible indeed are of physiological importance.

In the course of the years many accessory reactions, not featuring in the classical schemes have been demonstrated to be possible in vitro but it remains difficult to see which of them are of importance in vivo and which are not. For instance in 1976, Hurlet-Birk Jensen, Josso and Béguin [1] produced evidence for thrombin formation in the very early stage of hemostasis before clotting occurred. This was done by means of the measurement of the activation of factors V and VIII in the blood flowing from a wound in normal and congenitally deficient subjects i.e. in a setup that approaches in vivo conditions. It is one of the main tasks of clotting physiology today to find out what reactions are playing under this type of conditions. In general, the (patho)physiology of hemostasis and thrombosis has a wider scope than the study of interactions of isolated coagulation factors. This has to be kept in mind while reading a review on coagulation biochemistry.

The basis of the physiology of the coagulation were established in the second part of the XIXth century. After the discovery of thrombin (Buchanan 1836-1845, Schmidt 1861-1892) the definition of fibrinogen (Virchow 1856, Denis 1859) and its isolation by Hammarsten (1876-1880), the demonstration of the important role of calcium in coagulation (Arthus and Pages 1890) and finally the discovery of "prothrombin" by Pekelharing in 1895, Morawitz in 1905 proposed the first coherent model of coagulation, which will then be maintained during some forty years. In 1940 Seegers purified "prothrombin" (i.e. what is now known to be a mixture of the factors II, VII, IX and X). This opened the era of modern biochemical coagulation research. Yet, still in 1947, only two proteins of coagulation were sufficiently defined: fibrinogen and prothrombin. In that year Owren published his study on factor V (proaccelerin). Concomitantly Owren created a methodology which allowed the discovering of ten clotting factors. In 1964, the hypothesis of a "cascade" of enzymatic reactions was advanced by Macfarlane [2] and Davie and Ratnoff [3]. This was the trigger for many enzyme mechanistic studies that led to the establishment of a reaction sequence. We will first discuss the modern version of this reaction sequence (A), then the reactions by which the velocity of thrombin formation is maintained within the required limits (B), and finally the inhibitory reactions (C). We limit our discussion to the formation and leave out the actual clotting reaction, i.e. the action of thrombin on fibrinogen. Usually, these days fibrinogen is discussed in extenso in reviews of fibrinolysis.

A. The basic mechanisms of thrombin formation

Limited proteolysis

The backbone of the blood coagulation mechanism is a series of enzyme activations by limited proteolysis. Studies on digestive proteolytic enzymes [(chymo-)trypsin, pepsin, etc.] and their zymogens have made proenzyme → enzyme conversions of proteolytic enzymes one of the main subjects of classical enzymology [4-6]. The main chain of tissue thromboplastin induced proteolytic activations in blood is:

$$\text{VII} \Rightarrow \text{X} \Rightarrow \text{II}$$ [1]

1. In this and subsequent reaction schemes, the open arrow (⇒)represents proteolytic activation and not chemical conversion. Square brackets ([]) indicate enzymatically active complexes. PK=prekallikrein, TF=tissue factor, PL=phospholipid. Roman numerals indicate the factors: II=prothrombin, etc.

For intrinsic coagulation the main chain of actions is:

$$PK \Rightarrow XII \Rightarrow XI \Rightarrow IX \Rightarrow X \Rightarrow II$$

All the non-activated clotting factors participating in these chains are proenzymes of serine proteases, the activated enzymes consequently are serine proteases.

Biocatalysis at surfaces

In free aquous solution, the proteolytic activations shown above can be obtained, but they are accelerated up to 100,000 fold however by the presence of a phospholipid interface and specific protein cofactors. To illustrate this mechanism we will take the activation of prothrombin as an example. Factor X_a is capable to generate thrombin from prothrombin in free solution, but only in a very ineffective mechanism [7-9]. Hanahan and Papahadjopoulos [10] were the first to observe that an active prothrombinase exists only in preparations that contain the three components FX_a, FV_a and phospholipid. (The question of factor V activation will be discussed later.) Hemker et al [11] showed that the generation of prothrombinase activity can be described as the reversible formation of a complex of FX_a, FV, Ca^{++} and phospholipid. In series of very elegant experiments Rosing et al [12] later showed that phospholipids diminish the K_m for prothrombin conversion (a typical change would be from 3000 nM to 30 nM) whereas factor V_a increases the turnover number (k_{cat}) about 1000 fold.

Further investigations [13-19] showed that the change in K_m is caused by the fact that the lipid bound enzyme has a higher affinity for the substrate then the free enzyme has. The change in k_{cat} is probably brought about by an alignment of the active site of factor X_a to the vulnerable sites of factor II caused by their mutual interaction with factor V_a. In 1967 Hemker and Kahn [20] found that the factor X activating enzyme consists of the factors VIII_a and IX_a and phospholipid, forming a complex completely analogous to the prothrombinase complex. Later, van Dieijen et al [21] showed that in this complex the kinetic effects of phospholipids (on K_m) and factor VIII_a (on k_{cat}) were similar to those of phospholipid and factor V_a in the prothrombinase complex. Apart from their kinetic effect on k_{cat}, the factors V_a and VIII_a also serve to better bind their respective enzymes (FX_a and FIX_a) to phospholipid [22,23].

The available data, mainly from the laboratory of Nemerson [24] indicate clearly that factor VII and tissue thromboplastin form a complex that is again comparable to thrombinase. In this case the protein cofactor and the phospholipid are intimately bound but the mechanistic role of the protein cofactor, like factor V_a, seems to be to enhance the efficiency of the enzyme whereas the lipid serves to booster the affinity for the substrate. The most obvious difference with the other complexes resides in the fact that tissue thromboplastin does not arise from an on the spot combination of the protein cofactor and the lipid but is a tight lipoprotein complex, shed as such by wounded cells. We will not enlarge upon the surface reactions and cofactors of contact activation here for reasons that will be discussed later.

We can summarize the reactions of the classical coagulation pathways as follows:
Extrinsic pathway:

$$[\mathrm{VII, TF, PL}] \Rightarrow [\mathrm{X, Va, PL}] \Rightarrow \mathrm{II}$$

Intrinsic pathway:

$$\mathrm{PK} \Rightarrow \mathrm{XII} \Rightarrow \mathrm{XI} \Rightarrow [\mathrm{IX, VIIIa, PL}] \Rightarrow [\mathrm{X, Va, PL}] \Rightarrow \mathrm{II}$$

B. Control of the coagulation reactions

It is essential for the correct function of the hemostatic mechanism that thrombin formation be precisely controlled. The strong flow at the site of a wound, generated by the blood pressure, makes that thrombin that would be slowly formed, even in massive quantities, would be washed away. It therefore seems useful that thrombin formation occurs explosively after a given lag time. It is equally essential that this explosion is limited to the site of the trigger, i.e. to the site of the lesion. Else generalized thrombosis would be the logical consequence of the smallest wound. The strongly nonlinear generation kinetics of thrombin formation is caused by feedback activation, i.e. activation of thrombin formation by thrombin itself. The limitation of the explosion is due to inhibition of the active complexes. This inhibition is sometimes triggered by the activated products (factor X_a and thrombin). This means that besides feedback activation, feedback inhibition also plays an essential role in the coagulation mechanism.

Feedback activation

Activation of factor V and VIII by thrombin –

Both factor VIII and factor V have to be activated before they can play their role as a protein cofactor to the clotting enzymes. Thrombin is the enzyme that brings about these activations [25-28]. The activation of factor V has been described in terms of protein chemistry. The single chain molecule of factor V is cleaved in three places by thrombin and two of the four resulting fragments recombine under the influence of Ca^{++} to form factor V_a. The mode of interaction between factor VIII and thrombin is a similar process [29].

It has been described that in a human system factor X_a can activate factor VIII [30], but recently the importance of this phenomenon has been questioned on good grounds [31].

At this moment it is established beyond any reasonable doubt that activation of the factors V and VIII is obligatory for their taking part in the coagulation mechanism. From the work of Hurlet et al [1] it may be concluded that the activation of factor V and VIII does occur in vivo in the time course of normal hemostasis. An aberrant prothrombin that possibly yields a thrombin incapable of activating factor V, prothrombin Metz [32,33] causes a mild bleeding disorder. The feedback activation of factor VIII is rate limiting in the intrinsic pathway, whereas that of factor V is not rate limiting in the extrinsic one [34]. The results for this difference are not clear. It is the basis of the common laboratory observation that the aPTT is sensitive to the action of heparin whereas the prothrombin time is not.

Thrombin-activated factor V (FV_a) in a purified state, when kept under the right conditions is relatively stable. The active state of factor VIII always seems to be a transient phenomenon, ending in inactivation. Pentosan polysulphate, a heparin-like drug, acts by direct inhibition of factor VIII activation [35].

Activation of platelets by thrombin –

Thrombin is the most potent physiological platelet activator known [36], a concentration of 0.1 to 1.0 nM will suffice to trigger a half maximal release reaction. All other activators of human platelets need concentrations that are one or more orders of magnitude higher if they are to cause the same response.

Among the proteins released by platelets are factor V and heparin neutralizing proteins (platelet factor 4). The amount of factor V sequestered in the platelets is roughly 20% of the amount present in the plasma [37]. Thrombin, that causes the release reaction will also activate the released factor V. It has been shown that this activation rather then the release reaction itself is the rate limiting factor for the generation of factor V activity from triggered platelets [38].

The concentration of factor V in platelet poor plasma is about 25 nM whereas that of its partner, factor X is around 200 nM. This may lead one to think that the contribution of platelet factor V may be important in vivo. The aggregation of platelets at sites where the hemostatic mechanism is active will cause a futher increase in the ratio of platelet-factor V to plasma-factor V. Still patients with a storage pool deficiency that are unable to release factor V from their platelets do not have an important hemorrhagic diathesis [39]. It seems that only patients lacking factor V in both platelets and plasma do show a hemorrhagic syndrome [40]. This may be explained by the generally recognized fact that the normal level of any clotting factor represents a large functional excess. As a rule the level of any clotting factor must drop significantly below 10% before a decrease of the clotting function becomes apparent.

A second procoagulant function of platelets induced by thrombin together with collagen is the platelet "flip-flop" reaction discovered by Bevers et al [41]. This reaction consists of a transbilayer movement of the procoagulant, negatively charged phospholipids (primarily phosphatidylserine) that as a rule are to be found almost exclusively at the inner face of the cell membrane. In the presence of collagen and thrombin, platelets produce these procoagulant phospholipids at the outside of the cell without the cell being disrupted. The precise molecular mechanism of this reaction is not yet clear. Anyhow, platelets thus activated, offer large amounts of binding sites for the factors IX_a, VIII_a and V_a at their outer surface so that prothrombinase and the factor X activating enzyme can readily form there. One patient (Mrs. Scott, USA) has been described in which this mechanism is defective, she suffers from a mild hemorrhagic diathesis consequently known as Scotts syndrome [42].

It has been reported that collagen-activated platelets can start coagulation via a factor XI dependent mechanism and that ADP activation of platelets triggers coagulation via factor XII [43]. These findings remain to be confirmed. The recent observation that platelets release a potent inhibitor of factor XIa, so that factor IX activation by factor XI_a hardly proceeds in the presence of activated platelets [44] makes one doubt the importance of contact activation for in vivo thrombin generation.

The Josso loop –

In the classical view, contact factors and antihemophilic factors form the intrinsic pathway of thrombin formation and the importance of the role of the contact factors is derived from the recognized importance of the antihemophilic factors. The activating action of factor VII on factor IX invalidates this argument. The first indications that the action of the antihemophilic factors (FVIII and FIX) is not confined to the coagulation pathway started by the contact factors were obtained by Biggs and Nossel [45]. Josso [46] was the first to postulate that factor VII can activate factor IX so that the antihemophilic factors play a role in thromboplastin triggered coagulation. This means that factor X can be activated either directly by factor VII and tissue thromboplastin or indirectly by factor IX_a (together with factor VIII_a) that, in its turn has been activated by factor VII. It is easy to see that the function of this pathway will anyhow be dependent upon the amount of thromboplastin available. The contribution of the direct, one-step action of factor VII_a on factor X_a formation will be constant in time and roughly proportional to the concentration of thromboplastin.

The contribution via the pathway

$$VII \Rightarrow IX \Rightarrow X$$

will be small in the beginning of the reaction but will increase proportionally with time as the factor X activating enzyme (i.e. factor IX_a) builds up. The reinforcement loop constituted by the antihemophilic factors was called *the Josso loop* after its discoverer. As has been demonstrated by Xi et al it will gain in importance when clotting is started by increasingly smaller amounts of thromboplastin [47].

The early observations on the interconnections between the extrinsic and the intrinsic pathway did not get the attention they deserved until Osterud and Rappaport drew attention to the fact that the factor VII – thromboplastin complex is capable of activating factor IX in a partially purified system [48]. Later Zur and Nemerson [49], Jesty and Silverberg [50] and Marlar and Griffin [51] established this pathway without any reasonable doubt.

The physiological importance of the Josso loop is difficult to ascertain because of the thromboplastin dependent – and hence time – dependent effect discussed above. It is tempting to see the Josso-loop mechanism as an explanation for the clinical observation that hemophiliacs tend to bleed in thromboplastin poor organs such as joints, but this can hardly be accepted as a proof of its importance. Jesty and Silverberg [50] calculate that the activation of factor X by factor VII_a is six to seven times faster than the activation of factor IX. Zur and Nemerson [49] find a ratio of ten of the theoretical maximal velocities but argue that the actual ratio will be completely dependent upon the thromboplastin concentration. Van den Besselaar et al [52] conclude from observations in deficient human plasmas that the Josso loop is of no importance in human plasma. The work of Ma Xi demonstrates that in clotting plasma at low concentrations of tissue thromboplastin the Josso loop contributes significantly to thrombin generation [47]. Kalousek et al [53] have reported that factor X is able to activate factor IX. This would constitute a mutual activation interaction that could enhance factor X activation even without activation of factor IX by factor VII. Their experiments have been carried out in purified systems that did not contain protein cofactors (FV and FVIII). Any indication as to the physiological significance of this interaction is lacking at this moment.

Activation of factor VII –

The current view on the starting mechanism of coagulation is based on the observation that the proenzyme factor VII has a non-neglectible enzymatic activity [54,55]. Once it adsorbes onto tissue thromboplastin, the activity of factor VII is enhanced so as to become sufficiently important to start the clotting process. It has been observed however that there exists a more active form of factor VII, the two chain factor VII_a. This form can be generated from the one chain form in a number of different ways. Altman and Hemker [56] showed, as early as 1967, that the contact activation mechanism can enhance factor VII activity in vitro. The cold activation of factor VII, involving kallikrein and different other proteins has been well established. It has also been described that factor VII can be activated by factor IX_a and by factor X_a [58,59]. A very interesting suggestion is made by Morrisson-Silverberg and Jesty [59], when they claim that a complex of factor VII, tissue thromboplastin and factor X_a in the proteolytically active species.

If anywhere, then it is at the level of the activation of factor VII that every conceivable reciprocal interaction of clotting factors has been claimed whereas any indication of their physiological importance is lacking. It is evident that not all biochemical observations necessarily represent reactions that play a role in (patho-)physiology. This being said, it must also be mentioned that often conclusions are drawn too quickly from clinical observations. Tradition has it that the scarce observations of a factor VII deficiency or of any other rare clotting factor deficiency provoke speculations as to the physiological importance of a deficiency, of that specific factor. Some observe a low factor VII level (<5%) without clinical symptoms whereas others find these patients severely handicapped. The same holds for factor XI deficiencies and others. In trying to interprete these data one should not forget that:

a) Any really important bleeding syndrome will lead to death either before or shortly after birth. Only the relatively mild syndromes survive. We remind of the analogy in thrombophilia: antithrombin III (ATIII) and protein C deficiencies are very rarely seen in the homozygous states, probably because complete deficiencies are lethal to the foetus.

b) Any deficiency that does not lead to a clinically important syndrome will more often then not go unnoticed. It must be kept in mind that the physiological levels of clotting factors as a rule represent a large excess of that factor so that a decrease to as low as $\simeq$10% of the normal level will not cause any overt disease. The number of deficiencies that are recognized not to cause problems will therefore depend on chance findings and hence be under-estimated. This is illustrated by the fact that these disorders tend to cluster around laboratories that specialize in research on the blood coagulation and that are backed up by competent clinicians. We thus see that neither the really important deficiencies nor those without any clinical consequences will be recognized in routine medical practice. Therefore it is very hard – if not impossible – to draw conclusions on the mechanism of the blood coagulation process from the correlation between observed clinical symptoms and the accompanying clotting factor deficiencies.

Feedback inactivation

There are two important mechanisms that depend on the previous activation of a clotting factor and that leed to eventual inhibition of thrombin formation. There are a) protein C and S depedent inactivation of the factors V_a and VIII_a and b) the extrinsic pathway inhibitor mechanism.

a) Thrombomodulin triggered reactions

Downstream of a lesion in the vessel wall there will be a region with intact endothelium. It is physiologically important that thrombin formation does not extend too far in the intact vessel. One of the mechanisms responsible for this is the reaction sequence triggered by thrombomodulin [60]. This protein occurs at the surface of intact endothelial cells. Thrombin binds with high affinity to this molecule and, as the name indicates, undergoes a modulation of its specificity. It is no longer capable of any action on the clotting factors I, V, VIII, or XIII. Instead it becomes capable of activating protein C. Protein C [61] is a vitamin K dependent pre-serine protease that, once it is activated by the thrombin-thrombomodulin complex becomes a potent inactivator of factors V_a and VIII_a. This makes that the survival time of any prothrombinase and tenase action in a region lined by intact endothelium must be very short. The action of activated protein C is markedly enhanced by another vitamin K dependent factor, protein S. For further details see [62-64].

b) The extrinsic pathway inhibitor

The extrinsic pathway inhibitor is a circulating plasma protein that also is adsorbed on the endothelial wall. It has the capacity to bind to activated factor X and form a complex that is a strong inhibitor of the thromboplastin-factor VII_a complex. This mechanism makes that tissue factor induced factor X activation will stop as soon as a sufficient amount of factor X_a has been produced. The details of the kinetic consequences of this behaviour remain to be investigated.

For full details on the extrinsic pathway inhibitor the reader is referred to [65].

C. Inhibition of the coagulation reaction products

The inactivation of the active serine proteases of blood coagulation is a physiologically important mechanism. Antithrombin III (ATIII) is the main plasma protein responsible for this action [66-68]. Its importance is readily deduced from the fact that a 50% deficiency state already implies a major risk of thrombosis. Apart from ATIII, coagulation proteases can also be inactivated by α_2-macroglobulin and other antiproteases such as α_1-antitrypsin (see [69] for a review). We determined that ATIII in clotting plasma is responsible for the inhibition of 64% of the thrombin formed, α_2-macroglobulin for 23% and remaining inhibitors for 13%.

Among the anti-proteases, ATIII is extremely important because of the fact that its activity can be enhanced by heparins [28-30] which makes it the lever on which this important family of antithrombotic drugs acts. Heparin cofactor II (HCII) will not contribute to thrombin inactivation under normal circumstances [70]. In spite of its name it will neither be active in the presence of therapeutic heparin concentrations. It starts to play a role however when drugs like dermatan sulfate or pentosan polysulfate are present in the plasma. It is interesting to note that those drugs that act with HCII only cannot be overdosed, which might be the major cause of their alledgedly low hemorrhagic activity. The plasma concentrations of prothrombin is $\simeq$2 μM, that of ATIII $\simeq$3 μM and that of HCII $\simeq$1 μM. this makes that activated ATIII can kill all the thrombin that might ever be formed, but that in the case of HCII activation always half of the thrombin goes unharmed.

As we have discussed before, thrombin will enhance its own formation by activating the factors V and VIII as well as platelets. Any inhibition of thrombin formation and any reaction that inactivates thrombin therefore will interfere with this positive feedback. We have shown that inhibition of thrombin by heparin modulates the extend of activation of factor VIII in the intrinsic system [34]. Because heparin acts via ATIII, this means that heparin influences factor VIII dependent coagulation pathways indirectly by inhibiting the feedback activation of factor VIII.

Also diminution of the available amount of thrombin will cause a decreased rate of activation of platelets in platelet rich plasma. This will cause an increase of the lag time of the thrombin burst in platelet rich plasma. The amount of thrombin formed is surpisingly not influenced by the presence of heparin (<0.5 U/ml). This could be shown to be due to neutralization of the heparin by released platelet factor IV [71].

In clotting plasma one has also to reckon with competition for clotting proteases between procoagulant complexes and protease scavengers. It has been observed [72,73] that ATIII will attack factor X_a less readily in the presence of phospholipids then in free solution and even less if both phospholipids and factor $V_{(a)}$ are present. In vivo this protection seems even to be complete [34]. Anyhow inhibition of factor X_a by heparin, inclusive most low molecular weight heparins, seems, contrary to current believe, not to contribute importantly to their therapeutic action [34,74]. What holds for factor X_a and ATIII, in principle holds for all surface bound proteases and all antiproteases. Lipid binding of factor IX_a protects this enzyme too from ATIII-heparin action. Surprisingly we have the impression that factor IX_a inhibition does play a role in the action of heparins (unpublished).

References

1. Hurlet-Birk Jensen A, Béguin S, Josso F. Factor V and VIII activation "in vivo" during bleeding. Evidence of thrombin formation at the early stage of hemostasis. Path Biol 1976;24:6-10.
2. MacFarlane RG. An enzyme cascade in the blood clotting mechanism and its function as a biochemical amplifier. Nature 1964;202:498.
3. Davie EW, Ratnoff OD. Waterfall sequence for intrinsic bloodclotting. Science 1964;145:1310.
4. Boyer P (ed). The enzymes. III. Hydrolysis. New York: Peptide Bonds Academic Press 1970.
5. Neurath H. Structure and function of proteolytic enzymes. In: Sela M (ed). New perspectives in biology. New York: Elsevier 1964:28-79.
6. Griffin JH, Cochrane CG. Recent advances in the understanding of contact activation reactions. Seminars in Thromb Hemostas 1979;Vol.V:254-73.
7. Esmon CT, Jackson CM. The conversion of prothrombin. III. The factor X_a, catalyzed activation of prothrombin. J Biol Chem 1974;249:7782-90.
8. Jobin F, Esnouf MP. Studies on the formation of the prothrombin converting complex. Biochem J 1967;102:666-74.
9. Esmon CT, Owen WG, Jackson CM. A plausible mechanism for prothrombin activation by factor X_a, Factor V_a, phospholipid and calcium ions. J Biol Chem 1974;249:8045-7.
10. Papahadjopoulos DP, Hanahan DJ. Observations on the interaction of phospholipids and certain clotting factors in prothrombin activator formation. Biochim Biophys Acta 1964;90:436-9.
11. Hemker HC, Esnouf MP, Hemker PW, Swart ACW, MacFarlane RG. Formation of prothrombin converting activity. Nature 1967;215:248-51.
12. Rosing J, Tans G, Govers-Riemslag JWP, Zwaal RFA, Hemker HC. The role of phospholipids and factor V_a in the prothrombinase complex. J Biol Chem 1980;255:274-83.
13. Nesheim ME, Eid S, Mann KG. Assembly of the prothrombinase complex in the absence of prothrombin. J Biol Chem 1981;256:9874-82.
14. Van Rijn JLML, Govers-Riemslag JWP, Zwaal RFA, Rosing J. Kinetic studies of prothrombin activation: Effect of factor V_a, phospholipids on the formation of the enzyme-substrate complex. Biochem 1984;23:4557-64.
15. Nelsestuen GL, Kisiel W, Di Scipio RG. Interaction of vitamin K dependent proteins with membranes. Biochem 1978;17:2134-8.
16. Nesheim ME, Mann KG. The kinetics and cofactor dependence of the two cleavages involved in prothrombin activation. J Biol Chem 1983;258: 5386-91.
17. Nesheim ME, Taswell JB, Mann KG. The contribution of bovine factor V and factor V_a to the activity of prothrombinase. J Biol Chem 1979;254: 10952-62.
18. Rosing J, Tans G, Govers-Riemslag JWP, Zwaal RFA, Hemker HC. The role of phospholipids and factor V_a in the mechanism of prothrombin activation. Thromb Haemostas 1979;42:177(abstract).
19. Tans G, Rosing J, van Dieijen G, Hemker HC. Conjectures on the mode of action of factor V and VIII. In: Mann KG, Taylor FB (eds). The regulation of coagulation. New York/Amsterdam: Elsevier North Holland 1980: 173-85.

20. Hemker HC, Kahn MJP. Reaction sequence of blood coagulation. Nature 1967;215:1201-2.
21. Van Dieijen G, Tans G, Rosing J, Hemker HC. The role of phospholipid and factorVIII$_a$ in the activation of bovine factor X. J Biol Chem 1981; 256:3433-42.
22. Lindhout T, Govers-Riemslag JWP, v.d. Waart P, Hemker HC, Rosing J. Factor V$_a$-factor X$_a$ interaction. Effects of phospholipid vesicles of varying composition. Biochem 1982;21:5494-502.
23. Van Dieijen G, van Rijn JLML, Govers-Riemslag JWP, Hemker HC, Rosing J. Assembly of the intrinsic factor X activating complex: Interactions between factor IX$_a$, factor VIII$_a$ and phospholipid. Thromb Haemostas 1985; 53:396-400.
24. Silverberg SA, Nemerson Y, Zur M, Ostapchuk P. Kinetics of the activation of bovine coagulation factor X by components of the extrinsic pathway. Kinetic behavior of two-chain factor VII in the presence and absence of tissue factor. J Biol Chem 1977;252:8481-8.
25. Newcomb TF, Hoshida M. Factor V and thrombin. Scand J Clin Lab Invest 1965;17(Suppl.84):61-9.
26. Bergsagel DE, Nockolds ER. The activation of proaccelerin. Br J Haematol 1965;11:395-410.
27. Biggs R, MacFarlane RG, Denson KWE, Ash BJ. Thrombin and the interaction of factors VIII and IX. Br J Haematol 1965;11:276-95.
28. Suzuki K, Dahlbäck B, Stenflo J. Thrombin catalyzed activation of human coagulation factor V. J Biol Chem 1982;257:6556-64.
29. Vehar GA, Davie EW. preparation and properties of bovine factor VIII (antihemophilic factor). Biochem 1980;19:401-10.
30. Mertens K, Bertina RM. Activation of human coagulation factor VIII by activated factor X, the common product of the intrinsic and the extrinsic pathway of blood coagulation. Thromb Haemostas 1982;47:96-100.
31. Pieters J, Lindhout T. The limited importance of factor X$_a$ inhibition to the anticoagulant property of heparin in thromboplastin-activated plasma. Blood 1988;72:2048-52.
32. Rabiet MJ, Jandrot-Perrus M, Boissel JP, Elion J, Josso F. Thrombin Metz: Characterization of the dysfunctional thrombin derived from a variant of human prothrombin. Blood 1984;63:927-34.
33. Josso F, Rio Y, Béguin S. A new variant of human prothrombin: Prothrombin Metz, demonstration in a family showing double heterozygosity for congenital hypoprothrombinemia and dysprothrombinemia. Haemostasis 1982;12:309-16.
34. Béguin S, Lindhout T, Hemker HC. The mode of action of heparin in plasma. Thromb Haemostas 1988;60:457-62.
35. Wagenvoord R, Hendrix H, Soria C, Hemker HC. Localization of the inhibitory site(s) of pentosan polysulphate in blood coagulation. Thromb Haemostas 1988;60:220-5.
36. Zucker MB, Nachmias VT. Platelets activation. Arteriosclerosis 1985; 5:218.
37. Tracy PB, Eid LL, Bowie EJW, Mann KG. Radioimmunoassay of factor V in human plasma and platelets. Blood 1982;60:59-63.
38. Baruch D, Hemker HC, Lindhout T. Kinetics of thrombin induced release and activation of platelet factor V. Eur J Biochem 1986;154:213-8.

39. Weiss HJ, Witte LD, Kaplan KL, et al. Heterogenecity in storage pool deficiency studies of granule bound substances in 18 patients including variants deficient in alpha granules platelet factor 4, thromboglobulin and platelet derived growth factor. Blood 1979;54:1296-319.
40. Tracy PB, Giles AR, Mann KG, Eid LL, Hoogendoorn H, Rivard GE. Factor V (Quebec) a bleeding diathesis associated with a qualitative platelet factor V deficiency. J Clin Invest 1984;74:1221-8.
41. Bevers EM, Comfurius P, van Rijn JLML, Hemker HC, Zwaal RFA. Generation of prothrombin-converting activity and the exposure of phosphatidylserine at the outer surface of platelets. Eur J Biochem 1982;122: 429-36.
42. Rosing J, Bevers EM, Comfurius P, et al. Impaired factor X and prothrombin activation associated with decreased phospholipid exposure in platelets from a patient with a bleeding disorder. Blood 1985;65:1557-61.
43. Walsh PN, Griffin JH. Contributions of human platelets to the proteolytic activation of blood coagulation factors XII and XI. Blood 1981;57:106-18.
44. Soons H. Personal communication.
45. Biggs R, Nossel HL. Tissue extract and the contact reaction in blood coagulation. Thromb Diath Haemorrh 1961;6:1-14.
46. Josso F, Prou-Wartelle O. Interaction of tissue factor and factor VII at the earliest phase of coagulation. Thromb Diath Haemorrh 1965;(Suppl.17): 35-44.
47. Xi M, Béguin S, Hemker HC. Importance of factor IX-dependent prothrombinase formation – The Josso Pathway – in clotting plasma. Haemostasis 1989;19:301-8.
48. Osterud B, Rapaport SI. Activation of factor IX by the reaction product of tissue factor and factor VII: Additional pathway for initiating blood coagulation. Proc Natl Acad Sci USA 1977;74:5260-4.
49. Zur M, Nemerson Y. Kinetics of factor IX activation via the extrinsic pathway. J Biol Chem 1980;255:5703-7.
50. Jesty J, Silverberg SA. Kinetics of the tissue factor-dependent activation of coagulation factors IX and X in a bovine plasma system. J Biol Chem 1979;254:12337-45.
51. Marlar RA, Griffin JH. Alternative pathways of thromboplastin-dependent activation of human factor X plasma. Ann NY Acad Sci 1981;370:325-35.
52. Van den Besselaar AMHP, Ram IE, Alderkamp GHJ, Bertina RM. The role of factor IX in tissue thromboplastin induced coagulation. Thromb Haemostas 1982;48:54-8.
53. Kalousek F, Konigsberg W, Nemerson Y. Activation of factor IX by activated factor X: A link between the extrinsic and intrinsic coagulation systems. Febs lett 1975;50:382-5.
54. Jesty J, Nemerson Y. Purification of factor VII from bovine plasma. Reaction with tissue factor and activation of factor X. J Biol Chem 1974;249: 509-15.
55. Nemerson Y. Regulation of the initiation of coagulation by factor VII. Haemostas 1983;13:150-5.
56. Altman R, Hemker HC. Contact activation in the extrinsic blood clotting systems. Thromb Diath Haemorrh 1967;18:525-31.
57. Nemerson Y. Biological control of factor VII. Thromb Haemostas 1976; 35:96-100.

58. Radcliffe R, Nemerson Y. Activation and control of factor VII by activated factor X and thrombin. Isolation and characterization of a single chain form of factor VII. J Biol Chem 1975;250:388-95.
59. Morrisson-Silverberg SA, Jesty J. The role of activated factor X in the control of bovine coagulation factor VII. J Biol Chem 1981;256:1625-30.
60. Esmon CT, Owen WG. Identification of an endothelial cell cofactor for thrombin-catalyzed activation of protein C. Proc Natl Acad Sci USA 1981; 78:2249-52.
61. Stenflo J. A new vitamin K-dependent protein. Purification from bovine plasma and preliminary characterization. J Biol Chem 1976;251:355-63.
62. Stenflo J, Jonsson M. Protein S. A new vitamin K-dependent protein from bovine plasma. Febs Lett 1979;101:377-81.
63. Marlar RA, Kleiss AJ, Griffin JH. Human protein C inactivation of factors V and VIII in plasma by activated molecule. Ann NY Acad Sci 1981; 370:303-10.
64. Suzuki K, Stenflo J, Dahlbäck B, Teodorsson B. Inactivation of human coagulation factor V by activated protein C. J Biol Chem 1983;258:1914-20.
65. Rapaport SI. Inhibition of factor VII_a/tissue factor-induced blood coagulation: With particular emphasis upon a factor X_a-dependent inhibitory mechanism. Blood 1989;73:359-65.
66. Abildgaard U. Highly purified antithrombin III with heparin cofactor activity prepared by disc electrophoresis. Scand J Clin Lab Invest 1968;21: 89-91.
67. Biggs R, Denson KWE, Akman N, Borrett R, Hadden M. Antithrombin III, antifactor X_a, and heparin. Br J Haematol 1970;19:283-305.
68. Rosenberg RD, Damus PS. The purification and mechanism of action of human anti-thrombin-heparin cofactor. J Biol Chem 1973;248:6490-505.
69. Travis J, Salvesen GS. Human plasma proteinase inhibitors. Ann Rev Biochem 1984;52:655-709.
70. Tollefsen DM, Majerus DW, Blank MK. Heparin cofactor II. Purification and properties of a heparin-dependent inhibitor of thrombin in human plasma. J Biol Chem 1982;257:2162-9.
71. Béguin S, Lindhout T, Hemker HC. The effect of trace amounts of tissue factor on thrombin generation in platelet rich plasma. Its inhibition by heparin. Thromb Haemostas 1989;61:25-9.
72. Marciniak E. Factor X_a inactivation by antithrombin III. Evidence for biological stabilization of factor V. J Biol Chem 1973;256:1625-30.
73. Josso F, Béguin S. Changes in the antithrombin III activity at the interface plasma-phospholipids. Thromb Haemostas 1981;46:285(abstract).
74. Hemker HC. The mode of action of herparin in plasma. In: Verstraete M, Vermylen J, Lijnen HR, Arnout J (eds). Thrombosis and haemostasis. Leuven: International Society on Thrombosis and Haemostasis and Leuven University Press, 1987:17-36.

STRUCTURE-FUNCTION RELATIONSHIPS OF HUMAN COAGULATION PROTEINS[1]

L.W. Hoyer

Introduction

Coagulation proteins interact to amplify and localize the response to blood vessel damage so that fibrin is deposited at the appropriate site. Progress in protein chemistry and molecular biology has clarified the ways in which the structural properties of coagulation proteins influence function. As enzyme-cofactor-substrate complexes are key to normal plasma coagulation, this chapter will emphasize studies of the vitamin K-dependent proteins and the cofactor proteins (factors V and VIII) that participate in the "tenase" and "prothrombinase" complexes.

The purification of human coagulation proteins, the cloning of the relevant genes, and the expression of modified proteins through site-directed mutagenesis have progressed remarkably during the past decade. In addition, the molecular characterization of "experiments of nature", the hereditary coagulation disorders hemophilia A and hemophilia B, has contributed to our understanding of coagulation factor structure-function. Because factor VIII and factor IX are coded by X chromosome genes, most mutations cause a bleeding disorder in hemizygous males. For this reason, factor VIII and factor IX deficiencies are much more common than are deficiencies of coagulation factors coded by autosomal genes. For the latter proteins, heterozygous individuals have plasma coagulation protein levels approximately 50% of normal, adequate in almost all cases for normal hemostasis. Only homozygous individuals are symptomatic from these coagulation factor deficiences.

Amplification during the coagulation cascade is essential if a small signal generated by a surface reaction or release of tissue factor is to lead to the conversion of significant quantities of fibrinogen to fibrin. This series of reactions also localizes fibrin formation to the site of injury. The escape from this localization in "disseminated intravascular

1. Supported in part by NIH grants HL 36099 and RR 05737.

coagulation" illustrates the consequences of a more general activation. A third characteristic of the coagulation cascade is the inherent capacity to modulate the reaction. This includes feedback inhibition through the protein C/protein S pathway.

Within the coagulation cascade, it is essential to differentiate the family of zymogens, the vitamin K-dependent factors, and the protein cofactors, large glycoproteins that accelerate the enzymatic reactions. The former group includes factors VII, IX, X, and prothrombin; factors V and VIII and the protein cofactors. Although different in structure and localization, tissue factor also has a cofactor role. This chapter will emphasize recent structure-function studies of factor IX, a vitamin K-dependent enzyme, and factor VIII, a protein cofactor.

Coagulation factor serine proteases

Two common domains are characteristic of the mature vitamin K-dependent coagulation proteins. Each has a highly conserved region containing 9-12 γ-carboxyglutamic acid residues at the amino terminus. It is designated the "Gla domain". At the carboxy terminus, approximately half the mass of each protein is a highly conserved serine protease domain that is generally similar to the comparable region in chymotrypsin and trypsin.

In addition to the Gla and catalytic domains, these coagulation protein enzymes have additional polypeptide domains that are responsible for their unique substrate subspecificities and for their abilities to specifically associate with appropriate cofactors. For example, prothrombin has two "kringle" structures while factors VII, IX and X contain two "epidermal growth factor-like" domains. In factor IX and factor X, the first epidermal growth factor domain contains a posttranslationally modified amino acid, β-hydroxy aspartic acid. Prothrombin, factor VII and factor IX circulate in plasma as single chain zymogens. Plasma factor X is a 2-chain zymogen as a consequence of proteolytic cleavages that occur during, or shortly after, secretion from the liver. Recent reviews should be consulted for a more detailed discussion of the properties of the vitamin K-dependent proteins [1,2].

Because of its relative abundance in normal plasma (100 μg/ml), most of our early knowledge of vitamin K-dependent proteins came from detailed studies of prothrombin and its fragments. Thus, associations of these proteins with metal ions and acidic phospholipids were first demonstrated for prothrombin [2]. Recently, Tulinsky's laboratory has published X-ray crystallographic data for prothrombin fragment 1 stabilized by calcium [3]. These studies document the conformation transition that is required to generate a metal ion-stabilized form. This requires posttranslational carboxylation of almost all of the glutamates in the Gla region, for prothrombin molecules lacking as few as two Gla residues do not undergo the conformational change or bind to an acidic phospholipid [4]. For this reason, the inhibition of the carboxylation by dietary vitamin K deficiency or by antagonists leads to the release of molecules that are not able to develop the necessary stabilized structure with divalent cations. As a result, the incompletely processed proteins cannot participate as substrates or enzymes in the formation of the macromolecular complexes.

Factor IX structure-function: Information obtained from the study of molecular defects in hemophilia B

The cDNA and the entire 34 kb factor IX gene have been sequenced [5]. The coding DNA is divided into eight exons that generally corresponds to the several functional domains (Figure 1). Extensive genetic heterogeneity in hemophilia B has been established by the wide range of different mutations that has been identified by analysis of patient DNA. The defects include gross gene alterations, micro-deletions that usually have a frameshift effect leading to premature termination of translation, and single base substitutions. In addition, 5′ regulatory region changes have been detected as have mutations affecting splice junctions. Within the coding sequences, both nonsense (new stop codon) and missense (amino acid substitution) mutations have been identified. Although each hemophilia B family has its own specific defect, some mutations have been identified in a number of unrelated families, especially those in which transitions affect CG dinucleotides.

The gross gene alterations, frameshift mutations, and nonsense mutations all prevent factor IX formation. As a consequence, they provide no new information about factor IX structure-function. The missense mutations have contributed greatly, however, and these data will be reviewed here. For a complete list of factor IX defects in hemophilia B, the reader is referred to a recent database publication [6] and, reviews by Thompson [7,8].

To date, over 30 different missense mutations have been detected in hemophilia B patients, a few of them in as many as 20 different families. Each affects the factor IX primary structure in a way that has been determined by comparing the amino acid or the factor IX gene nucleotide sequence for the patient with that of normal factor IX (Figure 1).

As yet, no mutations have been detected within the factor IX signal peptide. There are, however, mutations at propeptide arginine residues –1 and –4 that cause hemophilia B. These mutations prevent cleavage, so that the 18 amino acid propeptide remains attached to the amino terminus of the mature, circulating factor IX. Impaired IX function in these patients is associated with incomplete γ-carboxylation of some [9,10], but not all of the mutant proteins [11,12]. In addition, the unprocessed peptide may interfere with the calcium-dependent conformational change within the adjacent Gla domain [11]. The apparently different effect of the glutamine for arginine –4 substitution

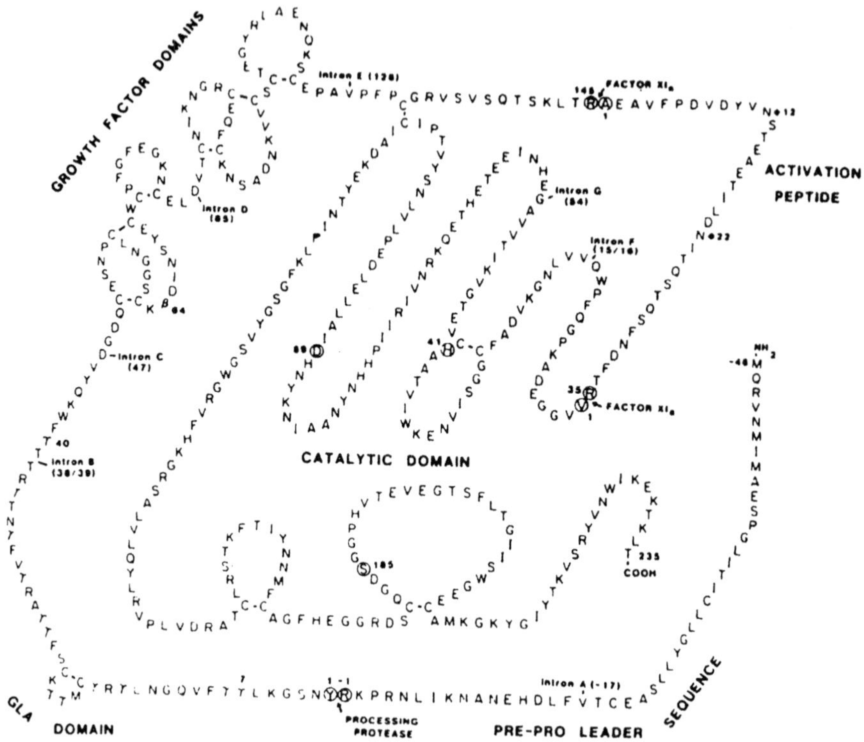

Figure 1. The amino acid sequence of human prepro factor IX. The amino acid sequence is given in the single letter code and the locations of seven introns (A-G) are indicated. The prepro leader sequence (–46 to –1) is removed during biosynthesis by a signal peptidase and a processing protease that cleaves the R-Y bond between –1 and +1. The light chain includes the Gla and growth factor domains (residues 1 through 145). A 35 amino acid activation peptide is released during cleavage by factor XI_a , and the amino acids at the cleavage sites are circled. The 235 amino acids of the heavy chain catalytic domain are numbered from 1-235 in this figure. They correspond to residues 181-415 for the entire protein, the nomenclature used in the text. The three principal amino acids participating in catalysis are circled: histidine 221 (H 41 in this figure); aspartic acid 269 (D 89); and serine 365 (S 85). Two potential glycosylation sites are indicated by solid diamonds; γ indicates γ-carboxyglutamic acid; and β indicates β-hydroxyaspartic acid. [From reference 5, with prmission].

in factor IX San Dimas [10] (incomplete γ-carboxylation) from that in factor IX Oxford 3 [11] and factor IX Kawachinagano [12] (normal γ-carboxylation) has not been resolved. While this may be the result of differences in methodology, it is also possible that the patients differ by polymorphisms that usually have no effect.

The Gla domain itself is coded by exons 2 and 3, and individual molecular defects causing hemophilia B have been identified for four of the twelve Gla residues [8]. A different kind of mutation within the Gla domain, substitution of arginine for cysteine 19, prevents the formation of an intramolecular disulfide bond, and the hemophilic protein circulates with an attached peptide that is disulfide bound to cysteine 23 [8,13].

The two growth factor-like domains are coded by exons 4 and 5, and 10 different missense mutations have been identified within these regions. Mutations at asparagines 47 and 64 cause mild hemophilia B with normal circulating antigen [8], suggesting that they, together with asparagine 49, contribute an important high affinity calcium-binding site that is independent of the Gla domain. To date, this is the only information about the growth factor-like domains that has emerged from studies of dysfunctional hemophilia B proteins.

The factor IX heavy and light chains remain together after activation through a disulfide bond involving cysteine 132. This bond is essential, for a cysteine to arginine mutation at that site causes severe hemophilia B with no detectable plasma factor IX antigen [8]. Mutations at the "alpha" cleavage site (arginine 145) produce moderately severe or mild hemophilia B that is caused by impaired factor XI_a cleavage of the light chain-activation peptide bond. In contrast, cleavage at arginine 180-valine 181 is essential for activity, and substitutions for either residue cause severe hemophilia B [14]. As is generally the case for cleavage site mutations, the amount of immunoreactive factor IX-like protein is normal in these individuals.

Many different molecular defects have been identified within the catalytic domain of the factor IX chain (exons 6-8). The function of this trypsin-like serine protease requires the formation of an ion pair between valine 180 –after β-activation cleavage– and the side chain of asparagine 364, adjacent to the active center serine 365. Thus, when the arginine 180-valine 181 bond is not cleaved, ion pair formation is prevented. Similarly, the mutation, asparagine 364 to valine, causes severe hemophilia B [8]. Another defect that appears to disrupt ion pair formation is the substitution of valine for glycine 309. Though this residue is remote on the linear sequence, it is actually within a few Ångstroms of the ion pair so that a side chain substitution for the glycine hydrogen prevents the necessary ion pair interaction [15]. As expected, mutations of the active center serine –or adjacent, conserved residues– produce severe hemophilia B [8].

Mutations that interfere with the third element of catalysis, substrate binding, also cause hemophilia B. A positively charged substrate protein arginine is thought to interact with a pocket in which asparagine 359 provides an essential negative charge. While there are no recognized mutations at this residue, several other substitutions appear to affect factor IX function by blocking substrate binding. These include the substitution of arginine for glycine 396, the replacement of isoleucine with threonine at 397, and mutations at alanine 390 [8].

Several other catalytic region mutations also demonstrate critical structure-function properties. For example, the mutation of alanine 233 to threonine and arginine 248 to glutamine cause hemophilia B with mild or moderate reduction in factor IX activity and comparable reductions in factor IX antigen [8,16]. The normal specific activity of these mutant proteins suggests that mRNA or protein instability cause hemophilia B in these patients. Moreover, the small amount of factor IX-like protein in these plasmas does not react with monoclonal antibodies that bind a specific catalytic region surface conformational epitope [16]. Thus, these defects modify the protein structure in a way that does not interfere with factor IX function.

Cofactor proteins

The structures of the soluble plasma protein cofactors, factor V and factor VIII, are highly homologous. There is approximately 30% sequence identity, and both proteins are synthesized as high molecular weight procofactors. In the case of factor V, the circulating protein is a single chain species, while factor VIII is a mixture of noncovalently associated polypeptide fragments that are bound, in turn, to the von Willebrand factor. Factors V and VIII share a common structural configuration of triplicated A domains and duplicated C domains (Figure 2). The B domain that connects the A2 and A3 domains has no

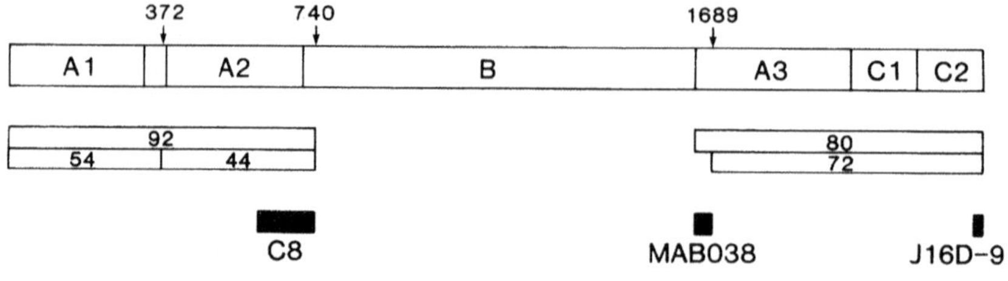

Figure 2. Human factor VIII.
The domain structure of human factor VIII and three thrombin cleavage sites (arrows). Below this are shown the thrombin cleavage fragments, with mass values in kDa. The solid boxes represent the regions containing epitopes for the monoclonal antibodies used to detect factor VIII fragments.

homology, however, and during proteolytic activation this segment is excised. Thus, the active cofactor is composed of the amino terminal-derived heavy chain and the carboxy terminal-derived light chain. In the case of factor VIII, the heavy chain is further cleaved by thrombin so that a heterotrimer is formed, and a peptide fragment is cleaved from the A3 domain (at residue 1689) so that factor VIII becomes separated from von Willebrand factor.

Because the plasma factor V concentration is so much greater than that of factor VIII, most of the early structure-function studies were done with factor V. While most of them were done with bovine factor VIII, the conclusions have been verified using human factor V and, more recently, human factor VIII. For example, it is rigorously established that both factor V and factor VIII circulate in plasma as procofactors, with thrombin or factor X_a cleavage necessary for activation. When activated, both cofactors have been shown to bind tightly to membranes containing acidic phospholipids [2]. Moreover, the protein-membrane interaction involves the cofactor light chain in both cases. There is a subtle difference, however, in that the predominant phospholipid binding of factor V_a is the A3 domain [17], while the factor VIII membrane binding site appears to be within the C domain [18]. The heavey chain functions, interaction with the enzyme and the substrate to form a coagulant complex, have been documented for factor V [19], but there are as yet no comparable data for the interaction of factor VIII with the enzyme and substrate that participate with it in "tenase" complex.

Factor VIII structure-function: Information obtained from molecular defects in hemophilia A

The gene that codes for factor VIII is one of the largest known, occupying 186 kb on the X chromosome. The coding DNA is divided into 26 exons, including several of nearly 3 kb. They are separated by 25 introns, some as big as 32 kb. The cDNA codes for a 19 amino acid signal peptide and a 2332 amino acid mature factor VIII molecule that is synthesized as a single chain [20,21]. Including carbohydrate, the factor VIII molecular weight is estimated to be over 300,000.

It is likely that the greater frequency of factor VIII deficiency than factor IX deficiency is due to the greater size of the factor VIII gene, hence the greater likelihood of a mutation causing a significant molecular defect. However, the size of the factor VIII gene also makes it much more difficult to identify a specific molecular defect. While deletions, missense mutations and nonsense mutations have been identified in some patients, the characterization of molecular defects in hemophilia A has been less successful than in hemophilia B. To date, a specific defect has been determined in less than 10% of the families that have been studied [22,23].

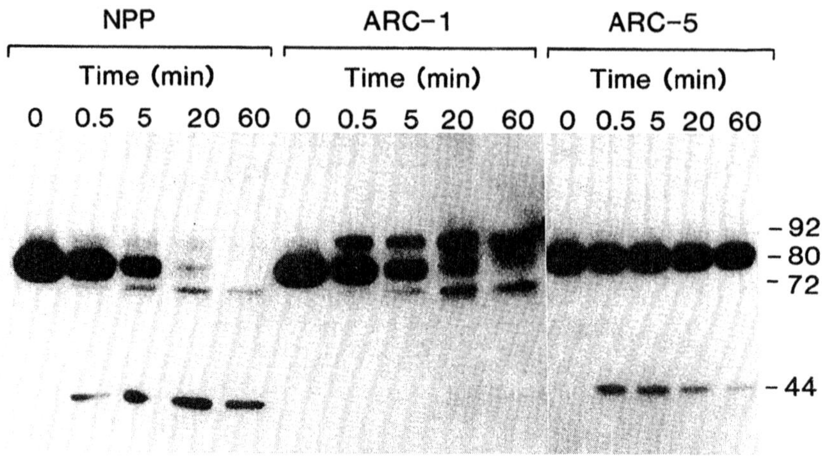

Figure 3. Identification of thrombin cleavage site mutation. Immunoadsorbed normal (NPP) and CRM-positive (ARC-1 and ARC-5) factor VIII is detected by immunoblotting using monoclonal antibodies (Figure 2) that react with the factor VIII heavy chain (92 kDa and its 44 kDa fragment) and the factor VIII light chain (80 kDa and its 72 kDa fragment). Factor VIII eluted from the immunoadsorbent beads (time 0) and immunopurified factor VIII incubated with thrombin for 0.5-60 min is identified by autoradiography after incubation with the three monoclona anti-factor VIII and I^{125}-labeled anti-mouse immunoglobulin. The ARC-1 factor VIII heavy chain (92 kDa) and the ARC-5 factor VIII light chain (80 kDa) are not cleaved.

In contrast to the correspondence of specific mutations with functional defects in hemophilia B, most factor VIII point mutations cause hemophilia A in which there is no detectable plasma factor VIII by immunoassay. Only 5% of factor VIII deficient patients have sufficient mutant protein to permit characterization. These individuals, designated cross-reacting material (CRM)-positive, have normal or increased amounts of plasma factor VIII-like protein by immunoassays [24].

As most factor VIII point mutations cause CRM-negative hemophilia A, they must be interpreted indirectly as affecting parts of the protein that, if modified, are changed in a way that either prevents synthesis or release, or markedly affects protein stability. Useful direct structure-function information comes only from the 5% of patients who are CRM-positive.

Several of these CRM-positive patients have been studied intensively, and interesting recent data suggest that many of them have thrombin cleavage site mutations. As thrombin cleavage at amino acids 372 and 1689 is crucial for factor VIII procoagulant function, it is not surprising that mutations at these sites cause hemophilia. The essential role of thrombin activation in factor VIII function has been recognized for some time [26] –and was directly demonstrated by Pittman and Kaufman using site-directed mutagenesis [25].

Two strategies have been used to identify these thrombin cleavage site mutations. One approach, that of Gitschier and coworkers, has been to amplify selected factor VIII regions by the polymerase chain reactions (PCR) [27]. The PCR-amplified DNA is then screened for mutations by discriminate hybridization using oligonucleotide probes. When 215 hemophilia A DNA samples were analyzed, two defects were identified, a nonsense mutation (stop codon) at amino acid 336, and a substitution of cysteine for arginine at amino acid residue 1689 [27]. The latter defect affects the critical factor VIII light chain thrombin cleavage site.

A different approach has been taken by Arai and coworkers: direct identification of thrombin cleavage site mutations in CRM-positive hemophilia A plasmas [28]. In this analysis, the nonfunctional protein is immunoadsorbed, treated with thrombin, and then characterized by immunoblotting to determine if thrombin cleavage has occured (Figure 3). Three of the first twelve CRM-positive plasmas examined in this way had missense mutations preventing thrombin cleavage [28,29]. In one patient (ARC-1 in Figure 3), the molecular defect was a substitute of histidine for arginine 372. This protein, factor VIII-Kumamoto, lacks procoagulant function because the heavy chain is not cleaved by thrombin to separate the A and A2 domains. In two other patients, unrelated individuals with the identical missense mutation, arginine 1689 to cysteine, the coagulation defect was the result of impaired factor VIII light chain cleavage. The factor VIII from one of these patients (ARC-5) is also shown in Figure 3. It is of interest that the factor VIII activity levels in these two patients are higher than those of the patient with the same molecular defect that was reported by Gitschier and coworkers [27]. All three patients have normal or elevated factor VIII antigen levels [27,29,30]. However, one patient has no detectable factor VIII activity and his severe hemophilia has caused frequent, recurrent hemarthroses [27]. The other two have low, but easily detectable, factor VIII activity (2-5% of normal). This caused mild hemophilia with very infrequent factor VIII treatment and no arthropathy in one patient, and a more severe disorder, with joint destruction and frequent factor VIII replacement therapy, in the other [29]. Again, we do not understand the basis for the distinct clinical and biochemical differences for patients with apparently identical molecular defects.

A second approach to structure-function analysis, the use of antibodies to factor VIII, has also been productive. As noted previously, many human antibodies to factor VIII react with factor VIII light chain C2 domain epitopes. As these antibodies block factor VIII binding to phospholipid, it appears that the factor VIII-phospholipid interaction is the carboxy-terminus (C2 domain) of the light chain [18].

Monoclonal antibodies to factor VIII are also useful in characterizing structure-function relationships. Monoclonal antibodies to the extreme amino terminal region of the factor VIII light chain react with the peptide cleaved from the light chain by thrombin and they block factor VIII binding to von Willebrand factor [31,32]. Thus, they define the region of factor VIII that is critical for the covalent noninteraction of factor VIII with von Willebrand factor.

Summary

Information about the structure-function relationships of human coagulation proteins has come from several different kinds of analysis. In some cases, standard purification and protein analysis has led to useful insights. More recently, characterization of the molecular defects responsible for hemophilia A and hemophilia B has provided information about typical vitamin K-dependent and procofactor proteins. These experiments of nature are being supplemented by data obtained using site-directed mutagenesis to generate modified proteins. Finally, antibodies to coagulation factors have been very useful in localizing some factor VIII and factor IX functions. Together, these approaches are clarifying the sequential reactions that occur in plasma coagulation. They will guide further efforts in recombinant technology toward the goal of preparing modified proteins that have increased therapeutic potential.

Acknowledgements

Studies from the author's laboratory reported here have been supported by grants HL 36099 and RR 05737 from the National Institutes of Health. The contributions of Drs. Morio Arai and Ashraf Aly to these studies is gratefully acknowledged as is the technical assistance of Maria Scott and Norma Trabold and the secretarial assistance of Debbie Wilder. Dr. Arthur Thompson kindly shared data for a number of hemophilia B studies prior to their publication.

References

1. Furie B, Furie BC. The molecular basis of blood coagulation. Cell 1988;53: 505-18.

2. Mann KG, Nesheim ME, Church WR, Haley P, Krishnaswamy S. Surface-dependent reactions of the vitamin K-dependent enzyme complexes. Blood 1990;76:1-16.
3. Soriano-Garcia M, Park CH, Tulinsky A, Ravichandran KG, Skrzypczak-Jankun E. Structure of Ca^{2+} prothrombin fragment 1 including the conformation of the Gla domain. Biochemistry 1989;28:6805-10.
4. Malhotra OP, Nesheim ME, Mann KG. The kinetics of activation of normal and gamma-carboxyglutamic acid-deficient prothrombins. J Biol Chem 1985;260:279-87.
5. Yoshitake S, Schach BG, Foster DC, Davie EW, Kurachi K. Nucleotide sequence of the gene for human factor IX (antihemophilic factor B). Biochem 1985;24:3736-50.
6. Giannelli F, Green PM, High KA, et al. Hemophilia B data base of point mutations and short additions and deletions. Nucl Acids Res 1990;18:4053-9.
7. Thompson AR. Structure and biology of factor IX. In: Benz EJ, Cohen JH, Furie B, Hoffman R, Shatil SJ (eds). Hematology: Basic principles and practice. New York: Churchill Livingston, 1990:1308-16.
8. Thompson AR. Molecular biology of the hemophilias. In: Coller BS (ed). Progress in hemostasis and thrombosis. Vol.10. Philadelphia: Plenum 1991: 175-214.
9. Diuguid DL, Rabiet MJ, Furie BC, Liebman HA, Furie B. Molecular basis of hemophilia B: A defective enzyme due to an unprocessed propeptide is caused by a point mutation in the factor IX precursor. Proc Natl Acad Sci USA 1986;83:5803-7.
10. Ware J, Diuguid DL, Liebman HA, et al. Factor IX San Dimas. Substitution of glutamine for ARG^{-4} in the propeptide leads to incomplete γ-carboxylation and latered phospholipid binding properties. J Biol Chem 1989;264: 11401-6.
11. Bentley AK, Rees JG, Rizza C, Brownlee GG. Defective propeptide processing of blood clotting factor IX caused by mutation of arginine to glutamine at position –4. Cell 1986;45:343-8.
12. Sugimoto M, Miyata T, Kawabata S, et al. Factor IX Kawachinagano: Impaired function of the Gla-domain caused by attached propeptide region due to substitution of arginine by glutamine at position –4. Br J Haematol 1989;72:216-21.
13. Bertina RM, van der Linden IK. Factor IX Zutphen. A genetic variant of blood coagulation factor IX with an abnormally high molecular weight. J Lab Clin Med 1982;100:695-704.
14. Huang M-N, Kasper CK, Roberts HR, Stafford DW, High KA. Molecular defect in factor IX_{Hilo}, a hemophilia B_m variant: Arg → Gln at the carboxyterminal cleavage site of the activation peptide. Blood 1989;73:718-21.
15. Thompson AR, Chen S-H, Brayer GD. Severe hemophilia B due to a G to T transversion changing Gly 309 to Val and inhibiting active protease conformation by preventing ion pair formation. Blood 1989;74:134a.
16. Chen S-H, Thompson AR, Zhang M, Scott CR. Three point mutations in the factor IX genes of five hemophilia B patients: Identification strategy using localization by altered epitopes in their hemophilic proteins. J Clin Invest 1989;84:113-8.
17. Krishnaswamy S, Mann KG. The binding of factor V_a to phospholipid vesicles. J Biol Chem 1988;263:5714-23.

18. Arai M, Scandella D, Hoyer LW. Molecular basis of factor VIII inhibition by human antibodies: Antibodies that bind to the factor VIII light chain prevent the interaction of factor VIII with phospholipid. J Clin Invest 1989;83:1978-84.
19. Guinto ER, Esmon CT. Loss of prothrombin and of factor X_a-factor V_a interactions upon inactivation of factor V_a by activated protein C. J Biol Chem 1984; 259:13986-92.
20. Gitschier J, Wood WI, Goralka TM, et al. Characterization of the human factor VIII gene. Nature 1984;312:326-30.
21. Toole JJ, Knopf JL, Wozney JM, et al. Molecular cloning of a cDNA encoding human antihemophilic factor. Nature 1984;312:342-7.
22. Antonarakis SE. The molecular genetics of hemophilia A and B in man. Factor VIII and factor IX deficiency. Adv in Hum Gene 1988;17:27-59.
23. White GC, Shoemaker CB. Factor VIII gene and hemophilia A. Blood 1989;73:1-12.
24. Hoyer LW, Breckenridge RT. Immunologic studies of antihemophilic factor (AHF, factor VIII): Cross-reacting material in a genetic variant of hemophilia A. Blood 1968;32:962-71.
25. Pittman DD, Kaufman RJ. Proteolytic requirements for thrombin activation of anti-hemophilic factor (factor VIII). Proc Natl Acad Sci USA 1988;85: 2429-33.
26. Rapaport SI, Schiffman S, Patch MJ, Ames SB. The importance of activation of antihemophilic globulin and proaccelerin by traces of thrombin in the generation of intrinsic prothrombinase activity. Blood 1963;21:221-35.
27. Gitschier J, Kogan S, Levinson B, Tuddenham EGD. Mutations of factor VIII cleavage sites in hemophilia A. Blood 1988;72:1022-8.
28. Arai M, Inaba H, Higuchi M, et al. Direct characterization of factor VIII in plasma: Detection of a mutation altering a thrombin cleavage site (Arginine-372 - Histidine). Proc Natl Acad Sci USA 1989;86:4277-81.
29. Arai M, Higuchi M, Antonarakis SE, et al. Characterization of a thrombin cleavage site mutation (Arg 1689 to Cys) in the factor VIII gene of two unrelated patients with cross-reacting material positive hemophilia A. Blood 1990;75:384-9.
30. O'Brien DP, Pattinson JK, Tuddenham EGD. Purification and characterization of factor VIII 372-Cys: A hypofunctional cofactor from a patient with moderately severe hemophilia A. Blood 1990;75:1664-72.
31. Bahou WF, Ginsburg D, Sikkink R, Litwiller R, Fass DN. A monoclonal antibody to von Willebrand factor (vWF) inhibits factor VIII binding. Localization of its antigenic determinant to a nonadecapeptide at the amino terminus of the mature vWF polypeptide. J Clin Invest 1989;84:56-61.
32. Leyte A, Verbeet MP, Brodniewicz-Proba T, van Mourik JA, Mertens K. The interaction between human blood-coagulation factor VIII and von Willebrand factor. Biochem J 1989;257:679-83.

THE ROLE OF CALCIUM IN COAGULATION AND ANTICOAGULATION

M.E. Mikaelsson

The quality of the coagulation-related blood-derived products is markedly affected by the manner in which blood is collected. Standard anticoagulation solutions contain citrate which efficiently prevents blood clotting by chelation of calcium and other metal ions. However, there are two sides to the matter, which is often overlooked. For instance, chelation of calcium leads to conformational changes of the coagulation factors V and VIII which results in loss of the procoagulant activity.

This paper will highlight the fundamental role of calcium in coagulation and the consequences of anticoagulation. After an overview of the wide variety of interactions where calcium is essential (Figure 1), attention is focused on factor VIII and the importance of calcium for its function and stability.

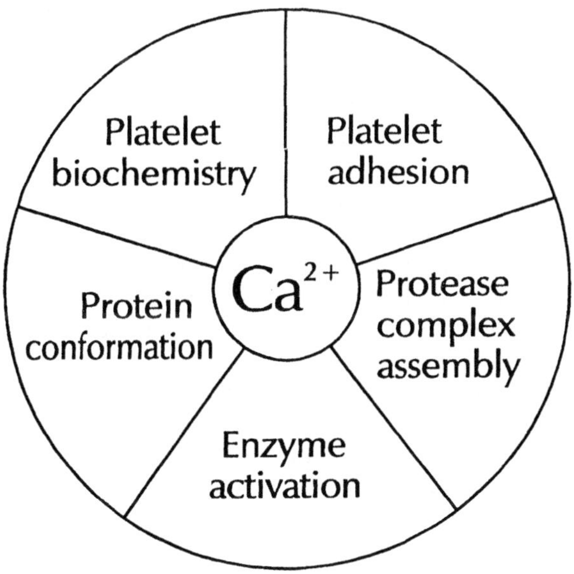

Figure 1. The role of calcium in blood coagulation.

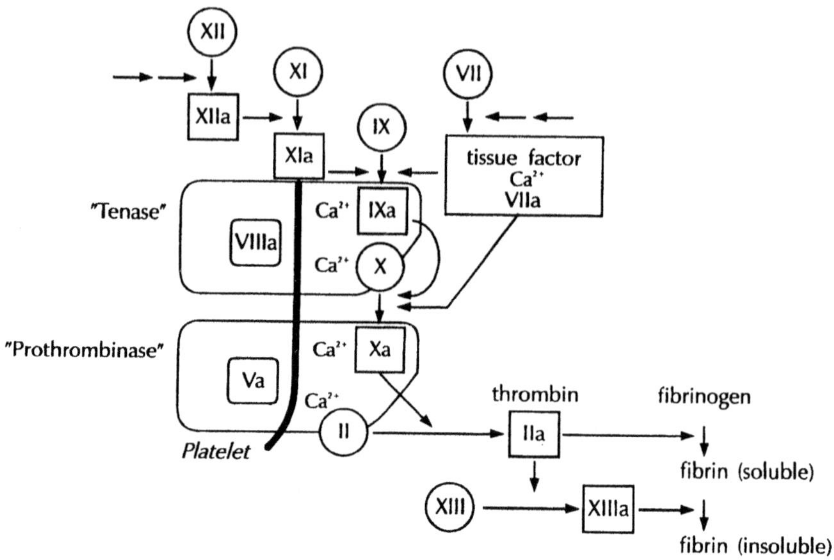

Figure 2. Blood coagulation.

Normal hemostasis requires free ionized calcium for the initial platelet plug formation and also for most events in the blood coagulation process. Baumgartner, Sakariassen, Sixma and others have studied the adherence of platelets to exposed subendothelium using various perfusion chamber models [1-3]. They found that calcium and von Willebrand factor are essential for normal platelet adherence and for the subsequent spreading of platelets on the subendothelium. Since von Willebrand factor does not interact with platelets in the circulating blood, it has been postulated that binding of von Willebrand factor to subendothelium leads to a conformational change that unmasks a calcium dependent, platelet binding domain. These von Willebrand factor mediated reactions are shear rate dependent. At the satellite symposium on cell adhesion after the SSC meeting in Barcelona (1990) several studies were presented which indicated that the adherence of platelets was totally dependent on von Willebrand factor at high wall shear rates but not at low shear rates. Furthermore, Dr. Ikeda demonstrated that binding of von Willebrand factor to platelets triggered an increase in the intracellular calcium concentration. This calcium influx occurred only at high shear rates and in the presence of von Willebrand factor.

In the platelet several intracellular events are modulated by the calcium ion concentration [5]. An increase of the intracellular calcium levels upon stimulation of platelets leads to activation of a number of calcium dependent enzymes and processes that regulate the platelet metabolism as well as the secretion of many active substances. The platelet function and preservation aspects will be discussed in detail in another session.

Turning to coagulation (Figure 2), the presence of calcium is fundamental in several ways; on one hand it is essential for the protein conformation of most coagulation factors and on the other hand it acts as a linker and cofactor in several enzymatic events in the coagulation process.

Blood coagulation takes place on the membrane surface exposed upon activation of platelets, a feature well adapted to its purpose. The cascade of zymogen activations requires the proximity that membrane-binding offers in order to enhance the velocity. The assembly of the enzyme complexes tenase and prothrombinase on the membrane surface is dependent on calcium as a linker between charged groups on serine proteases and acidic membrane phospholipids [6-8]. Moreover, these vitamin K-dependent enzymes are unable to interact with acidic phospholipids unless they are in the calcium stabilized form [6,9]. Elimination of Gla-residues produces enzyme variants which cannot undergo the conformational transition that is required for membrane binding.

Calcium has a similar function in the factor VII-tissue thromboplastin complex with activates factor X via the extrinsic pathway and factor IX via the Josso pathway [10]. In the coagulation process there are also some membrane-independent enzyme activations which require calcium ions, namely the activation of factor IX [11] and factor XIII [12]. Finally the regulating mechanisms which involve antithrombin and other inhibitors as well as activated protein C, are also influenced by the calcium level.

Enzyme complex formation on membrane surfaces has a dramatic impact on the catalytic efficiency in comparison with free enzyme in solution. Mertens and coworkers [13] have shown that the relative rate for activation of factor X by factor IX_a is enhanced five orders of magnitude when the complete tenase complex is assembled. Although not understood in every detail, membrane binding provides higher local concentrations, optimal steric orientation and opportunities of regulation. In addition, the reactants are protected from circulating inhibitors and other substances in the environment.

The vitamin K-dependent serine proteases are characterized by a highly conserved domain at the N-terminus. This Gla domain contains about ten Gla, γ-carboxyglutamic acid, a rare amino acid with two carboxyl groups [14]. Calcium ions act as linkers between the Gla residues sticking out from the protease and acidic phospholipids exposed on the platelet membrane.

In general, interactions with divalent linkers are counteracted by high concentrations of the linker due to blocking of the binding sites.

Figure 3 shows the influence of the calcium level on the clotting time in a one-stage factor VIII assay [15]. Increased amounts of calcium ions result in prolonged clotting times. In fact, Crawford and coworkers [16] have demonstrated that calcium chloride can be used as an anticoagulant at high concentrations.

For several decades, factor V and factor VIII have been known as the most labile coagulation proteins. In 1965, Weiss published a study on the cation and pH dependence [17] and drew the conclusion that calcium is the plasma cation which protects these proteins against inactivation. This finding, however, has been neglected in general practice; at blood banks as well as in research laboratories where citrate still is the standard anticoagulant.

In the late 1970s Gail Rock rediscovered the essential role of calcium ions for the integrity of factor VIII [18]. By collecting blood in heparin instead of CPD she found a markedly improved stability and recovery of factor VIII in plasma. In Groningen Dr. Smit Sibinga has implemented the use of heparin as anticoagulant in the production of factor VIII concentrates and reported high yields [19]. Also in Aarhus in Denmark citrate has been replaced by heparin with good results.

In order to study the effect of calcium we reclacified fresh CPD plasma and added heparin to prevent activation. As shown in Figure 4 the initial decay rate was much lower in the recalcified plasma than in the control CPD plasma. The stability of heparin plasma was identical to

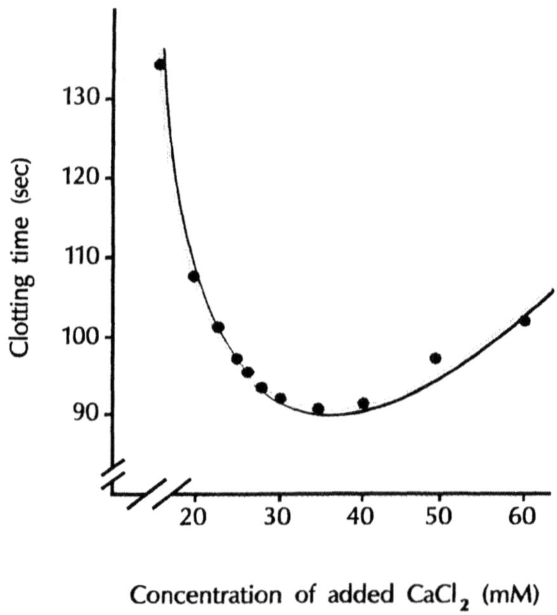

Figure 3. Influence of Ca^{2+} on the clotting time in a one-stage FVIII:C assay.

that shown here for the recalcified plasma. Since pH rose during the incubation we ascribed the accelerated decay after six hours to this drift in pH. By addition of the buffer HEPES we managed to keep pH in the range 7.1-7.3 which resulted in a significant improvement. Well buffered, recalcified plasma was virtually completely stable for 24 hours at +37°C. One-stage and two-stage assays as well as chromogenic substrate assays gave identical results. Addition of inhibitors did not affect the principal results.

Fibrinopeptide A (FPA) is a sensitive indicator of thrombin formation and was therefore chosen as marker of coagulation activation. However, no generation of FPA was detected during the incubation of plasma at 37°C, either in the recalcified plasma or in the ordinary CPD plasma.

The results of the stability studies suggested that the factor VIII/von Willebrand factor complex contains metal ion bridges. In order to identify any intrinsic metal ions, purified factor VIII/von Willebrand factor preparations were subjected to atomic absorption spectrophotometric analysis. Prior to the metal determination, buffer exchange was performed by gelfiltration on Sephadex G25 in an ultra-pure buffer in order to remove all free or loosely associated metal ions.

On average our preparations contained one mole calcium per mole von Willebrand factor subunit [20]. All the other metals tested for, were below the detection limit. When the purified factor VIII complex

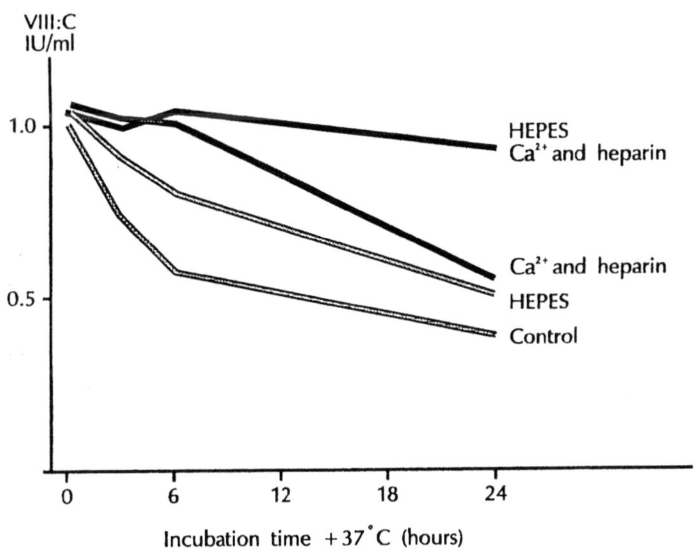

Figure 4. Stability of FVIII:C in CPD plasma (control) HEPES-buffered CPD plasma, recalcified heparinized CPD plasma and recalcified heparinized HEPES-buffered CPD plasma. FVIII:C was assessed by a one-stage assay after treatment with Heparsorb (General Diagnostics, US) to remove heparin.

was incubated with EDTA prior to the buffer exchange, no calcium was found in the protein peak. Moreover, all the coagulant activity was lost. It is an interesting observation that factor V, which is structurally very similar to factor VIII, also has been shown to contain calcium [21]. Factor V also contains copper [22] and it has been speculated whether factor VIII also contains copper ions.

Fass and coworkers [23] have shown that the heavy and light chains of factor VIII dissociate upon treatment with EDTA. The precise location of the metal bridges is not yet elucidated. However, it is conceivable that calcium stabilizes factor VIII by linking on the one hand the heavy and light chains within factor VIII and on the other hand by linking the light chain of factor VIII to von Willebrand factor.

Recent experiments published by Nordfang and Fay [24,25] have demonstrated that the assembly of active factor VIII from isolated inactive subunits requires the presence of calcium or manganese ions. Copper ions did not promote the reassembly. Several other factors e.g. von Willebrand factor have influence on the regeneration of active factor VIII.

In blood and plasma collection for fractionation the driving force is the production of factor VIII concentrates. The citrate anticoagulants used for whole blood collection have been chosen primarily for their benefits to red cell preservation. In Scotland, Prowse and coworkers [26] have investigated the possibility of reducing the citrate strength. When blood was collected in half-strength citrate the stability of FVIII:C in plasma was improved, but the recovery in cryoprecipitate was unaffected as long as fresh frozen plasma was used. In contrast, the use of half-strength citrate improved the yield significantly when cyroprecipitate was prepared from overnight-stored plasma. The final concentration of citrate was 10 mM in the half-strength citrate plasma. Further reduction of the citrate concentration did not provide sufficient protection against clotting. Generation of fibrinopeptide A (FPA) and platelet activation start at a citrate level of approximately 8 mM. The plasma level of ionized calcium was only 0.1 mM when blood was collected in half-strength citrate.

Earlier studies in our laboratory have shown that half-strength citrate improves the stability of FVIII:C but not to the same extent as heparin [20]. Physiological plasma levels of ionized calcium, around 1 mM, are required to completely protect factor VIII against inactivation. Therefore another alternative, namely recalcification of CPD plasma, immediately after harvesting, was explored. Heparin was added to inhibit clotting. ordinary CPD plasma collected by double plasmapheresis was reaclcified and heparinized to a final concentration of 10 mM calcium chloride and 10 units per ml of heparin. After the recalcification the level of ionized calcium was about 1.0 mM. Alternately, the first or second plasma unit was left untreated to serve as control. Treated and untreated units were frozen within one hour from the plasmapheresis. When processed, a lyophilized intermediate purity concentrate was prepared from 3-8 kg plasma pools. The cryo-paste was divided into two parts which were dissolved in Tris buffer or Tris-citrate buffer. The markedly improved stability of FVIII:C in plasma obtained by recalcification was not reflected in a statistically significant improvement of the yield of VIII:C in cryo or final product (Figure 5). The explanation is that all the stabilized factor VIII was not recovered in the cryoprecipitate. Further testing revealed that the cryosupernatant from recalcified plasma had a higher content of FVIII:C than the CPD plasma supernatant.

The addition of citrate to the process buffer led to a significant in-activation of factor VIII for both types of plasma (Figure 5). The final yield was 510 units per kg when recalcified plasma was processed in the presence of calcium ions, but only 290 units per kg when citrate was present throughout the process.

This last finding has been exploited in the new generation of manu-facturing processes for factor VIII, based on immunoaffinity chroma-tography. Citrated buffers have been abandoned and the level of ionized calcium is controlled throughout the process.

In summary, calcium ions play an important role in platelet reac-tions, in preserving the structure and function of coagulation factors, in the assembly of enzyme complexes on membranes and also in some other enzyme reactions.

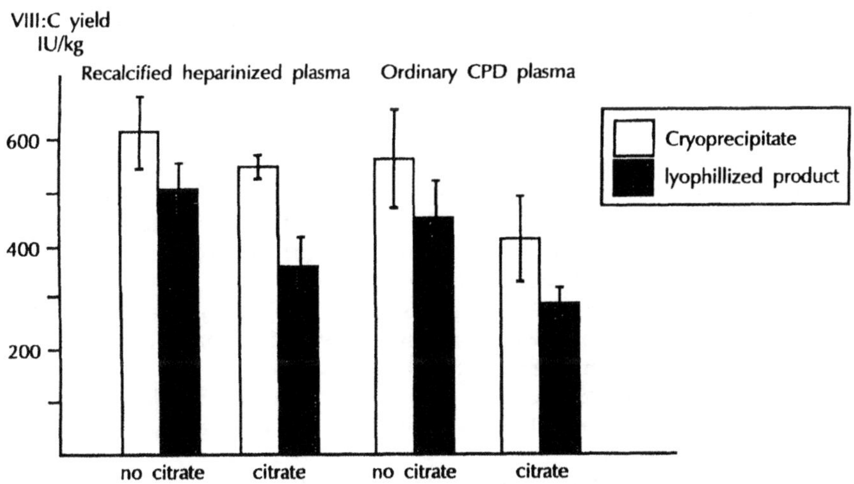

Figure 5. Yields of FVIII:C during the preparation of an intermediate purity factor VIII concentrate from small pools of recalcified heparinized CPD plasma or ordinary CPD plasma. FVIII:C was assessed by a one-stage assay. The data represent mean ± standard deviation for each group.

Finally anticoagulation by means of citrate has a detrimental effect on the structure of factor VIII which results in loss of activity. In the production of factor VIII concentrates the yields can be improved by controlling the level of ionized calcium throughout the process.

Acknowledgements

Part of the work on Ca^{2+}-stabilization of factor VIII was supported by a grant from the National Swedish Board for Technical Development.

References

1. Baumgartner HR. The role blood flow in platelet adhesion, fibrin deposition and formation of mural thrombi. Microvasc Res 1973;5:167-79.
2. Sakariassen KS, Bolhuis PA, Sixma JJ. Platelet adherence to subendothelium of human arteries in pulsatile and steady flow. Thromb Res 1980;19: 547-59.
3. Muggli R, Baumgartner HR, Tschopp TB, Keller H. Automated microdensitometry and protein assays as a measure for platelet adhesion and aggregation on collagen-coated slides under controlled flow conditions. J Lab Clin Med 1980;95:195-207.
4. Sakariassen KS, Ottenhof-Rovers M, Sixma JJ, Factor VIII-von Willebrand factor requires calcium for facilitation of platelet adherence. Blood 1984; 63:996-1003.
5. Crawford N, Scrutton MC. Biochemistry of the blood platelet. In: Bloom AL, Thomas DP (eds). Hemostasis and thrombosis. Eddinburgh: Churchill and Livingstone, 1987:47-77.
6. Nelsestuen GL, Broderius M, Martin G. Role of γ-carboxyglutamic acid. An unusual transition required for calcium-dependent binding of prothrombin to phospholipid. J Biol Chem 1976;251:5648-56.
7. Nelsestuen GL. Interaction of vitamin K-dependent proteins with calcium and phospholipid membranes. Fed Proc 1978;37:2621-5.
8. Esmon CT, Suttie JW, Jackson CM. The functional significance of vitamin K action. Difference in phospholipid binding between normal and abnormal prothrombin. J Biol Chem 1975;250:4095-9.
9. Borowski M, Furie BC, Bauminger S, Furie B. Prothrombin requires two sequential metal-dependent conformational transitions to bind phospholipid. J Biol Chem 1986;261:14969-75.
10. Xi Ma, Béguin S, Hemker HC. Importance of factor IX-dependent prothrombinase formation –the Josso pathway– in clotting plasma. Haemostasis 1989;19:301-8.
11. Kingdon HS, Davie EW, Ratnoff OD. The reaction between activated plasma thromboplastin antecedent and diisopropylphosphofluoridate. Biochemistry 1964;3:166-73.
12. Cook RD, Holbrok JJ. Calcium and the assays of human plasma clotting factor XIII. Biochem J 1974;141:71-8.
13. Mertens K, Wijngaarden A van, Bertina RM. The role of factor VIII in the activation of human blood coagulation factor X by activated factor IX. Thromb Haemostas 1985;54:654-60.

14. Stenflo J, Fernlund P, Egan W, Roepstorff P. vitamin K-dependent modifications of glutamic acid residues in prothrombin. Proc Natl Acad Sci USA 1974;71:2730-3.
15. Mikaelsson ME, Oswaldsson UM. Standardization of VIII:C assays: A manufacturer's view. Scand J Haematol 1984;33(Suppl.40):79-86.
16. Crawford N, Crook M, Dawes J, Gray CRW. The sole use of magnesium chloride for blood anticoagulation: Preservation of platelet surface-bound "proteinaceous halo". (Abstract). Thromb Haemostas 1987;58:245.
17. Weiss HJ. A study on the cation and pH dependent stability of factors V and VIII in plasma. Thromb Diath Haemorrh 1965;14:32-51.
18. Rock G, Tittley P, Fuller V. Effect of citrate anticoagulants on factor VIII levels in plasma. Transfusion 1988;28:248-52.
19. Smit Sibinga CTh, Das PC. Heparin and factor VIII. Scand J Haematol 1984;33(Suppl.40):111-22.
20. Mikaelsson ME, Forsman N, Oswaldsson UM. Human factor VIII: A calcium-linked protein complex. Blood 1983;62:1006-15.
21. Hibbard LS, Mann KG. The calcium-binding properties of bovine factor V. J Biol Chem 1980;255:638-45.
22. Mann KG, Lawler CM, Vehar GA, Church WR. Coagulation factor V contains copper ion. J Biol Chem 1984;259:12949-51.
23. Fass DN, Knutson GJ, Katzmann JA. Monoclonal antibodies to porcine factor VIII coagulant and their use in the isolation of active coagulant protein. Blood 1982;59:594-600.
24. Nordfang O, Ezban M. Generation of active coagulation factor VIII from isolated subunits. J Biol Chem 1988;263:1115-8.
25. Fay PJ. Reconstitution of human factor VIII from isolated subunits. Arch Biochem Biophys 1988;262:525-31.
26. Prowse C, Waterston YG, Dawes J, Farrugia A. Studies on the procurement of blood coagulation factor VIII. In vitro studies on blood components prepared in half-strength citrate anticoagulant. Vox Sang 1987;52:257-64.

EFFECT OF BLOOD COLLECTION ON THE HEMOSTATIC POTENTIAL OF COAGULATION PROTEINS

R. Pflugshaupt, G. Kurt

Proteins with hemostatic properties are among the most important components of human plasma. Although FVIII:C will soon be available as a recombinant product, FVIII:C isolated from donor blood plasma will not be completely replaced in the following decade. Therefore, blood transfusion services and producers of therapeutic plasma products have the obligation to use the donated blood as efficiently as possible. World-wide efforts are made to optimize quality and yields of these components, not only because of the extremely high price of the subsequent products, but also due to the voluntary nature of the blood donation. The loss of quantity and quality of the hemostatic components takes place not only during the purification process, but is most importantly influenced by a number of factors prior, during and after the blood donation.

These factors are:

- psychological situation of the blood donor;
- technique of venipuncture;
- way of mixing of blood and anticoagulant;
- duration of donation;
- time-lag between donation end and the stripping of the tubing;
- duration and temperature of blood storage before separation of cells;
- technique of separation of plasma from blood cells;
- freezing and storage of plasma before cryoprecipitation.

In the follwoing it will be shown how some of the above mentioned points can be influenced in a positive way by adequate procedures.

A difficult venipuncture may cause contamination of the blood with tissue factor; such donations and also those in which blood flow was unusually slow should not be used as a source of fresh frozen plasma or for the manufacturing of coagulation factors [1]. This is –beside proper technique of venipuncture– mainly a problem of the condition of the donor, a fact which can not be influenced by the phlebotomist.

Improper mixing of blood with anticoagulant results in insufficient anticoagulation and hence in the formation of traces of the proteolytic enzyme thrombin. One of the functions of thrombin consists of activating FVIII:C, resulting in a feedback mechanism which enhances the formation of more thrombin. In fact, it seems that the first traces of thrombin are mainly involved in this mechanism [2]. The more visible activity of thrombin is its action on fibrinogen which enables this plasma protein to polymerize to insoluble fibrin, observable as blood clotting. The first action of thrombin on fibrinogen is to cleave arginine-glycine bonds at the N-terminal end of the two alpha chains of the molecule releasing two fibrinopeptides A (FPA); after a short time two other arginine-glycine bonds, at the beta chains, are cleaved releasing two fibrinopeptides B. If the coagulation system is activated during blood donation, the amount of formed thrombin can be estimated by measuring the FPA content of a given sample, with indirect information on the activation of FVIII:C. This activation is followed by a loss of stability of this factor [3-5]. Some years ago we have studied the influence of mixing blood and anticoagulant during donation [6]. We asked ourselves, if the FPA content of donors plasma is influenced by the method of blood collection and if high FPA content of the starting fresh frozen plasma impairs the quality of factor VIII preparation.

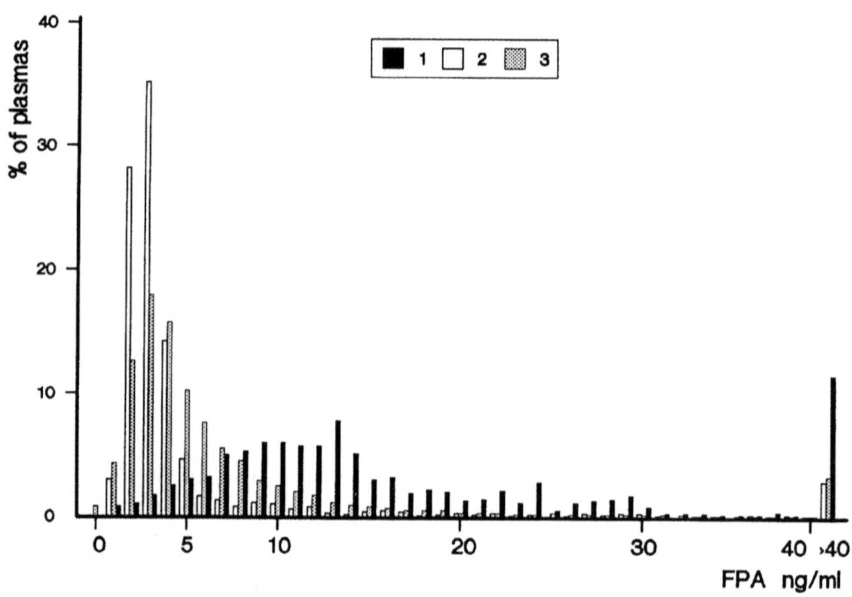

Figure 1. Distribution of FPA content in three experiments: 1) Collection I, before intensive instruction, n=1,185; 2) Collection II, after intensive instruction, n=1,179; 3) Samples collected during 21 month, according to variant 2 (Table 3), n=25,165.

In a first experiment we studied the influence of mixing blood and anticoagulant in a small series of blood donation. Perfect mixing, by automatic mixing balance or turning the bag upside down every 30 to 45 seconds, yielded low FPA values (3.6 ± 1.9 ng/ml; 2.9 + 0.80 ng/ml resp.); on the other hand, leaving the bag hanging without special mixing gave very high FPA content (57.3 ± 53.3 ng/ml). We decided to test, in a large experiment, the FPA values of our routinely collected blood. Plasma from 1,185 bottles containing material from 2-3 donors were analyzed for FPA content. The amount of FPA varied in a wide range and more than 10% of samples contained more than 40 ng/ml FPA (collection I). The distribution of FPA content of the plasmas is shown in Figure 1. From our experiments showing the effect of mixing blood and anticoagulant we knew that the results could be far better. The personnel of our mobile teams were duly informed and instructed about our experiments, and they were asked to exactly follow our mixing instructions. We then tested 1,179 small pools from the new collection for FPA (collection II). The distribution of the results is also shown in Figure 1; the difference between the two collections is highly significant and there remains no doubt that perfect mixing during donation is an important point of the collection protocol.

From these two plasma collections we produced six lots of factor VIII concentrates [7]. The plasmas of the lots were chosen according to their FPA content (>30; <30; <7 ng/ml). Some of the analytical results of the three most informative lots are presented in Table 1. The most striking result was the lot with plasmas containing more than 30 ng/ml FPA clotted after dissolution and could not be processed. Just

Table 1. Analytical results of the most informative three lots of factor VIII concentrates with different FPA content of the starting plasma.

	FPA content of starting plasma (ng/ml)		
	>30 **n=171/x=62.9** **SD=18.92**	**<30** **n=1014/x=13.12** **SD=6.46**	**<7** **n=1021/x=3.38** **SD=0.98**
FVIII:C (IU/ml) of cryoprecipitate	5.0 clotted	4.2	3.9
FVIII:C after process before lyophilisation	–	23.5	19.0
Solubility (min)	–	2.5	1.5
Stability at RT (no clotting, h)	–	>48	>48
FVIII:C after dissol. (IU/ml)	–	21.8	26.5
FVIII:C (24 h at RT) (IU/ml)	–	33.0	25.3
Maximum thrombin activation	–	13 ×	30×

Table 2. Analytical results of three groups of cryoprecipitates with different FPA content of the starting plasma.

	n	FPA content of starting plasma	FVIII:C U/ml	Solubility min	Clotted after 24 h
Group 1	8	2.5 ± 0.24	3.05 ± 1.59	5.47 ± 2.5	1
Group 2	9	21.2 ± 6.65	2.97 ± 1.36	4.28 ± 1.1	0
Group 3	8	183.2 ± 151.10	3.01 ± 0.70	11.57 ± 5.0	4

after dissolution we found a higher activity of factor VIII than in the other lots, probably due to activation. The striking difference between the other two lots were the improved stability and the better thrombin activation in the final product of the lot with less than 7 ng/ml FPA.

In another experiment we produced some small pool cryoprecipitates (AHF SRK) from plasma with defined FPA contents. The findings are shown in Table 2. It is obvious that high FPA content influences

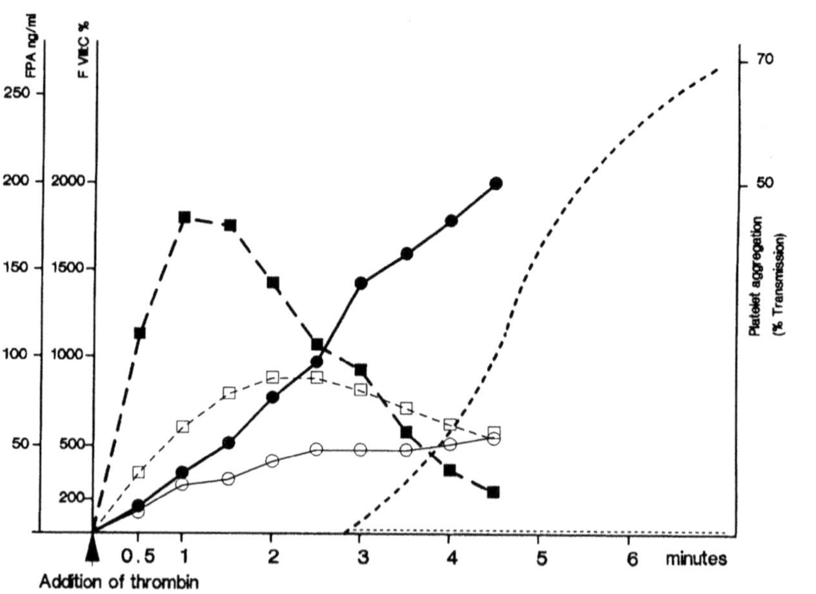

Figure 2. Activation and inactivation of FVIII:C, generation of FPA and aggregation of platelets after addition of thrombin in two different concentrations. ■–■ = FVIII:C % 0.0125 U/ml thrombin; □–□ = FVIII:C %, 0.0031 U/ml thrombin; ●–● = FPA ng/ml, 0.0125 U/ml thrombin; ○–○ = FPA ng/ml, 0.0031 U/ml thrombin; -------- = platelet aggregation %, 0.0125 U/ml thrombin; .... = platelet aggregation %, 0.0031 U/ml thrombin.

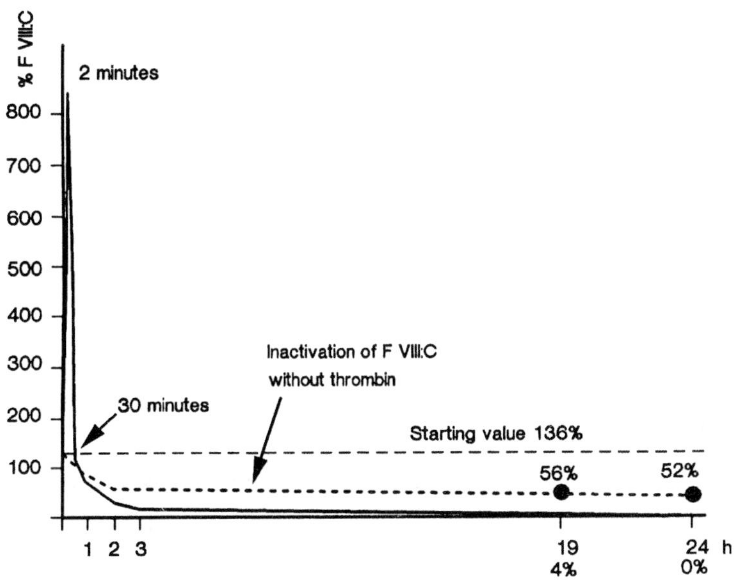

Figure 3. Activation and inactivation of FVIII:C by thrombin (0.0031 U/ml) in a plasma sample of a healthy donor.

the solubility and stability of such products, while –surprisingly– the FVIII:C activity seems to be approximately the same in all samples. This was also found by others [1,8,9].
During these investigations we made some studies on factor VIII activation and inactivation by thrombin. It is well-known that thrombin activation is important for factor VIII procoagulant function [2,10-12]. Activation of factor VIII results in a loss of stability of this factor [3,4]. Figure 2 shows the activation and subsequent inactivation of factor VIII, the generation of FPA in platelet poor plasma and the aggregation of platelets in platelet rich plasma of the same donation after addition of thrombin in two different concentrations. Factor VIII activity and FPA content were measured every 30 seconds. The maximum of factor VIII activity was reached one minute after addition of thrombin in the higher (0.0125 U/ml) and approximately two minutes in the lower (0.0031 U/ml) concentration. FPA generation is linear during the first five minutes and depends as expected on the thrombin concentration. The aggregation of platelets starts later and is only seen with the higher concentration of thrombin.

In two other experiments we studied the inactivation of factor VIII after thrombin activation. Figure 3 shows the result when a fresh plasma sample of a healthy donor was activated with 0.0031 U/ml thrombin. Measurement was started only two minutes after thrombin

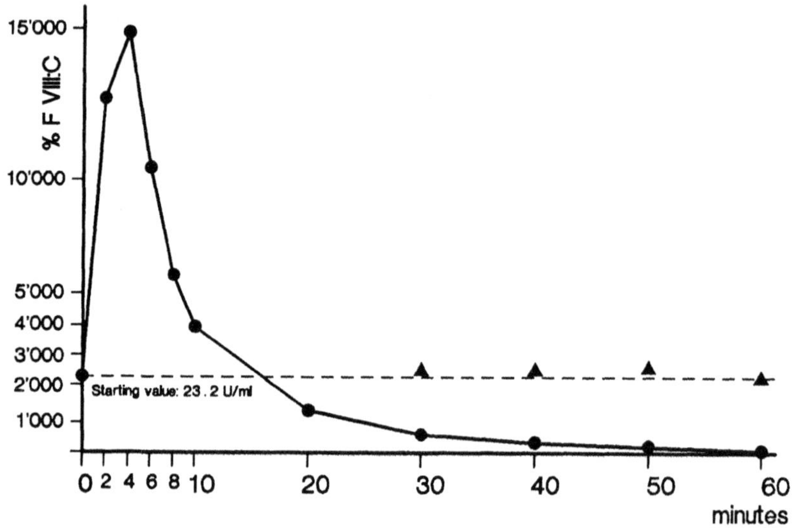

Figure 4. Activation and inactivation of FVIII:C by thrombin (0.0031 U/ml in a factor VIII concentrate.

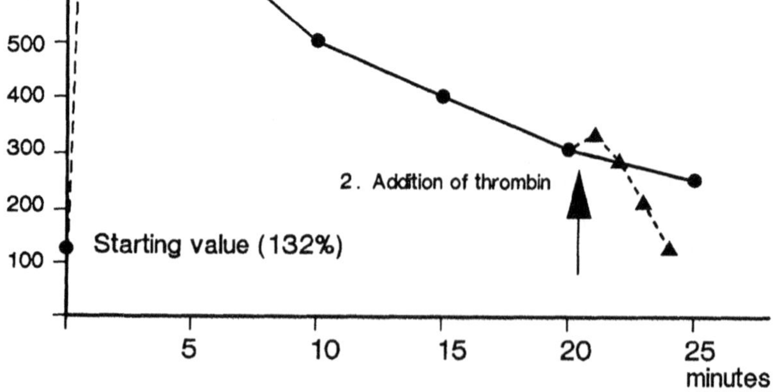

Figure 5. Trail to reactivate FVIII:C by thrombin after a first activation and subsequent inactivation.

addition, when inactivation already took place. After 30 minutes the starting value of 136% was reached, after one hour only 50% and after 24 hours no factor VIII activity was left. A plasma sample without activation stored under the same conditions showed still 40% of the starting value after 24 hours.

A similar experiment was undertaken by activating a factor VIII concentrate with 0.0031 U/ml thrombin. Figure 4 shows the activation and inactivation diagram. After four minutes a seven-fold activation was reached, after one hour no activity was left. A sample without activation did not appreciably lose any activity in the same time.

Factor VIII which has been activated and inactivated by thrombin cannot be activated a second time. The addition of thrombin a second time only accelerates the inactivation (Figure 5).

Some other experiments showed the kinetics of FPA generation during blood donation. Forty-eight tubes (or plastic tubings as used in donation sets) were filled with four ml of blood without any anticoagulant. The FPA generation was stopped by heparin/trasylol in intervals each prolonged by five seconds from one tube to the other. Figure 6 shows the results of two of these experiments. The generation of FPA starts after approximately two minutes, but we must take in consideration that the activation of factor VIII has already started at that time. The first visible clot appears between four and five minutes; concomitantly FPA content is over 700 ng/ml. This finding supports the observation

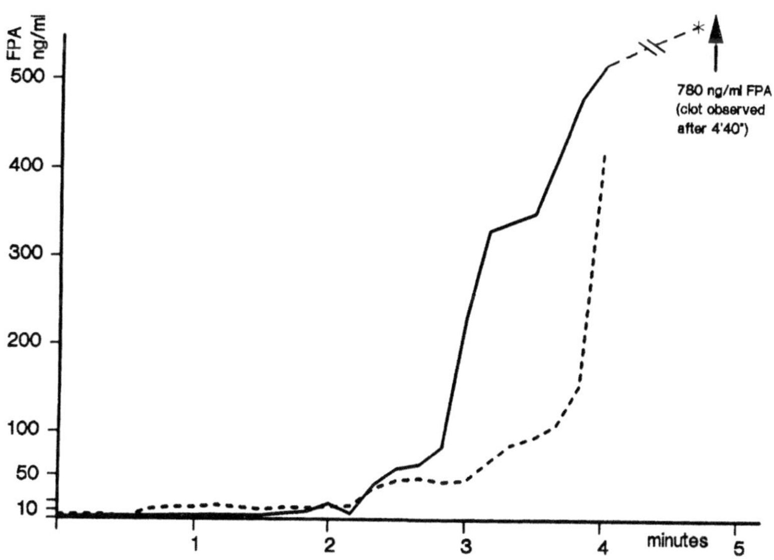

Figure 6. Kinetics of FPA generation in blood donation lines.

that late stripping of the content of the collection tubing in the blood bag could result in high FPA values [1,13].

The Central Laboratory of the Dutch Red Cross Blood Transfusion Service has recently changed its blood collection protocol by adding the following procedure: Each blood collection is ended by transferring the needle from the vein into the rubber stopper of an evacuated sampling tube, all blood in the blood line is thus removed and replaced by anticoagulated blood from the blood bag [14]. In the sequel of our FPA study we proposed to our board to use our findings for the improvement of the quality of plasma for the production of coagulation factor concentrates. The three proposals submitted to the board are summarized in Table 3. The board decided to follow variant 2 with the slight modification that only ten samples per mobile team were examined (= 80 samples a day, analyzed in lots of 240 twice a week). Venipuncture personnel were instructed via written protocols and diagrams on the correct venipuncture and mixing of blood with anticoagulant. During 21 months we tested 25,165 plasma samples for FPA content. The overall results are shown in Figure 1. The results were far better than before any instruction was given but did not reach the quality seen after the very intensive instruction during the second collection.

Improper venipuncture, long time of donation, insufficient mixing of blood and anticoagulant, late stripping of the tubing, might be reasons for activation of the coagulation system. The measurement of FPA is a sensitive tool to evaluate such an activation regardless the cause.

The highest quality of plasma could be reached by screening all samples for activation, and eliminating those with high values. The FPA test is until now the most investigated tool; the limit for elimination of plasma samples would probably lay around 20 ng/ml. In practice the

Table 3. Three variants to use the findings for the improvement of the quality of plasma for the production of coagulation factor concentrates.

	Variant 1	**Variant 2**	**Variant 3**
FPA determination	all donations	20 samples per mobile team (= 160 per day)	100 samples per day, without identification
Frequency of tests	every day	2-3 times per week	1-2 times per week
Evaluation of results	plasmas with high FPA can be eliminated	plasmas with high FPA can be eliminated (partially)	no elimination of plasmas with high FPA
Estimation of quality of blood collection	good	possible	possible
Personnel requirement	0.5-1 person (automatization)	0.5 person	0.1 person

Table 4. Comparison of the results of FPA and TAT determination in 20 blood donations.

	FPA (ng/ml) donors value	good mixing	poor mixing	TAT (ug/ml) donors value	good mixing	poor mixing
X	3.34	8.06	12.95	2.28	5.53	12.36
SD	1.26	5.78	13.26	0.73	3.46	9.55
n	20	10	10	20	10	10

FPA test seems not very suitable for mass screening because of its laborious and time consuming procedure. Some time ago, a new test became available which measures thrombin/antithrombin III-complexes (Enzygnost-TAT, Behring Ag, Germany). Antithrombin III is the most relevant inhibitor of thrombin by formation of complexes which are sensitive parameters of a latent activation of the plasmatic coagulation system [15]. The test uses an ELISA technique and could probably be automated. We made some preliminary experiments with the kit which is available commercially. The results are shown in Table 4 and Figure 7. The good correlation between FPA and TAT suggests that TAT might be a tool for screening of plasma protein activation during blood collection, extended studies are planned.

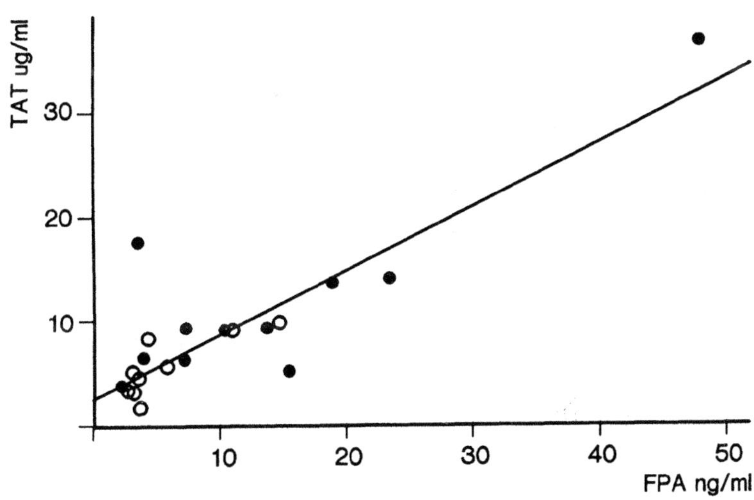

Figure 7. Correlation between FPA and TAT content in donor plasmas after improper and good mixing of blood and anticoagulant during donation (r^2=0.78). ○ = good mixing; ● = improper mixing.

References

1. Prowse CV, Bessos H, Farrugia A, Smith A, Gabra J. Donation procedure, fibrinopeptide A, and factor VIII. Vox Sang 1984;46:55-7.
2. Brod) K, Anderson LO, Sandberg H. Kinetics of activation of human factor VIII by thrombin. Thromb Res 1980;19:299-307.
3. Rick ME, Hoyer LW. Thrombin activation of factor VIII. I. The effect of inhibitors. Br J Haematol 1977;36:585-97.
4. Rick ME, Hoyer LW. Thrombin activation of factor VIII. II. a comparison of purified factor VIII and the low molecular weight factor VIII procoagulant. Br J Haematol 1978;38:107-19.
5. Hoyer LW, Trabold NC. The effect of thrombin on human factor VIII. J Lab Clin Med 1981;97:50-64.
6. Pflugshaupt R, Kurt G. FPA content: A criterion of quality for plasma as factor VIII source. Vox Sang 1983;45:224-32.
7. Wickerhauser M. Large-scale preparation of factor VIII concentrate from frozen cryoethanol precipitate. Throm Diath Haemorrh 1971;43(Suppl.): 165-73.
8. Carlebjörk G, Blombäck M, Akerblom O. Improvement of plasma quality as raw material for factor VIII:C concentrates. Storage of whole blood and plasma and interindividual plasma levels of fibrinopeptide A. Vox Sang 1983;45:233-42.
9. Törmä E, Myllylä G. Parameters affecting the fractionation of factor-VIII:C activity in production of very high purity AHF concentrates. Scand J Haematol 1984;33(Suppl.40):123-6.
10. Rapaport SI, Schiffman S, Patch MJ, Ames SB. The importance of activation of antihemophilic globulin and proaccelerin by traces of thrombin in the generation of intrinsic prothrombinase activity. Blood 1963;21:221.
11. Rapaport SI, Hjort PF, Patch MJ. Further evidence that thrombin-activation of factor VIII is an essential step in intrinsic clotting. Scand J Clin Lab Invest 1965;84:88.
12. Osterud B, Rapaport SI, Schiffman S, Chong MMY. Formation of intrinsic factor-X-activator activity, with special reference to the role of thrombin. Br J Haematol 1971;21:643.
13. Skjonsberg OH, Kierulf P, Fagerhol MK, Godal HC. Thrombin generation during collection and storage of blood. Vox Sang 1986;50:33-7.
14. Over J. Personal communication.
15. Pelzer H, Schwarz A, Heimburger N. Determination of human thrombin-antithrombin III complex in plasma with an enzyme-linked immunosorbent assay. Thromb Haemostasis 1988;59:101-6.

FACTOR VIII YIELDS FROM ANTICOAGULANT EXCHANGED HAEMONETICS ULTRALITE™ PLASMA

J. Speak, A.M. Cumming, R.T. Wensley

Introduction

Hemophilia A, which results from a lack of procoagulant factor VIII (FVIII), is the commonest severe hemostasis disorder. It is inherited as a sex-linked recessive characteristic, affecting approximately 1:10,000 males. The main therapy for Hemophilia A is FVIII replacement using FVIII concentrate. Cryoprecipitate is no longer recommended as a primary treatment of Hemophilia A for reasons of viral safety. Cryoprecipitation however remains the first step in the production of the great majority of FVIII concentrates derived from human plasma. Recoveries of FVIII in concentrates are low and the need for viral inactivation has further reduced the yields. We now describe work in progress to improve the recovery of FVIII in cryoprecipitates based upon the principle of anticoagulant exchange using heparin and calcium chloride.

It is believed that the two chain FVIII molecule is linked by calcium ion bridges [1]. Citrate based anticoagulants chelate the calcium bridges causing the FVIII molecule to lose stability with consequent loss of FVIII activity (FVIII:C). This stability can be restored by recalcification (addition of calcium chloride) together with heparin [1-4].

We have previously reported a 23% increase in FVIII yields in concentrates prepared from plasma derived from the Baxter Autopheresis C™ cell separator [5]. Plasma obtained by this system is platelet free.

The initial aim of the present study was to investigate the potential for improved yields of FVIII in single donation cryoprecipitates in which anticoagulant exchange reagent was added to citrated plasma containing significant numbers of platelets, to give a final concentration of heparin 1.0 IU/ml and approximately 50% of physiological levels of ionized calcium. The Haemonetics Ultralite™ is in routine use at the Regional Blood Transfusion Centre in Manchester, UK, and gives platelet counts in the derived plasma of approximately 30-40×10^9/l.

Earlier work by our group [unpublished] using Haemonetics Ultralite™ derived plasma showed that recalcification to greater than physicological levels of ionized calcium resulted in clot formation, after freezing and thawing of the plasma had taken place. We believe that this may be due to calcium-induced platelet activation. It was necessary to see if sub-physiological levels of ionized calcium would stabilize FVIII without activation of coagulation.

Materials and methods

Plasma-ionized calcium concentration and anticoagulant exchange

Unfractionated mucous sodium heparin (5,000 IU/ml with chlorobutol 0.5%) was purchased from Leo laboratories, UK. A solution of 1 molar calcium chloride was obtaind from BDH Chemicals Ltd, Poole, UK. Ionized calcium was measured using a calcium ion selective electrode (ISE), Russell pH Ltd, Fife, Scotland, in conjunction with a Corning model Delta 150 pH/ion meter, Corning Ltd, Essex, UK, in accordance with the manufacturer's instructions.
Heparin was added to a final concentration of 1.0 IU/ml to half strength citrate phosphate dextrose (CPD 50) anticoagulated plasma, along with 1 molar calcium chloride, titrated using the ISE. In subsequent work with single donation cryoprecipitates, a fixed volume of anticoagulant exchange reagent was used. The required volume to add was calculated from the volume of calcium chloride required for titration of the citrated plasma to 0.5 mM free ionized calcium concentration.

Measurement of FVIII:C in heparinized plasma

A microtitre chromogenic FVIII assay (Coatest®, Kabi Diagnostics, Uxbridge, London), was used according to manufacturers instructions, and with appropriate plasma dilutions to negate the heparin effect.

Radioimmunoassay for platelet factor 4 (PF4), and fibrinopeptide A (FPA)

PF4 analysis was undertaken using a kit obtained from Abbott Diagnostics, Maidenhead, UK. The plasma derived from the Haemonetics Ultralite™ was anticoagulated with CPD 50, or anticoagulant exchanged with heparin and recalcified to 0.5 mM ionized calcium by titration using the ISE. Following incubation at 21°C for 0, and 4, and 24 hours, aliquots of plasma were placed in Thrombotect™ tubes (Abbott Diagnostics) to inhibit in vitro release of PF4. FPA was similarly analysed using a radioimmunoassay obtained from Biodiagnostics, Upton upon Severn, UK.

Preparation of single donation cryoprecipitates

The Haemonetics Ultralite™ was used to collect 600 ml plasma donations (CPD 50 anticoagulated). Two 180 ml aliquots were prepared, one left in CPD 50 (control), and the other anticoagulant exchanged (heparin added to a final concentration of 1.0 IU/ml and recalcification to approximately 50% of physiological levels (0.5 mM of ionized calcium). Following freezing at –70°C, a rapid thaw (90 min at 22°C) for extraction of the cryoprecipitate in the CPD 50 control and anticoagulant exchange variant (n=11) was undertaken. On the later extractions (n=9) a slow thaw (12 h at 4°C) was carried out.

Results

The microtitre Coatest® chromogenic FVIII assay was assessed for validity when using plasma containing heparin at a final concentration of 1.0 IU/ml. Ten donations, each split into control CPD 50 and a heparin variant were assayed for FVIII:C. Using a paired t test, no significant difference between the two groups was found at the 20% level.

An experiment was divided in order to see if ionized calcium concentrations of 0.5 mM would stabilize the FVIII without evidence of clotting. FVIII:C, FPA, and PF4 were measured at collection, and 4, and 24 hours following incubation of the plasma at 21°C. Loss of FVIII:C was minimal after 24 hours compared to control CPD 50 anticoagulated plasma, and the levels of FPA (reflecting thrombin activity) and PF4 (indicating platelet activity) were low, suggesting that no problems with clotting would occur at this concentration of ionized calcium (Table 1). It was then necessary to see if the observed increase in FVIII stability in plasma would result in increased yields of FVIII:C in cryoprecipitates.

Using eleven individual donations, a mean increase of 8.3% in FVIII yields was observed in the extracted cryoprecipitates in the anticoagulant exchange variant compared to CPD 50 control, when cryoprecipi-

Table 1. FVIII:C, FPA, and PF4 measured in plasma containing ionized calcium at 0.5 mM vs CPD 50 control incubated at 21°C for 24 hours.

	Time 0 hour		Time 4 hour		Time 24 hour	
	CPD	Ca2+	CPD	Ca2+	CPD	Ca2+
FVIII:C (% remaining)	100	100	100	104 (n=4)	68	97
FpA (ng/ml)	3.2	2.8	4.0	3.2	4.0	6.0
PF4 (ng/ml)	72.6	89.8	105.3	119.3	154.1	171.9

Each result represents the mean of five experiments unless otherwise stated.

Table 2. Total FVIII yields in cryoprecipitates (IU, n=11).

	CPD 50	Anticoagulant exchanged
1	62	81
2	195	186
3	119	132
4	62	56
5	142	179
6	105	106
7	72	95
8	192	186
9	112	140
10	102	126
11	160	147
$\bar{X}$	120	130

Fast thaw cryoprecipitate extraction (22°C for 2 hours). X = mean
Anticoagulant exchange reagent (heparin to 1.0 IU/ml, ionized calcium to 0.5 mM).
There was no significant difference at the 10% level using a paired t test.

Table 3. Total FVIII yields in cryoprecipitates (IU, n=9).

	CPD 50	Anticoagulant exchanged
1	130	150
2	127	156
3	114	136
4	56	84
5	141	167
6	142	174
7	134	165
8	122	145
9	113	114
$\bar{X}$	119.9	143.4

Slow thaw cryoprecipitate extraction (4°C for 12 hours). X = mean
Anticoagulant exchange reagent (heparin to 1.0 IU/ml, ionized calcium to 0.5 mM).
There was a significant difference at the 0.2% level (p=<0.002) using a paired t test.

tation was carried out at 22°C for 90 min (Table 2). By paired t test this was not significant at the 10% level.

However, when the same experiment was carried out with cryoprecipitation at 4°C for 12 h (n=9), a 19.6% increase in FVIII yield was observed in the anticoagulant exchange variant versus the CPD 50 control (Table 3). By paired t test this was significant at the 0.2% level.

Discussion

The first requirement of this study was to investigate the validity of the FVIII assay in the presence of heparin at a final concentration of 1.0 IU/ml in plasma. The use of Polybrene® and in particular Protamine has its drawbacks, due to the anticoagulant and possible procoagulant nature of the polycations [6]. The heparin effect can be removed completely by dilution using the Coatest® microtitre chromogenic assay.

We have previously shown that recalcification of citrated plasma to physiological levels of ionized calcium caused no problems with clotting of platelet-free plasma [5]. However unpublished work with Haemonetics Ultralite™ plasma which contains significant numbers of platelets showed that recalcification to physiological and supra-physiological levels of ionized calcium resulted in platelet aggregation and clot formation following freezing and thawing of the plasma. This may be due to calcium-induced platelet activation. The aim of this study was to investigate the potential for improved yields of FVIII from plasma containing significant numbers of platelets. We considered the possibility that sub-physiological levels of ionized calcium would stabilize the FVIII without activation of coagulation. At 0.5 mM ionized calcium (approximately half normal plasma levels) the FVIII activity was stabilized and FPA (reflecting thrombin activity) and PF4 (indicating platelet activation) showed no signs of initiation of coagulation (Table 1).

Having optimized the anticoagulant exchange reagent, it was necessary to see if the increased stability of FVIII seen in anticoagulantexchanged plasma, compared with CPD 50 control plasma would result in increased yields of FVIII in cryoprecipitates derived from that plasma.

The results of our experiments showed that increasing the cryoprecipitate thaw time resulted in a relative increase in FVIII yields in the anticoagulant exchange cryoprecipitates compared to the control CPD 50 anticoagulated cryoprecipitates. An 8% increase was observed when the thawing conditions were 22°C for 90 min and 19% when 4°C for 12 h was utilized (Tables 2 and 3). These findings may be due to the FVIII remaining stable during preparation of cryoprecipitates from anticoagulant-exchanged plasma whereas loss of FVIII:C occurs during preparation of citrated cryoprecipitates. Greater losses occurring when the thawing time is prolonged.

References

1. Mikaelsson ME, Forsman N, Oswaldson U. Human blood factor VIII: A calcium linked protein complex. Blood 1983;62:1006-15.
2. Krachmalnikoff A, Thomas DP. The stability of factor VIII in heparinized plasma. Thromb Haemost 1983;49:224-7.

3. Cumming AM, Wensley RT, Power DM, Delamore IW. The influence of anticoagulant on the in vitro level and stability of factor VIII procoagulant activity. Thromb Res 1987;46:391-5.
4. Rock GA, Cruickshank WH, Tackaberry ES, Ganz PR, Palmer DS. Stability of FVIII:C in plasma: The dependence on protease activity and calcium. Thromb Res 1983;29:521-35.
5. Cumming AM, Wensley RT, Winkleman L, Lane RS. A simple plasma anticoagulant-exchange method to increase the recovery of factor VIII in therapeutic concentrates. Vox Sang 1990;58:264-9.
6. Cumming AM, Jones GR, Wensley RT, Dundall RB. In vitro neutralization of heparin in plasma prior to the activated partial thromboplastin time test. An assessment of four heparin antagonists and two anion exchange resins. Thromb Res 1986;41:43-56.

DISCUSSION

P.M. Mannucci, C.Th. Smit Sibinga

C.Th. Smit Sibinga (Groningen, NL): Dr. Hoyer, how does the EGF fit into the four domains which you mentioned in the beginning, the Gla domain, the growth factor domain, the activation peptide domain and the catalytic domain?

L.W. Hoyer (Rockville, MD, USA): I am afraid I may have used an abbreviation in one case and not in the other. The second domain is the EGF or epidermal growth factor, so that those are the same; it is coded by the third and fourth factor IX exons. It is a very interesting calcium-dependent binding area, which is separate from Gla, but seems essential for function, though probably very differently.

A question for both Dr. Lindhout and Dr. Mikaelsson. The question is how the calcium interaction with Gla is effective. You suggest that it serves as a bridge between the phospholipid and the Gla, but also it is possible to show by physical techniques that there is a conformational change within the vitamin K dependent protein when calcium interacts. So, I am wondering how calcium causes a change in the protein shape and also is available to interact with phospholipid on the surface of the platelet. That would imply that it is really doing two things; I am curious about your thoughts on this matter.

M. Mikaelsson (Stockholm, S): I think that when calcium is present, there is a conformational change and transition of the vitamin K dependent proteases. Since there is a whole series of Gla residues, it is quite possible an internal change in the conformation that leads to exposure of the other carboxy groups, namely the Gla residues that participate in the association with phospholipids. They have to be in a proper arrangement.

T. Lindhout (Maastricht, NL): In addition, work by the group of Zwaal[1] has indicated that clotting factors also bind to positively

1. Rosing J, Tans G, Speijer H, Zwaal RFA. Calcium independent activation of prothrombin on membranes with positively charged lipids. Biochemistry 1988;27:9048-55.

charged phospholipids. The role of calcium ions is not completely understood, but a calcium-induced conformational change in the protein might be a primary step.

L.W. Hoyer: Another mechanism that we emphasized is the interaction of factor VIII with phospholipids that occur at the far terminal region of a C2 domain, which is not calcium dependent. So, there are probably many ways in which proteins can interact with lipid surfaces.

L.H. Siegenbeek van Heukelom (Alkmaar, NL): Dr. Mikaelsson, as a clinician may I ask you a simple question? You have talked much about calcium in vitro. However, in the hospital we find many situations of hypercalcemia and hypocalcemia, but I have never seen the coagulation system disturbed. What is the situation in vivo, in a patient with hypercalcemia or hypocalcemia?

M. Mikaelsson: I think that the variatons that you may see in vivo are rather small, because changes that effect the clotting are much larger and would have other effects on the heart rate etc. There is also another reason; the coagulation process as we have stressed here is a very local process at the site of injury, where there is a local regulation of the calcium levels.

C.F. Högman Uppsala, S): As was mentioned in some of the lectures, Prowse et al[2,3] have shown that reducing the concentration of citrate in the anticoagulant does improve the stability of factor VIII, when stored in whole blood and at room temperature. I think that we have to balance between a risk of thrombin formation because of the decreased concentration of citrate and an improved stability of factor VIII. I wonder if you have any comments about the possibility to use this in practical transfusion work.

M. Mikaelsson: As I mentioned, we have studied the possibility of reducing the citrate strength. But in our hands we do not find this optimal. You cannot reduce the citrate concentration further, because then the protection against clotting is not sufficient. So, that is the reason why we chose the alternative to recalcify the citrated plasma to be able to reach higher levels of free calcium. In half-strength citrate the calcium level is only 0.1 mM, when you have to reach a level definitely

2. Prowse C, Waterston YG, Dawes J, Farrugia A. Studies on the procurement of blood coagulation factor VIII: In vitro studies on blood components prepared in half-strength citrate anticoagulant. Vox Sang 1987;52:257-64.
3. Griffin B, Bell JK, Prowse C. Studies on the procurement of blood coagulation factor VIII. In vivo studies on blood components prepared in half-strength citrate coagulant. Vox Sang 1988;54:193-8.

above 0.5 mM. If you stress the conditions at which you test the instability, you have to reach physiological levels of 1 mM calcium, to render factor VIII completely stable.

T. Lindhout: I am puzzled by what you are calling a different instability of factor VIII. The question is whether factor VIII during storage becomes (partially) activated or not. There is a large homology between factor V and factor VIII. We all know that factor V and factor V_a are very stable proteins in the presence of calcium ions. But in contrast to activated factor V, activated factor VIII rapidly looses its activity. How is that possible? Are there other factors involved, such as the pH?

M. Mikaelsson: What I have discussed sofar is the stability of FVIII:C. I have not discussed activated factor VIII at all, that is quite different.

C.Th. Smit Sibinga: Dr. Pflugshaupt, a comment related to your observation that thrombin does not have the ability to reactivate factor VIII: I think it might do that only once!

R. Pflugshaupt (Bern, CH): I think in plasma or in this concentrate it is unstable at the moment it is activated. That may be different in an absolutely purified product; there it might be stable after activation.

T. Lindhout: Yes, I can remember a paper,[4] not that long ago, showing that when you decrease the pH to 6.5, factor VIII remains perfectly stable.

L.W. Hoyer: You recall a very nice paper by Pete Lollar. But I think it may not be directly applicable here. He was studying porcine factor VIII and it may be different from human. However, the major difference is that he was working with highly purified activated factor VIII and showed the instability of the A2 domain. That may be very different from what happens in plasma, with all of the proteases that could affect factor VIII. So, it is going to be a little while before we know what this elegant observation means for clinical concentrates.

C.Th. Smit Sibinga: I think you are right.

R. Wensley (Manchester, UK): Dr. Mikaelsson, we heard about the assembly of the clotting factors on the surface of platelets and about "flip-flop". Now, other phospholipids present in plasma may be in

4. Lollar P, Parker CG. pH-dependent denaturation of thrombin-activated porcine factor VIII. J Biol Chem 1990;265:1688-92.

cheilomicrons and lipoproteins; is there any evidence that these may participate in similar reactions? In other words should we take the alimentary state of the patient into account, whether they are postprandial or not?

M. Mikaelsson: Studies performed by Andersson and Brown[5] have shown that other lipids also have a procoagulant activity in in vitro systems. However, I think that in vivo the local coagulation process is mainly dependent on the platelet phospholipids exposed upon activation.

R. Wensley: What is the right combination of phospholipids acting for "flip-flop"?

T. Lindhout: The situation is complicated. Recent studies have shown that when platelets are activated, they form small vesicles, causing platelet dust in the circulation. Those vesicles may serve as a procoagulant surface. On the other hand it has also been shown that for instance factor X activation at the surface of endothelial cells is quite well possible, although you do not have negatively charged lipids there. So, I think there is more than only the surface of an activated platelet that is functioning here.

L.W. Hoyer: One of the important features of coagulation is the fact that it is concentrated in a specific location. Von Willebrand factor plays a very important role in bringing factor VIII to the platelet surface so that the very small concentration of factor VIII in the circulation becomes an adequate level at the site of injury. I wonder, does this platelet dust have glycoprotein IB?

T. Lindhout: That is right, so it can form microaggregates too.

J.K. Smith (Oxford, UK): There are good reasons why fractionators have not appeared to take advantage of all the discoveries about calcium and heparin over the last ten years. I would like to share a few of them with you. One is that there are other important proteins than factor VIII recoverable from plasma. It is also true that the protective effects of calcium on citrated plasma, with or without the addition of heparin do tend to take some time to show up. You need to harvest the plasma perhaps after about six hours to show any improvement. Many centres can ensure that plasma is separated within the time in which calcium would have an advantage. We have actually fractionated plasma

5. Andersson L-D, Brown JE. Interaction of factor VIII/von Willebrand factor with phospholipid vesicles. Biochem J 1981;200:161-7.

taken into ACD-B which gives a citrate concentration near to that of half-strength citrate and found, first of all, that it was the only plasma we have met which routinely gave FPA above 20 pmol/ml. Secondly, although the plasma fractionated did well for factor VIII, the factor IX was unusable, because of activation. So, I think we would not be in a great hurry to bring the effective plasma citrate down much below about 10 mmol/l even in plasmapheresis plasma, where you do not have long exposure before freezing the plasma. We have found that the variation in delivery of anticoagulant is so great that you have to have an anticoagulant delivery system designed for at least 14 mmol/l citrate to be sure that some of your donations are not well below 10 mmol/l and to prevent activation of factor IX.

Well, perhaps Dr. Pflugshaupt would say if he managed to fractionate factor IX from his various plasmas with high levels of FPA for instance. Kabi has done so.

M. Mikaelsson: We have done some experiments where we recalcified plasma and found that heparin affects the purification of other factors like factor IX. It is, however, possible to remove heparin after cryoprecipitation, if you add citrate again as anticoagulant once you have removed the cryoprecipitate. Heparin can be removed on ion exchange matrices.

H.J.C. de Wit (Leeuwarden, NL): Perhaps I might give a short comment on this topic. We tried to process half-strength citrate anticoagulated blood in the buffy coat method as described first by Prins[6] and produce platelet concentrate from buffy coats as described by Pietersz.[7] In validating those products we could see that making platelet concentrates by buffy coat method from half-strength citrate anticoagulated blood is virtually impossible, where the validation of red cells in SAG-M seems to be all right. But because of the impossibility of making platelets from that whole blood we stopped doing any further research.

S. Stienstra (Nijmegen, NL): Dr. Pflugshaupt. I can imagine that you changed from the fibrinogen marker fibrinopeptide A to the thrombin marker thrombin-antithrombin III complex. Why did you choose for the thrombin-antithrombin III ELISA, since this is a rather indirect parameter for measuring thrombin activation. There is also from the same company an ELISA available for measuring fragment 1 + 2 from thrombin. That is a direct marker for the thrombin activation.

6. Prins HK, de Bruijn JCGH, Henrichs HPJ, Loos JA. Prevention of microaggregate formation by removal of "buffy-coats'. Vox Sang 1980;39:48-51.
7. Pietersz RNI, Loos JA, Reesink HW. Platelet concentrates stored in plasma for 72 hours at 22°C prepared from buffy coats of CPD blood collected in a quadruple-bag SAGM system. Vox Sang 1985;49:81-5.

R. Pflugshaupt: We just tried with the TAT, because this was available when we did the study in the past.

J.Ph.H.B. Sybesma (Dordrecht, NL): Dr. Pflugshaupt told us that it is important to have a good mixing procedure, but I want to know what are the instructions nowadays: What is the frequency of your mixing?

R. Pflugshaupt: The instruction says that it should be mixed every 30-45 seconds by turning the bag up and down.

C.Th. Smit Sibinga: Dr. Speak, the title of your presentation actually gave me the expectation that there would be a very specific role of the Haemonetics Ultralite in the recovery of your cryoprecipitate. But I did not really grasp that out of your data. What would have been the results, if you would have used for instance Autopheresis-C or any other machine.

J. Speak (Manchester, UK): It was necessary to overcome the problem inherent in the Ultralite system, the presence of platelets in the plasma, when using an anticoagulant exchange reagent. It would obviously be of benefit to go from 0.5 mM upto physiological levels of ionized calcium, this unfortunately was not possible. By employing the Autopheresis-C there would be minimum platelet contamination and we would not have run into the problems. To overcome the relatively high platelet counts in the Ultralite system we lowered the ionized calcium concentration, maintaining factor VIII stability without running into problems with clotting or insolubility.

C.Th. Smit Sibinga: But filtration recovered plasma for instance is supposed to be cell-free, because of the filtration process.

J. Speak: Well, I can assure you that platelet counts were performed on plasma derived from the Ultralite and all counts were greater than 30×10^9/l probably due to the fact that we are dealing with a system that separates only by centrifugation. The Autopheresis-C uses a mixture of centrifugation and filtration and is probably more effective at complete cell removal.

C.Th. Smit Sibinga: You do not have the comparison yet. Can we anticipate that for the future?

J. Speak: Dr. Cumming observed a 23% increase in factor VIII yields in the anticoagulant-exchange variant when compared to a citrate control using plasma derived from the Autopheresis-C. We intend to do a 4 kg model of fractionation using plasma derived from the Ultralite.

C.Th. Smit Sibinga: I could draw attention to another problem. When a pure filtration technique, for instance, in hollow fibre is involved, the contact of the blood with the membrane over the length of the tubing is such intense, that it might lead to activation and that might eventually jeopardize the whole story of recovery.

R. Wensley: I do not think we have much experience of the hollow fibre machines or systems and indeed in the UK we have not brought them into blood banking use; 99% of our plasma comes from the Haemonetics centrifugal systems. I do not think we could use the pure filtration systems, because they are so traumatic. We do not have any figures for activation from these machines, but it is my guess that they would probably produce quite activated materials. I shall be interested to know if anybody has got any data.

C.Th. Smit Sibinga: Mr. de Wit uses hollow fibre filtration principle predominantly in his centre. He might comment.

H.J.C. de Wit: We, indeed, use the hollow fibre device. We did quite a large study testing the quality of plasma that came from the Organon Teknika machine. Results will be published soon in Transfusion Science[8] and I can tell you that although we measured lots of parameters for activation like TAT and other complexes, plasma quality was good and coagulation activation could not be measured.

I.M. Nilsson (Malmö, S): Dr. Hoyer, would you like to discuss the possibility by determining gene defect in families with hemophilia B to predict if these patients are going to develop antibodies or not.

L.W. Hoyer: To my knowledge, in hemophilia B the experience is a little more consistent in that most of the patients who have developed inhibitors have had deletions. I think the original reports suggested there was an almost 1 to 1 relationship. My feeling about inhibitors is that you need to have two things to develop an inhibitor. You have to have a molecular defect in the factor VIII or factor IX gene, that results in the lack of circulating protein so that there is an immunologic response to the transfused protein. You also have to have the correct immune response genes, so that your are able to respond to this foreign protein. It is for this reason that the formation of inhibitors is always going to be complicated and probably not predictable just from the coagulation factor gene defect. It will be an interaction between that and the immune response capacity.

8. Eijkhout HW, van Driessche P, Schade JH, Hack CE, de Wit HJC. Evaluation of the Organon Teknika plasmapur plasmapheresis system with new software and two types of filter. Transfusion Science: in press.

I.M. Nilsson: Yes thank you. We have determined the gene defect in 44 Swedish families with hemophilia B and none of the patients with point mutations has developed any antibodies.

L.W. Hoyer: I think that suggests that those point mutations almost always allow the synthesis of a small amount of factor IX-like protein. I wonder if some of those point mutations were nonsense, causing a stop code on or are you only talking about amino acid changes? When a point mutation causes a stop code on, it may have the same effect as a deletion.

I.M. Nilsson: All our patients with antibodies had deletions. But we also have patients with deletions without having antibodies.

L.W. Hoyer: That emphasizes the immune response issues.

M. Mikaelsson: I want to add some information to my previous reply to Dr. Lindhout. When we studied the stability of factor VIII in plasma, we also used gel filtration to see whether factor VIII was associated with von Willebrand factor or not. In fresh plasma collected in citrate or heparin, factor VIII is completely associated with von Willebrand factor, the carrier protein. But if you collect blood in EDTA or add EDTA to heparin plasma factor VIII dissociates from von Willebrand factor. Furthermore, factor VIII itself dissociates into the different chains. If you use high concentration of calcium, factor VIII also dissociates from von Willebrand factor, which is in agreement with the hypothesis that there are metal ion bridges linking these two proteins.

L.W. Hoyer: Except that you can also dissociate the two with high concentrations of sodium chloride. So, I wonder if the effect might not be more electrostatic than specifically calcium-related.

M. Mikaelsson: Maybe both. There are also further speculations that in addition there may be hydrophobic interaction as a secondary linkage between the heavy chain and von Willebrand factor. But the hydrophobic interaction should be promoted by high ionic strength. It is very difficult to speculate on this in detail.

I would like to emphasize that changes in the anticoagulation has rather limited effect on factor VIII provided you handle the plasma collection and freezing promptly. The main problem in plasma fractionation and the production of therapeutic factor VIII concentrates is the poor yield in the cryoprecipitation. The yield in that step – even if you have 1 IU/ml in the starting plasma – is below 50%; that is the major question we should address.

C.Th. Smit Sibinga: That is very true; that actually was a major question during the symposium last year when we spoke about low temperature biology in relation to the recovery of factor VIII specifically but other cold insoluble globulins as well.[9] However, we did not come to the right answer, yet. So we come back to the same question.

9. Smit Sibinga CTh, Das PC. Separation and purification of cold insoluble globulines. In: Smit Sibinga CTh, Das PC, Meryman HT (eds). Cryopreservation and low temperature biology in blood transfusion. Dordrecht: Kluwer Academic Publ, 1990;129-44.

II. PRESERVATION ASPECTS

PLATELET FUNCTION PRESERVATION

S. Holme

Introduction

Due to more aggressive anti-cancer therapy in recent years, with thrombocytopenia as a principal side effect, the production of platelet concentrates (PC) by the American Red Cross Blood Services rose by 150% during the period from 1978 to 1988 [1]. Significantly less increase in production of RBC, only 24%, was seen during the same time period. As a result of the increased demand for platelets, there have been substantial efforts to make platelet transfusions more cost effective (i.e., to improve platelet yield and quality so that less units need to be transfused, while reducing the costs of processing and storage).

There also have been other factors which have affected new developments and research in platelet processing and preservation. With the general knowledge in 1983 that HIV could be transmitted by transfusion, there has been a shift toward utilization of single donor (apheresis) products to limit donor exposure, and in the development of systems to remove or inactivate viruses. Furthermore, as the need for long-term support of PC for the multi-transfused patient has grown, new techniques to remove or inactivate leukocytes have been developed to delay or prevent platelet refractoriness.

Even with the current "state of the art" conditions for processing and storage, there is a substantial loss of platelet viability during storage [2]. The nature of this lesion is not known, although there is increasing evidence that platelet activation during storage may play a role [3].

There is also some concern about the hemostatic function of stored platelets. It is well known that the platelets rapidly lose their responsiveness to aggregation agents during storage [4]. The lesion has been related to defects in arachidonate [5] and phosphatidylinositol metabolism [6], and to failure in regulation of intracellular free calcium [7]. Little is known, however, about the reversal of this defect in vivo postinfusion and the hemostatic consequences for the transfused patient.

In this paper, the new developments in platelet collection, processing, and storage will be reviewed. Additionally, recent advances in the research to elucidate the nature of loss of platelet function and viability during storage and discussion of possible approaches to prevent this loss will be described.

Developments in collection, processing, and storage of PC

Collection and processing

In routine blood bank processing of PC, whole blood is collected from the donor into the anticoagulant CPD or CPDA-1 and subjected to a soft centrifugation to obtain supernatant platelet-rich plasma (PRP). The PRP is then transfused to a special platelet container with suitable gas permeability and subjected to a hard spin to pellet the platelets. All but approximately 50 ml of plasma is removed with resuspension of platelets after a one to two our rest period. Storage is carried out on an agitator at a temperature of 20-24°C.

The inclusion of phosphate, adenine, and high dextrose levels in the anticoagulant is essential for red cell storage; for platelet processing and storage, the critical factor is the reduction in whole blood unit pH levels from 7.4 to 7.0 by the acid citrate and acid phosphate. At pH levels above 7.4, platelets are easily activated, resulting in difficulties with resuspension after the second hard spin. Recent studies have suggested that use of half-strength citrate in the anticoagulant, which improves factor VIII preservation, has minimal effect on platelet yield and quality [8].

Besides centrifugation speed and time, which has been reviewed in several papers [9-11], there are several other factors that are critical for good platelet harvest.

Recent studies have suggested that the period of hold of the whole blood units before processing is of importance for optimal platelet separation and yield [11,12]. Initiating the centrifugation within one to two hours after collection appears to result in poorer yields and perhaps poorer platelet quality than allowing for a hold period of eight hours. The likely cause for this, as will be discussed later, is that platelets are highly sensitive to activation immediately after collection. However, they rapidly lose their sensitivity to aggregating stimuli with storage, thereby reducing the possibility for activation and clumping with a longer hold period. Another factor that may contribute to the higher yield and better separation with a longer hold is that the red cells appear to undergo some changes in their rheological properties after collection, resulting in better packing during centrifugaton.

In Europe, an alternative method for component separation has recently been introduced. This is the so-called buffy coat (BC) method [13]. In this procedure, the whole blood units undergo a hard centrifugation with the platelets sedimented together with the white cells onto a cushion of red cells (the white cell layer is often referred to as the "buffy coat"). The platelet-rich BC, with approximately 30 ml of plasma, is then transferred to a separate satellite container and subjected to a soft spin to sediment contaminating white and red cells. The advantages of this method are that both the red cells and the BC-PC have greatly reduced white cell contamination compared to conventional PRP-derived components, the platelets may be less activated due to the pelleting against the red cells instead of the container wall, and finally, this method offers better possibilities for more cost-effective automatic processing with use of plasma-free synthetic media. Disadvantages of this technique are a reduced platelet harvest and the loss of approximately 30 ml of red cells in the buffy coat.

We have recently conducted a paired study, using ten donors, where PC obtained by using standard PRP or by using buffy coat-derived techniques were compared [14]. The buffy coat was prepared after a 6-hour hold of the whole blood unit, transferred into a Neocell plastic container, and held overnight. It was then subjected to a soft spin and the supernatant platelet concentrates transferred into a CLX platelet container for storage. PRP-PC were also processed after a 6-hour hold using standard ARC methods. BC-PC had significantly lower platelet yield (0.62 ± 0.2 versus $0.87 \pm 0.2 \times 10^{11}$ plts/unit; although WBC contamination was significantly reduced (19 ± 11 versus $364 \pm 156 \times 10^{6}$ WBC/unit). At day 1 of storage, BC-PC platelets demonstrated less β-TG release and were more discoid-shaped; however, after five days of storage, there were no significant differences between BC-PC and in various platelet properties including in vivo post transfusion percentage recoveries and survivals, ATP levels, GPIb levels, β-TG and LDH release, lactate production, and respiratory activity. This suggests that, although BC-PC may be less activated during the PC-processing phase, with storage the same lesions occur as for PRP-PC. These findings confirm previous studies reported by Fijnheer et al [15]. Of interest was that we could not demonstrate any effect of WBC on either the metabolic activity or platelet quality such as had been suggested previously in studies by Pieterz et al [16] and Sloane et al [17]. This discrepancy may be that the amount of contaminating WBC in our study was lower than in the earlier studies.

Buffy coat processing is very suitable for use in automated processing systems, and are now in routine use in The Netherlands, Sweden, and Italy. A system used by Högman in Uppsala involves simultaneous automatic squeezing out of red cells from the bottom of the container and plasma from the top, while the platelet-rich buffy coat remains in the container [18]. The squeezing is regulated by optic sensors. Four of these buffy coats are then pooled into a transfer bag using a sterile docking device. A platelet additive solution is then added and the pooled BC subjected to a soft spin to remove red and white cells. The supernatant PC, approximately 200 ml, is then transferred to a PL-732 container for storage. Similar platelet yield to that obtained by using conventional PRP separation techniques has been reported using this processing system.

In the USA, the use of automatic blood cell separators has increased substantially during the last decade. As mentioned previously, the concern about transmitting diseases and the problem with alloimmunization are the main reasons for this. Plateletapheresis machines routinely allow for separation of 3-5 $\times 10^{11}$ platelets, which corresponds to 5-8 single random donor units, within a period of two hours.

Most apheresis machines are continuous-flow instruments by which blood from the donor is continuously collected from one vein and processed in a centrifugational field, with return of red cells and plasma to the donor through a different line into another vein. New instruments such as Haemonetics M-30, V-50, and Baxter Plateletcell now utilize single-vein access with collection of blood and return of processed blood through the same line. The IBM 2997 and its successor, the COBE SPECTRA, have two-stage processing of the platelet-rich plasma, which allows for a substantial reduction of contaminating leukocytes [19-22]. Studies have demonstrated that the quality of platelets obtained by apheresis machines is similar to that obtained by manual apheresis; however, of concern is the high degree of complement activation which occurs during machine processing with blood continuously centrifuged against the centrifugation bowl. In a study recently conducted in our laboratory, we observed that the amount of plasma C3a was 15 to 20 times higher with PC obtained from the CS-3000 than was found with manual apheresis-prepared PC [unpublished observations]. Further studies need to be conducted to examine this issue.

In view of the potential loss of market of random donor whole blood-derived PC to single donor apheresis platelets, there are efforts within the ARC to investigate the potential for a pooled platelet product for the hospitals. This product, consisting of 4-5 units of ABO-compatible platelets, pooled with the help of a sterile connecting system and stored in 1000 ml gas-permeable containers, may also be filtered for leukocyte removal prior to storage and used with a platelet additive solution. Recently, Snyder has evaluated properties of pooled platelets and found no differences as compared to PC stored as individual units [23].

Some recent studies have suggested that the presence of contaminating leukocytes in the platelet concentrates may cause not only febrile transfusion reactions and refractoriness in the multi-transfused patient, but also may reduce the platelet quality. First, the leukocytes may have a deleterious effect by competing with platelets for oxygen, thereby causing anaerobic conditions with risk of pH fall due to increased lactate output [16,24]. Second, release of leukocyte enzymes during storage may affect platelet surface glycoproteins essential for platelet function and viability [17]. The removal of leukocytes may also reduce the potential for virally transmitted diseases, since many viruses are associated with leukocytes.

With leukocyte removal or inactivation becoming more common in transfusion practice, there is substantial research going on to develop effective devices and systems. Currently, three different technologies are utilized; selective leukocyte depletion filters, double-stage apheresis systems, and irradiation. Studies on the newest development of filters such as PALL-100, Sepacell, and Asahi indicate that they are capable of a 4-log reduction with minimal effect on platelet quality [25-29]. There is, however, some platelet loss, in the range of 10-20%, with filtration. Studies in our laboratory have suggested that there is also a selective removal of large platelets. Furthermore, paired post-transfusion survival studies conducted in our laboratory with the cotton wool filter have shown a small, but significant, loss in survival of filtered platelets, indicating some injury caused by filtration [30,31].

Another approach currently being explored to deal with the problem of alloimmunization is inactivation of the immunogenicity of the white cells using ultraviolet (UV) irradiation [32]. It has been shown that UV-irradiated white cells are unable to induce an antibody response. Recent studies by Pamphilon et al [33] and Andreu et al [34] have suggested that the quality of platelets is not affected by the doses required to prevent a MLR and that this UV-irradiation method is feasible in practice. Clinical studies are currently being conducted at several laboratories to examine whether UV-irradiation is the preferred method for avoiding alloimmunization in the multi-transfused patient.

The risks of transmitting viral diseases with platelet transfusions have led to research concerning elimination or inactivation of viral agents. The use of photochemicals such as 8-methoxypsoralen (8-MOP) [35], aminomethyltrimethylpsoralen (AMT), and merocyanine-540 in combination with UV light have been described in recent studies [36]. Using doses that allowed for a 6-log viral kill, no gross damage to the platelet function and morphology has been observed with subsequent storage, although it was noted that UV-treated platelets were more activated as shown by increased lactate production and by the glycoprotein GMP-140 activation assay. It is apparent that further studies are needed in order to describe the effect of these photochemicals on platelet storage capabilities and to define the optimum treatment conditions.

Storage

Studies have shown that parameters such as storage temperature, the container, agitation, and the suspending medium must be carefully controlled in order to allow for optimal platelet preservation [for recent reviews see 4,37,38].

Early studies by Murphy demonstrated that platelet viability was substantially compromized at cold temperatures (1-6°C) which is used for red cell storage, as compared to room temperature storage (20-24°C) [39]. Recent studies by Gottshall and Aster have confirmed the lower limit of 20°C [40]. The cause for the loss of viability with storage at lower temperatures is not known; the most striking alteration is a shape change from disc to sphere, which has been associated with loss of microtubuli and cytoskeletal proteins [41].

Our laboratory, in collaboration with Moroff at Holland Laboratories (Rockville, MD), has recently examined the nature of platelet storage lesions which may occur as a result of a brief exposure (3-17 hours) to temperatures of either 4, 12, or 16°C [42]. These are conditions that may occur during shipping of platelet concentrates. In preliminary studies, it was observed that irreversible morphological change with tendency toward sphering took place with PC exposed to 4°C for only 3-5 hours, or to 12°C or 16°C for only 5-17 hours during a standard 5-day storage period at 22°C. In subsequent extensive in vivo and in vitro studies, it was investigated whether this morphological change caused by brief exposure to either 12°C or 16°C for 17 hours also affected in vivo survival and other platelet properties related to function and physiology. Using a paired study design, two units of PC from the same donor, obtained by double plateletapheresis, were mixed and divided into test/control units. The test units were exposed to either 12°C or 16°C for 17 hours between day 1 and day 2 of a standard 5-day period while the control unit was stored at 20-22°C throughout the 5-day storage period. Test and control units were labeled with different isotopes (In-111 or Cr-51) with simultaneous infusion. Test platelets showed a substantial loss in post-tranfusion survival which correlated highly with loss of discoid shape. Less reduction in both parameters was found with exposure to 16°C as compared to 12°C. The loss of viability, however, was not associated with any differences in platelet counts, pH, respiratory activity, glycolytic rates, adenine nucleotide metabolism, LDH, or β-thromboglobulin release, aggregation response, or surface glycoprotein Ib (by flow cytometry). Thus, this study shows that a very short exposure of platelets to temperature below 20°C has affected their viability, although no apparent alterations in their in vitro function and metabolism were detected.

Besides the effect of storage temperature on platelet viability, another factor that has had major impact on platelet preservation is the gas permeability of the container. The shift from the first-generation, thick-walled, polyvinylchloride container such as the PL-146 with low oxygen transport capabilities, the second-generation, highly gas-permeable containers has extended the platelet shelf life from 1-3 days to 5-7 days. The reason for this is that approximately 85% of platelet

ATP production during storage is by respiration [43]; a sufficient transport of oxygen through the container walls during storage is, therefore, essential for preservation. With insufficient oxygen availability during storage, accelerated anaerobic lactic acid production occurs, resulting in fall in pH and loss of viability [4]. PC with high platelet counts will require a higher rate of transport than PC with low counts. The relationship between the gas permeability of the container and the maximum platelet count that can be tolerated before anaerobic conditions occur has been discussed in several papers [37,43,44]. The 300 ml platelet container such as PL-732, 400 ml containers such as PL-1240, PL-2209 (Baxter), and CLX (Cutter), and the 600 ml Teruflex (Terumo) all have sufficient gas transport capabilities, with little risk of causing anaerobic conditions in PC with counts in the normal range. However, the use of larger containers to increase the oxygen transport poses the risk of increased platelet activation and damage [3].

The recent demand for single donor apheresis PC has resulted in need for storage of this product. Since the platelet counts in apheresis PC are in the range of $3\text{-}6 \times 10^{11}$, large size containers with high gas permeability are used for storage to ensure aerobic conditions. In most studies with 5-day stored apheresis PC, post-transfusion survival results comparable to that of manually prepared random donor PC have been reported [45-47]. However, recent studies by Slichter et al. have questioned the viability of apheresis stored platelets [48].

The type of plastic and plasticizer used in currently available second-generation containers appears to have minimal effect on platelet viability. Table 1 shows studies performed in our laboratory with 5-day stored platelet concentrates using PVC containers plasticized with diethylhexylphthalate (DEHP, XT-612 container); triethyl hexyl trimellitate (TEHTM, CLX container); butyryl trihexyl citrate (BTC, PL-2209); or polyolefin containers (PL-732). The plasticizer DEHP used in the PL-146 and the Teruflex PVC (XT-612) appears, however, to increase the loss of platelet functional properties such as aggregation and hypotonic shock response with storage while having a positive effect in maintenance of platelet discoid shape [49]. The nature of the effect of DEHP on platelets and its implications are uncertain.

Table 1. In vivo viability of 5-day stored platelet concentrates using various second-generation containers.

Container	Plastic	Plasticizer	No. of studies	% Recovery	Survival (hours)
XT-612	PVC	DEHP	10	46 ± 6	155 ± 30
CLX	PVC	TEHTM	24	49 ± 10	158 ± 28
PL-2209	PVC	BTC	5	47 ± 10	139 ± 44
PL-732	Polyolefin	–	46	48 ± 10	165 ± 31

Agitation of the stored PC appears to be essential for satisfactory preservation. In the absence of agitation of the PC, even when highly gas-permeable containers such as PL-732 are used, fall in pH occurs with risk of loss of viability [50]. There have been numerous studies conducted to examine different forms of agitation. These have suggested that a "to and fro", horizontal type of agitation is the gentlest form, while the use of elliptical agitation appears to be deleterious and should not be used for long-term platelet storage [50-54].

In view of the new developments in the processing of platelet concentrates, it has become clear that use of a synthetic medium for resuspension and storage of platelets offers additional advantages. Not only does it offer the opportunity to save more plasma, but there are also other potential benefits in using a plasma-free synthetic medium including avoidance of transfusion reactions caused by non-compatible plasma proteins and improvement of platelet quality, which will lessen the number of units needed in transfusion.

The fact that platelets continue to produce a substantial amount of lactic acid by metabolism of glucose is a major problem within the development of platelet additive solution. A buffer system with a pH range of 6.8-7.2 is required to neutralize the lactic acid. At this pH range heat sterilization cannot be performed due to caramelization of glucose. In order to manage this problem, two approaches have been undertaken: 1) use of glucose-free medium, and 2) use of two-component synthetic medium consisting of an acid part containing glucose and an alkaline part containing the buffer. These parts are mixed immediately before resuspension of the platelets.

Adams and Rock have shown that platelet in vitro properties are well maintained with platelets stored in the glucose-free crystalloid solution, Plasmalyte A, with approximately 20-30% plasma carryover [55]. Using buffy coat-prepared PC resuspended and stored in Plasmalyte A, Bertolini et al. have found satifactory platelet count increments after infusion in thrombocytopenic patients [56]. Murphy has developed a glucose-free medium with 25 mM phosphate. PC stored in this medium demonstrated good platelet survivals in preliminary studies [57], however, in confirmatory paired design studies, poorer platelet in vivo viability results were obtained with this medium as compared to storage in CPD-plasma [58]. A drawback with glucose-lacking media is that some plasma carryover is needed to provide for glucose and perhaps other fuels for energy.

Our laboratory has developed a synthetic medium with glucose and bicarbonate as buffer [59]. This medium has advantages in that it allows for maximal plasma removal and also that it can be used for storage of red cells. Extensive in vitro and in vivo testing has demonstrated improved viability with storage of platelets in this medium as compared to storage in CPD-plasma [60].

Table 2. Loss of in vivo viability during processing and storage of platelet concentrates.

Infused platelets	No. of studies	% recovery	Survival (hours)
Fresh, ACD tube collected	29	58 ± 10	201 ± 22
4-17 hour, manually processed PC	10	55 ± 10	189 ± 24
4-18 hour, machine processed PC	10	56 ± 5	186 ± 27
5-day stored PC (PL-732 containers)	46	48 ± 10	165 ± 31

The nature of loss of platelet viability during storage at currently optimal conditions

Even with the current "state of the art" conditions for processing and storage, there is a significant loss of platelet viability during storage. Shown in Table 2 are autologous post-transfusion survival data with In-111-labeled fresh and stored platelets; 1-2 hour PRP from blood collected into tubes containing ACD; 6-18 hour and 5-day stored CPD-plasma PC prepared from whole blood units using standard blood bank procedures and stored in PL-732 containers; and 6-18 hour ACD-PC (stored in 1000 ml PL-732 containers) processed by machine apheresis using the CS-3000. From the data, it is clear that there is little evidence of any injury due to collection or processing of the platelet concentrates per se, prepared either manually or by apheresis PC. There is, however, a significant reduction in both percentage recoveries (16%) and survivals (18%) with five days of storage. The cause for this storage lesion is not known.

In vivo, platelets demonstrate an age-dependent removal from circulation with a life span of nine to ten days. It is likely that platelets also age in vitro; the loss of viability with increasing storage period consequently may represent a natural in vitro ageing phenomenon. Platelets are without nuclei and have, therefore, no means for repair and maintenance of enzymes and cellular structures. Unfavorable storage conditions causing activation/stimulation of the platelets may accelerate this ageing process. Recent studies conducted by our laboratory have shown that the survival curves of stored PC not only become shorter as a consequence of ageing, they become more curvilinear with increasing time of storage [60]. This suggests that part of the shortened survival after storage is also related to random platelet damage.

There are several platelet characteristics that change in parallel with the loss of viability during storage [61]. During a 5-day storage, platelets undergo morphological changes with change from discoid shape to more irregular spherical forms, formation of fragments and microvesicles, and loss of internal granules [3,4]. These changes are

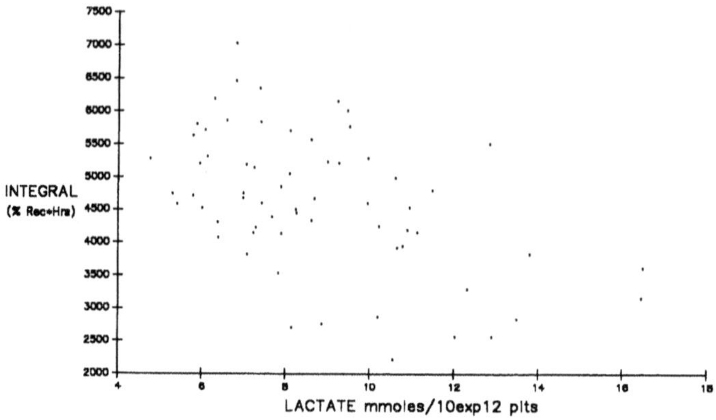

Figure 1. Integral versus lactate production in platelet concentrates stored in second-generation container for five days (n=64). Integral represents the area below the survival curve and was determined by calculation of the integral of the weighted mean function fit.

consistent with approximately 10-15% loss in mean size and reduction in density with five days of storage, LDH loss from platelet cytoplasma, loss of platelet factor 4 or β-thromboglobulin from α-granules. Fijnheer et al. have shown that the activation-dependent surface glycoprotein GMP-140 from the platelet α-granules becomes increasingly expressed on platelets during storage [62]. Furthermore, flow cytometric studies by Michelson have shown that there is an increasing number of platelets that have lost surface GPIb, another glycoprotein believed to be critical for platelet viability and function. These changes are consistent with morphological and physiological changes of platelets being continuously activated, as has been pointed out by Bode [4]. Potential mechanisms for activation during storage include thrombin generation and interaction of the platelet with the plastic surface of the bag. Furthermore, Bode has shown that, by addition of inhibitors of activation to the suspending medium, these storage-inflicted changes may be retarded [63-65].

Studies in our laboratory over the years where in vitro parameters of platelet morphology and biochemistry have been compared with in vivo viability, are also consistent with the hypothesis that platelet activation may speed up the in vitro ageing process and cause platelet injury. Shown in Figure 1 is the in vivo viability of 64 PC stored for five days in CPD or CPDA-1 plasma in second-generation containers versus platelet lactate production during the same period. Viability has been expressed as the sum of lifespans in circulation of the infused platelets, which was determined by the area below the survival curves (integral) [12]. It is clear that PC with high glycolytic activity during storage show reduced viability, perhaps as a result of activation. In addition, for the same PC, maintenance of platelet discoid shape (by photometric shape change measurements) and ATP levels were found to correlate significantly with percentage recoveries. Finally, as further support for the activation hypothesis, our laboratory, in collaboration with Bode, has recently shown that by storage of platelets in a plasma-free synthetic medium containing PGE_1 and theophylline, a substantial improvement in platelet in vivo viability could be demonstrated [66,67]. Furthermore, the improved viability was associated with markedly reduced lactate and thromboxane B_2 output and with improved preservation of discoid morphology and ATP and GPIb levels.

Loss of platelet function during storage and its reversal after infusion

It is well known that, during storage, platelets rapidly lose their responsiveness to aggregating agents such as ADP, epinephrine, collagen, and thrombin [4]. The decrease in responsiveness during storage is associated with a parallel decrease in platelet sensitivity to manifest the different stages of function such as shape change, aggregation, and secretion (release reaction), and thus appears to reflect a general loss in the ability to become activated or stimulated by the various agonists [51,68,69]. The nature of this lesion is not known. It has been shown that presence of the plasticizer DEHP accelerates the loss of aggregation response, that buffy coat-prepared platelets maintain a better responsiveness compared to PRP-derived platelets, and that use of inhibitors of platelet activation also offers a beneficial effect with regard to maintenance of aggregation. Several hypotheses have been suggested to explain the cause of loss in responsiveness to aggregating agents. These have been based on studies of biochemical processes believed to be essential in platelet activation that have also shown changes during storage, including arachidonate metabolism, phosphatidylinositol turnover, intracellular calcium regulation, and membrane lipid peroxidation [5-7,70]. However, a direct causal relation ship between the changes in these various biochemical processes and the loss of responsiveness during storage has not been demonstrated.

Little is known about exact hemostatic consequences of this functional defect of stored platelets. It has been suggested that there may be a reversal of the functional response after infusion [4,71]. Studies of infusion of 3-5 day stored platelet concentrates into thrombocytopenic patients have suggested that there was poor correction of bleeding time after one hour while, after 24 hours, substantial correction was observed [71,72]. In our laboratory, the ex vivo function of infused radiolabeled fresh and 5-day stored platelets into twelve donors has been investigated at various times post-infusion [73]. Fresh and stored platelets from the same donor were labeled with ^{111}In and ^{51}Cr, respectively, mixed, and simultaneously infused. ACD-anticoagulated blood samples were taken at 1 and 3 hours, 1, 3, and 5 days post-infusion and the functional behavior of the labeled platelets (test) was compared to that of the total circulating platelets (control) by various assays; percentage adhesion to collagen glass beads was quantitated as percentage decrease in radioactive counts (test) and platelet cell counts (control) of 5 ml samples added to a column of beads. The aggregability of the platelet to ADP (1 μM) and epinephrine (5 μM) in an aggregometer was measured by filtering aggregated samples through a column of cotton wool to remove the aggregates, and function was quantitated as percentage decrease in radioactive counts (test) and platelet cell counts (control) after filtration. Overall, ex vivo, infused, labeled fresh and stored platelets behaved very simularly to total circulating platelets, irrespective of time post-infusion. In testing of aggregation, stored platelets showed no response to ADP or epinephrine prior to infusion. Post-infusion, stored platelets showed a slight reduction in aggregation at 1 and 3 hours, with return to control levels at 24 hours. This shows that the loss in platelet aggregability observed during in vitro storage is not irreversible, but will be corrected upon infusion in vivo. Interestingly, no further change in ex vivo function was observed post-infusion with either fresh or stored platelets, which may indicate that viable circulating platelets maintain normal hemostatic function as they age in vivo.

References

1. American National Red Cross. Blood Services Opertions Report 1977-1978; 1982-1983; 1987-1988.
2. Holme S, Heaton WAL, Whitley P. Platelet storage lesion in second-generation containers: Correlation with in vivo behavior with storage up to 14 days. Vox Sang 1990;59:12-8.
3. Bode AP. Platelet activation may explain the storage lesion in platelet concentrates. Blood Cells 1990;16:109-26.
4. Murphy S. Platelet storage for transfusion. Seminars in Hematol 1985;22: 165-77.
5. Cesar JM, Navarro JL. Arachidonic acid metabolism in platelets stored for 5 days. Br J Haematol 1990;74:295-9.
6. Shukla SD, Morrison WJ, Klatchko DM. Response to platelet-activating factor in human platelets stored and aged in plasma, decrease in aggregation, phosphoinositide turnover, and receptor affinity. Transfusion 1989; 29:528-33.
7. Smith DJ, Odom DG, Cheney BA. Effect of diltiazem and a prostaglandin derivative (PGBX) on platelet function during long term storage. Transfusion 1989;29:153-8.
8. Griffin B, Bell K, Prowse C. Studies on the procurement of blood coagulation factor VIII. In vitro studies on blood components in half-strength citrate anticoagulant. Vox Sang 1988;54:193-8.

9. Kahn RA, Cossette I, Friedman LI. Optimum centrifugation conditions for the preparation of platelet and plasma products. Transfusion 1976;16:162-5.
10. Shimizu T, Kouketsu K, Kamiya T, Futagawa H, Hirose S. A novel second-generation polyolefin container for storage of single-donor apheresis platelets. Vox Sang 1989;56:174-80.
11. Solberg C, Hansen JB, Little C. Centrifugation of very freshly donated blood may yield platelets unstable to storage in the new generation of containers. Vox Sang 1989;56:25-31.
12. Holme S, Moroff G, Hallinen D, Hartman P, Heaton WAL. Properties of platelet concentrates (PC) prepared after extended whole blood holding time. Transfusion 1989;29:689-92.
13. Pietersz RNI, Reesink HW, Dekker WJA, Fijen FJ. Preparation of leukocyte-poor platelet concentrates from buffy coats. I. Special inserts for centrifuge cups. Vox Sang 1987;53:203-7.
14. Keegan T, Whitley P, Heaton A, et al. 5-Day stored buffy coat platelets show similar survival to paired PRP-derived concentrates. Abstract book Joint Congress of the International Society of Blood Transfusion and the American Association of Blood Banks, Los Angeles, 1990:59.
15. Fijnheer R, Pietersz RNI, Gouwerok CWN, et al. Platelet activation during preparation of platelet concentrates. Abstract. Transfusion 1989;29 (Suppl.): S142.
16. Pietersz RNI, de Korte D, Reesink HW, van den Ende A, Dekker WJA, Roos D. Preparation of leukocyte-poor platelet concentrates from buffy coats. III. Effect of leukocyte contamination on storage conditions. Vox Sang 1988;55:14-20.
17. Sloand EM, Klein HG. Effect of white cells on platelets during storage. Transfusion 1990;3-:333-8.
18. Högman CF, Eriksson L, Hedlund K, Wallvik J. The bottom and top system: A new technique for blood component preparation and storage. Vox Sang 1988;55:211-7.
19. Kurtz SR, McMican A, Carciero R, et al. Plateletpheresis experience with the Haemonetics blood processor 30, the IBM blood processor 2997, and the Fenwal CS-3000 blood processor. Vox Sang 1981;41:212-8.
20. Bertholf MF, Mintz PD. Comparison of plateletpheresis with two cell separators using identical donors. Transfusion 1989;29:521-5.
21. Schoendorfer DW, Williamson LH, Sheckler VL, Fitzgerald BP. Platelet collection with the Autopheresis-C® apheresis system. Vox Sang 1990;58: 100-5.
22. Rock G, Senack E, Tittley P. 5-Day storage of platelets collected on a blood cell separator. Transfusion 1989;29:626-8.
23. Snyder EL, Stack G, Napychank P, et al. Storage of pooled platelet concentrates. In vitro and in vivo analysis. Transfusion 1989;29:390-5.
24. Gottschall JL, Johnston VL, Rzadl, et al. Importance of white blood cells in platelet storage. Vox Sang 1984;47:101-7.
25. Kickler TS, Bell WR, Ness PM, Drew H, Pall DB. Leukocyte removal from platelet concentrates using a new leukocyte adsorption filter. Book of abstracts, XX Congress of the International Society of Blood Transfusion, London, 1988:280.
26. Vakkila J, Myllyla G. Amount and type of leukocytes in "leukocyte-free" red cell and platelet concentrates. Vox Sang 1987;53:76-82.

27. Miyamoto M, Sasakawa S, Ishikawa Y, Ogawa A, Nishimura T, Kuroda T. Leukocyte-poor platelet concentrates at the bedside by filtration through Sepacell-PL. Vox Sang 1989;57:164-7.
28. Van Marwijk Kooy M, van Prooijen HC, Borghuis L, Moes M, Akkerman JWN. Filtration: A method to prepare white cell-poor platelet concentrates with optimal preservation of platelet viability. Transfusion 1990;30:34-8.
29. Andreu G, Masse M, Lecrubier C. Evaluation of a new leukocyte removal filter for platelet concentrates: Sepacell-PL 10 N. Transfusion 1989;29 (Suppl.):S139.
30. Holme S, Ross D, Heaton WA. In vitro and in vivo evaluation of platelet concentrates after cotton wool filtration. Vox Sang 1989;57:112-5.
31. Holme S, Heaton A, Sawyer S, Whitley P. Investigation of in vivo viability and complement activity of infused pheresis platelet concentrates (PC) after cotton wool filtration. Abstract. Transfusion 1989;29(Suppl.):52S.
32. Lindberg JE, Slichter SJ, Murphy S, Schroeder DD, et al. In vitro function and in vivo viability of stored platelet concentrates. Transfusion 1983;23: 294-9.
33. Pamphilon DH, Potter M, Cutts M, et al. Platelet concentrates irradiated with ultraviolet light retain satisfactory in vitro storage characteristics and in vivo survival. Br J Haematol 1990;75:240-4.
34. Andreu G, Boccaccio C, Lecrubier C, et al. Ultraviolet irradiation of platelet concentrates: Feasibility in transfusion practice. Transfusion 1990;30: 401-6.
35. Lin L, Wieschahn GP, Morel PA, et al. Use of 8-methoxypsoralen and long-wavelength ultraviolet radiation for decontamination of platelet concentrates. Blood 1989;74:517-25.
36. Moroff G, Benade LE, Dabay M, et al. Use of photochemical procedures to inactivate viruses in platelet suspensions. Transfusion 1989;29:9S.
37. Heaton WA. Enhancement of cellular elements. In: McCarthy L, Wallas Ch (eds). New frontiers in blood banking. Arlington, Virginia: American Association of Blood Banks, 1986:89-125.
38. Bolin RB, Cheney BA, Simpliciano DA, Peck CC. In vitro evaluation of platelets stored in CPD-adenine formulations. Transfusion 1980;20:409-18.
39. Murphy S, Gardner FH. Platelet preservation. Effects of storage temperature on maintenance of platelet viability - deleterious effect of refrigerated storage. N Engl J Med 1969;280:1094-8.
40. Gottschall JL, Rzad L, Aster RH. Studies of the minimum temperature at which human platelets can be stored with full maintenance of viability. Transfusion 1986;26:460-7.
41. Prodouz KN, Walker LJ, White ML. Bacteriocidal properties of platelet concentrates. Transfusion 1974;14:116-9.
42. Holme S, Moroff G, Keegan T, George V, Heaton A. Platelet lesions caused by brief exposure (3-17 hours) to temperatures below 20°C. Abstract Joint Meeting of International Society of Hematology/American Society of Hematology, Boston MA. Blood 1990;76(Suppl.1):401a.
43. Kilkson H, Holme S, Murphy S. Platelet metabolism during storage of platelet concentrates at 22°C. Blood 1984;64:406-14.
44. Wallvik J, Akerblom O. The platelet storage capability of different plastic containers. Vox Sang 1990;58:40-4.

45. Shanwell A, Gulliksson H, Berg BK, Jansson BA, Svensson LA. Evaluation of platelets prepared by apheresis and stored for 5 days. In vitro and in vivo studies. Transfusion 1989;29:783-8.
46. Simon TL, Moore RC, Sierra E, Ferdinando B. Viability of 5-day apheresis platelets in a citrate plasticized bag using a new cell separator. Abstract. Transfusion 1987;27:536S.
47. Buchholz DH, Potter JH, Grode G, et al. Extended storage of single-donor platelet concentrate collected by a blood cell separator. Transfusion 1985; 25:557-62.
48. Slichter SJ, Price T. Viability of apheresis stored platelets (PLTS). Blood 1988;72(Suppl.):285a.
49. Holme S, Heaton A, Momoda G. Evaluation of a new, more oxygen-permeable polyvinylchloride container. Transfusion 1989;29:159-64.
50. Snyder EL, Koerner Jr TAW, Kakaiya R, Moore P, Kiraly T. Effect of mode of agitation on storage of platelet concentrates in PL-732 containers for 5 days. Vox Sang 1983;44:300-4.
51. Holme S, Vaidja K, Murphy S. Platelet storage at 22°C: Effect of type of agitation on morphology, viability, and function in vitro. Blood 1978;52:425-9.
52. Snyder EL, Bookbinder M, Kakaiya R, Ferri P, Kiraly T. 5-Day storage of platelet concentrates in CLX containers: Effect of type of agitation. Vox Sang 1983;45:432-7.
53. Bannai M, Mazda T, Sasakawa S. The effects of pH and agitation on platelet preservation. Transfusion 1985;25:57-9.
54. Snyder EL, Pope C, Ferri PM, Smith EO, Walter SD, Ezekowitz MD. The effect of mode of agitation and type of plastic bag on storage characteristics and in vivo kinetics of platelet concentrates. Transfusion 1986;26:125-30.
55. Adams GA, Rock G. Storage of human platelet concentrates in an artificial medium without dextrose. Transfusion 1988;28:217-20.
56. Bertolini F, Rebulla P, Riccardi D, Cortellaro M, Ranzi ML, Sirchia G. Evaluation of platelet concentrates prepared from buffy coats and stored in a glucose-free crystalloid medium. Transfusion 1989;29:605-9.
57. Murphy S, Grode G, Davisson W, et al. Platelet storage in a synthetic medium (PSM). Abstract. Transfusion 1986;26:568S.
58. Murphy S, Kagen L, Holme S, et al. Platelet storage in synthetic media lacking glucose and bicarbonate. Transfusion 1991;31:16-20.
59. Holme S, Heaton WA, Courtright M. Improved in vivo and in vitro viability of platelet concentrates stored for seven days in a platelet additive solution. Br J Haematol 1987;66:233-8.
60. Holme S, Heaton WAL, Whitley PL. Platelet storage lesions in second-generation containers: Correlation with in vivo behavior with storage up to 14 days. Vox Sang 1990;59:12-8.
61. Holme S, Heaton WA, Courtright M. Platelet storage lesion in second-generation containers: Correlation with platelet ATP levels. Vox Sang 1987;53:214-20.
62. Fijnheer R, Modderman PW, Veldman H, et al. Detection of platelet activation with monoclonal antibodies and flow cytometry. Transfusion 1990; 30:20-5.

63. Bode AP, Miller DT. Preservation of in vitro function of platelets stored in the presence of inhibitors of platelet activation and a specific inhibitor of thrombin. J Lab Clin Med 1988;111:118-24.
64. Bode AP, Miller DT. Metabolic status of platelet concentrates during extended storage: Improvement with pharmacological inhibitors and reduced surface-to-volume ratio. Vox Sang 1989;57:19-24.
65. Bode AP, Miller DT. The use of thrombin inhibitors and aprotinin in the preservation of platelets stored for transfusion. N Engl J Med 1989;113: 753-8.
66. Bode AP, Holme S, Heaton WA, Swanson MS. Extended storage of platelets in an artifical medium with the platelet activation inhibitors prostaglandin E-1 and theopylline. Vox Sang 1991;60:105-12.
67. Holme S, Bode A, Heaton A. Improved platelet in vivo viability following 14 days of storage using a synthetic medium with inhibitors. Abstract. Blood 1989;74(Suppl.):42a.
68. Scott NJ, Harris JR, Bolton AE. Effect of storage on platelet release and aggregation responses. Vox Sang 1983;45:359-66.
69. Kakaiya RM, Cable RG. The aggregation defect of platelets stored at room temperature in new formulation plastic containers. Vox Sang 1985;49: 368-9.
70. Fagiolo E, Lippa S, Mores N, et al. Peroxidative events in stored platelet concentrates. Vox Sang 1989;56:32-6.
71. Murphy S, Gardner FH. Platelet storage at 22°C; metabolic, morphologic, and functional studies. J Clin Invest 1971;50:370-7.
72. Murphy S, Kahn RA, Holme S, et al. Improved storage of platelets for transfusion in a new container. Blood 1982;60:194-200.
73. Holme S, Owens M, Sawyer S, Dunn S, Heaton A. Ex vivo function of infused radiolabeled fresh and 5-day stored platelets. Abstract Joint Meeting International Society of Hematology/American Society of Haematology, Boston, MA. Blood 1990;76(Suppl.1):401a.

PLATELET ADHESION TO THE VESSEL WALL

J.J. Sixma, Ph.G. de Groot

Introduction

Hemostasis is one of the most essential natural defense mechanisms. When a vessel is breached the hole is filled by a hemostatic plug. This plug consists of blood platelets. The formation of the hemostatic plug can be artificially subdivided in five different stages, representing the various mechanisms that are involved in this intricate process. These steps are: 1) adhesion; 2) activation; 3) secretion; 4) aggregation; and 5) thrombin formation.

The importance of each of these steps can be best explained by giving a simplified account of how a hemostatic plug is formed [for a more detailed review see ref. 1, 2 and 3]. When the blood vessel wall is breached, subendothelial or perivascular connective tissue is exposed to flowing blood. Blood platelets will adhere to this connective tissue. They will first make contact and then spread on this surface. This process is accompanied by activation of the blood platelets and secretion of small molecular products, proteins, and lysosomal enzymes. These products are released from the three types of secretory organels that are present in platelets: dense granula which contain serotonin, ATP, ADP, and calcium; α-granula which contain various adhesive proteins, growth factors, and other proteins that are involved in repair of the vessel wall or coagulation process; and lysosomes which in platelets act as secretory organels. As a consequence of this secretion process, ADP is liberated which will activate other platelets and this activation causes a change in the conformation of a receptor on the platelets. This receptor is glycoprotein IIb-IIIa (GPIIb-IIIa). When platelets are activated, GPIIb-IIIa becomes available as receptor for fibrinogen, fibronectin, vitronectin, and von Willebrand factor. At least three of these four proteins are dimeric or multimeric and platelet aggregation occurs because proteins such as fibrinogen, von Willebrand factor, and fibronectin will form a bridge between GPIIb-IIIa molecules on different platelets. This adhesion of blood platelets to one another is called platelet aggregation.

Aggregation continues untill an occlusive plug is formed. This plug is still friable and plasma may permeate through it. Through the action of tissue factor which is present in the connective tissue matrix of the vessel wall, the coagulation pathway is activated and thrombin forms. This thrombin leads to rapid local deposition of fibrin in the periphery of the hemostatic plug and to a thrombin dependent secretion process by which the platelet secretion granula are released also in more central areas of the hemostatic plug. This secretion process is accompanied by a strong interdigitation of the platelets that form the plug. Only when this last process has occurred a firm impermeable hemostatic plug is formed. The whole process of formation of the hemostatic plug usely takes between two and ten minutes in the human skin wounds. Over the following hours, the hemostatic plug changes gradually in appearance starting at the periphery where platelets obtain holes in their membrane and the cytoplasmic contents leaks out. The platelet remnants that remain form spheres and the spaces present between these platelet remnants are filled by thick dark staining fibrillar material which represents fibrin fibers. These fibrin fibers grow in thickness and these changes move from the periphery of the plug to more central areas. In this way, the platelet plug is transformed into a fibrin mass. This process has been called fibrinous transformation of the hemostatic plug. It may be accompanied by infiltration with leukocytes which may already begin to remove redundant parts of the plug. The formation of the fibrin network is essential for late hemostatis. When this fibrin network does not form in diseases such as hemophilia [4], the hemostatic plug becomes very vulnerable and a bleeding disorder exists which is characterized by a certain latency time between the initial lesion and the actual bleeding. Such a chain of events is typical for hemophilia A and B.

The formation of a thrombus is in many respects similar to the formation of a hemostatic plug. Also in thrombosis platelets attach to an injured vessel wall. In most instances there is no hole in the wall but just a simple denudation of the subendothelium or a rupture of an atherosclerotic lesion. Under normal conditions, such a small trauma, a very limited reaction occurs but under pathological conditions as occurs upon rupture of an atherosclerotic plaque, a much larger thrombus forms. The relative contribution of fibrin formation at the early stage of thrombosis is dependent on the shear rate. In veins, thrombosis occurs in static blood and much fibrin is formed from the start. In arteries with a low shear rate, a layer of fibrin is first deposited on the vessel wall and thrombi may form on top of this. Higher shear rate is seen in medium sized and small arteries and in arterioles. Platelets adhere directly to the subendothelium or connective tissue of the vessel walls and other platelets aggregate and form thrombi on it similar to the hemostatic plug formation. Fibrin threads often are seen to sprout from such trhombi [5].

Adhesion of blood platelets to the vessel wall

As seen above, adhesion of blood platelets to the connective tissue elements of the vessel wall is the first step in the formation of hemostatic plug or thrombus. Blood platelets first make a point contact with the basement membrane of the subendothelium or with a collagen fiber and they then spread along the surface of these connective tissue elements. The point contact is not dependent on metabolic energy, in contrast to platelet spreading as can be deduced from the inhibition observed at lower temperature or with metabolic energy inhibitors [6]. The spreading of platelets is accompanied by secretion. All our current knowledge has been obtained with the use of specially devised perfusion chambers in which vessel wall or connective tissue elements are studied under well standardized in vitro conditons. Most of the early data has been obtained using an annular perfusion chamber and rabbit aorta [6], but more recently human blood vessels such as renal arteries and more often the human umbilical artery have also been used with success [7]. Even more recently the extracellular matrix of cultured endothelial cells has been used as a good model of the vessel wall [8]. Studies using such models have provided insight in the adhesive molecules in the connective tissue, the receptors for them on the platelet membrane, and the factors which regulate platelet adhesion.

Adhesive molecules

The various connective tissue components to which blood platelets may adhere are summarized in Table 1. Various of these components such as: fibrinogen, fibronectin and von Willebrand factor are also present in plasma as well as in the secretion of α-granula of the blood platelet. Fibrinogen is by itself not a connective tissue component, but it may leak into the vessel wall from plasma. Platelet adhesion to fibrin plays an important role in the development of a thrombus.

The importance of plasma and platelet components can be deduced from experiments in which adhesion was studied under conditions where the relevant component was not present in plasma and/or absent from platelet secretion granula. In these studies, it has been shown that fibronectin in the vessel wall is by itself sufficient to support adhesion, whereas von Willebrand factor in the vessel wall is usely not sufficient. Sixty per cent or more of adhesion is supported by plasma von Willebrand factor which first binds to the vessel wall [9].

Table 1. Adhesive molecules.

Collagen I	Fibronectin	Thrombospondin
Collagen II	Fibrinogen	
von Willebrand factor	Laminin	

The contribution of platelet granulum proteins is more difficult to assess. Evidence has been provided that von Willebrand factor in platelet α-granula may have a contributary role in adhesion particularly when von Willebrand factor in plasma is low. This may explain why platelet adhesion in some patients with type I von Willebrand disease is higher than in others [10]. Patients with classic von Willebrand's disease, who have platelets with normal von Willebrand factor in their α-granula have a shorter bleeding time, than patients whose platelets lack it [11]. A possible role for platelet fibronectin can be deduced from experiments with isolated collagen in which it could be shown that very reactive collagens do not have a need for added fibronectin whereas less reactive forms do need it. It seems likely that the release reaction caused by the reactive collagens provide the fibronectin.

Collagen type I and III are unique as adhesion molecules in that they have a requirement for fibronectin and von Willebrand factor as supportive molecules for adhesion. Adhesion to other single proteins when coated on glass cover slips occurs at low shear rates without further support of other ligands. At high shear rates, adhesion is usely supported by the presence of von Willebrand factor which may come from plasma or from platelet α-granula. The reason for this is that for fibronectin, laminin, fibrinogen, and thrombospondin, platelet adhesion goes down at higher shear rates. For von Willebrand factor this is not the case. Von Willebrand factor becomes therefore the most important ligand at higher shear rates and adhesion to other single proteins is often supported by von Willebrand factor which is released from platelet α-granula or deposited from plasma. Recent studies have shown that this specific role of von Willebrand factor is caused by the very strong attachment of platelets to von Willebrand factor in comparison to e.g. fibronectin. Platelet adhesion to fibronectin appears to be reversible when adhered platelets are subjected to higher shear stresses, whereas this is not the case with platelets that have adhered to von Willebrand factor.

Platelet adhesion to laminin and thrombospondin is special in that they are both very strongly dependent on divalent cations. Platelet adhesion to laminin is partially dependent on magnesium, whereas calcium may play an inhibitory role. Platelet adhesion to thrombospondin is completely dependent on divalent cations. Both calcium and magnesium have an effect on adhesion.

The list of adhesion molecules in Table 1 is certainly not exhaustive. Platelet adhesion in a static system to vitronectin has been observed, but this ligand has not been studied in a flow system. Also various collagens like collagen type VI, VII, and VIII, and connective tissue molecules such as nidogen and SPARC (or osteonectin) have not been studied yet. Also the role of proteoglycans has not been explored. It is at present thus impossible to construct a composite picture of platelet adhesion to the vessel wall from the properties of the single matrix proteins that are contributing. Some interesting observations should be mentioned, however. Collagen as an isolated protein has a requirement for fibronectin when it is in a non-fibrillar form. Curiously enough, collagen as present in the vessel wall also needs fibronectin for adhesion and in this case collagen is fibrillar. This probably indicates that the collagen is shielded by other proteins and thus behaves as non-fibrillar. Another feature that should be mentioned is the cation dependence of adhesion to laminin and thrombospondin. Those proteins are abundantly present in the subendothelium, but adhesion to subendothelium is identical whether this occurs in heparinized blood or in blood that has been anticoagulated with citrate. This would suggest that laminin and thrombospondin are not essential for normal adhesion. They may play a contributory role or act as back-up molecules in exceptional situations.

Adhesion receptors

The mechanisms involved in the adhesion process of blood platelets to connective tissue substrate molecules is in many aspects similar to that of other cells. This is reflected in the receptors that are present on blood platelets. Adhesion receptors in general belong to a superfamily of so called integrins which consist of heterodimers with a specific α-subunit and a common β-subunit for each receptor [12]. The superfamily of integrins is subdivided into three main groups on the basis of their β-subunit. First, the VLA-proteins characterized by the presence of the β1-subunit. Second, the leukocyte adhesive molecules: Leucams, characterized by the presence of the β2-subunit. And third, the Cytoadhesins characterized by the presence of a β3-subunit.

The receptors on blood platelets are summarized in Table 2. Blood platelets have three VLA-molecules: VLA-2, on the platelet also called glycoprotein Ia-IIa, VLA-5, on the platelet called glycoprotein Ic-IIa, and VLA-6, on the platelet called glycoprotein Ic'-IIa. VLA-2 which on other cells is a laminin and a collagen receptor is a collagen receptor only on platelets. VLA-5 is a typical fibronectin receptor and VLA-6 is a laminin receptor. Leucams are as mentioned only present on leukocytes. Both of the cytoadhesins are found on platelets. GPIIb-IIIa is,

Table 2. Adhesion receptors.

Integrins	β-1 series	VLA-2 VLA-5 VLA-6
	β-3 series	GPIIb-IIIa VNR
Non-integrins		GPIb-α/β/GPIX GPIV ?

Table 3. Adhesive molecules and their receptors.

Collagen I and III	GPIa-IIa VLA-2 GPIV (?)
Fibronectin	GPIc-IIa VLA-5 GPIIb-IIIa GPIb (?)
von Willebrand factor	GPIb GPIIb-IIIa
Fibrinogen	GPIIb-IIIa
Laminin	GPIa-IIa (VLA-6)
Thrombospondin	GPIV ?

with 50-70,000 copies per platelet, the most abundant receptor on blood platelets. This complex is, as mentioned before, not only involved in adhesion, but also in aggregation. The other receptor that belongs to the cytoadhesins is the vitronectin receptor. This is also present on platelets, but only in about 100 copies per platelet. The physiological importance is probably minimal. Blood platelets have two other receptors, apart from the integrins. One is the glycoprotein Ibαβ-IX system which is a receptor for von Willebrand factor and perhaps also for fibronectin. This receptor is unique to the blood platelet. Characteristic for it is that it is only works under flow conditions. The other receptor which is not an integrin is glycoprotein IV on the blood platelet. It has been shown to be a thrombospondin and a collagen receptor [13,14]. Whether it also has a role as adhesion receptor for these ligands remains to be established. The various functions of the adhesion receptors on blood platelets is summarized in Table 3. A special case is fibronectin for which two and possibly three receptors are present. Under static conditions GPIIb-IIIa and VLA-5 are important with a major role for GPIIb-IIIa. Under flow conditions GPIIb-IIIa and VLA-5 have also been shown to be important when fibronectin is the single ligand, but GPIIb-IIIa is not essential for the fibronectin dependent adhesion to the endothelial cell matrix or to collagen. More recent studies have shown that GPIb may also play a similar role as adhesion receptor for fibronectin as it does for von Willebrand factor. For von Willebrand factor, GPIb is the primary receptor that forms a tight complex. At high shear rates, GPIIb-IIIa is also involved and this is responsible for the spreading that is essential at these high shear rates for a resistence to high shear stresses. The receptors for collagen and thrombospondin have not been identified completely.

Regulation of blood platelet adhesion

Insight in the regulation of blood platelet adhesion to the vessel wall by endothelial cells has been obtained from studies with cultured human endothelial cells. No systematic study has appeared of the culture conditions on platelet adhesion. In view of what is known of the influence of culture conditions on the composition of the extracellular matrix, it is evident that such conditions must be of great importance for adhesion too. Endothelial cells are polar in vivo. They may have only a limited time after confluence when they are polar in culture, however [15]. This is the time when they deposit a thick matrix. It seems likely that platelet adhesion will be much stronger to such a matrix. Comparison between non-confluent and confluent cells have shown that non-confluent cells make more thrombospondin and less collagen than confluent cells and also this will effect adhesion. Most of the adhesion studies in our laboratory have been performed with endothelial cells of the second passage that have just reached confluence. If such cells are stimulated with phorbol myristate acetate (PMA) or with more natural substances such as, thrombin, interleukin-1, tumor necrosis factor and endotoxin, specific changes occur in the extracellular matrix. These changes consist of a decrease in the von Willebrand factor and fibronectin content of the matrix [16] and an increase in the tissue factor [17]. Primary adhesion of blood platelets decreases and this can be corrected by the addition of extra von Willebrand factor. The decrease in fibronectin has no effect: addition of fibronectin does not correct adhesion. The extra tissue factor may lead to formation of much thrombin on subendothelium which is not usually found on the subendothelium with normal cultured human umbilical vein cells.

Most of the in vitro studies on the regulation of matrix composition have been performed with the fetal umbilical vein cells, but studies using adult endothelial cells have shown important differences. Such studies have shown the presence of much tissue factor in the extracellular matrix of adult cells which is not present in unactivated fetal cells. Also the amount of von Willebrand factor and fibronectin was much lower in the matrix of adult cells. These cells behave thus as if they were activated. This is apparently a tissue culture artifact, but it is not clear what causes this. Endogenous secretion of interleukin-1 from these cultured cells and autocrine stimulation seems a possible cause.

Endothelial cells also effect platelet adhesion via the product of natural inhibitors of adhesion. Such inhibitors are endothelial cell derived relaxing factor (EDRF) which is in its functional effects identical to nitric oxide and prostacyclin. Prostacyclin is an important inhibitor of platelet aggregation, but only inhibits adhesion at high concentration. Studies in which endothelial cells were treated with aspirin have indicated that such concentrations may occur locally and that prostacyclin may be effective in regulating adhesion. Nitric oxide is extremely shortlived in the circulation. One of the reasons for this is that it is scavenged by hemoglobin. Experimental studies have only succeeded in showing an effect of nitric oxide when this nitric oxide was introduced into the system locally at the injured vessel wall. Platelet adhesion to the matrix near still vital endothelial cells is enhanced by a competitive inhibitor of nitric oxide formation indicating that nitric oxide plays a regulatory role in adhesion. It seems likely that nitric oxide and prostacyclin are able to potentiate each other because their point of action is on either cyclic-GMP formation (nitric oxide) or on cyclic-AMP formation (prostacyclin), but this could not be shown in the experiments that were performed in our laboratory [De Graaf J., De Groot Ph.G., Moncada S., Palmer R., Sixma J.J., unpublished]. More work needs to be done to study these cross-talk (as they have been called) effects between endothelial cells and platelets.

Platelet storage and platelet adhesion

Little is known at present about the effect of platelet storage on platelet adhesion. It is not unlikely that there is a major effect because of cleavage of GP-Ib from the membrane has been found. This was compensated by the recruitment of new GP-Ib molecules from an intracellular store, probably from the surface connected membrane system [18]. Increased exposure of GP-140 and CD-63 was also observed indicating that platelet activation and platelet release had occurred [19]. In studies in our own laboratory, we compared the effect of filtration and centrifugation of platelet concentrates for the removal of leukocytes. Both procedures did not have an effect on platelet adhesion (Van Prooijen et al, unpublished]. It seems obvious that adhesion and thrombus formation studies using human blood vessel models can have a predictive role in the evaluation of blood platelet concentrates, because among all function tests, they are closest related to the in vivo situation. Their use as a general screening test will, however, be limited by their time-consuming nature.

References

1. Sixma JJ, Wester J. The hemostatic plug. Semin Hemat 1977;14:265-301.
2. Wester J, Sixma JJ, Geuze JJ, van der Veen J. Morphology of the early hemostasis in human skin wounds. Influence of acetyl salicylic acid. Lab Invest 1978;39:298-311.
3. Wester J, Sixma JJ, Geuze JJ, Heynen H. Morphology of the hemostatic plug in human skin wounds. Transformation of the plug. Lab Invest 1979;41:182-92.
4. Sixma JJ, van den Berg AA. The hemostatic plug in hemophilia A: A morphological study of hemostatic plug formation in bleeding time skin wounds of patients with severe hemophilia A. Br J Haematol 1984;58:741-53.
5. Zwaginga JJ, Sixma JJ, de Groot PhG. Activation of endothelial cells induces platelet thrombus formation on their matrix. Studies of a new in vitro thrombosis model with low molecular weight as anticoagulant. Arteriosclerosis 1990;10:49-62.

6. Baumgartner HR, Muggli R. Adhesion and aggregation: Morphologic demonstration, quantitation in vivo and in vitro. In: Gordon JL (ed). Platelets in biology and pathology. Amsterdam: North Holland, 1976:23-60.
7. Sakariassen KS, Banga JD, de Groot PhG, Sixma JJ. Comparison of platelet interaction of subendothelium of human renal and umbilical arteries on the extracellular matrix produced by human venous endothelial cells. Thromb Haemostas 1984;52:60-5.
8. Sixma JJ, Nievelstein PFEM, Zwaginga JJ, de Groot PhG. Adhesion of blood platelets to the extracellular matrix of cultured human endothelial cells. Ann N Y Acad Sci 1987;516:39-51.
9. Stel HV, Sakariassen KS, de Groot PhG, van Mourik JA, Sixma JJ. The von Willebrand factor in the vessel wall mediates platelet adherence. Blood 1985;65:823-31.
10. D'Alessio PA, Zwaginga JJ, de Boer HC, et al. Platelet adhesion to collagen in subtypes of type I von Willebrand's disease is dependent on platelet von Willebrand factor. Thromb Haemostas 1990;64:227-31.
11. Gralnick HR, Rick ME, McKeown LP, et al. Platelet von Willebrand factor: An important determinant of the bleeding time in type I von Willebrand's disease. Blood 1986;68:58-61.
12. Hynes RO. Integrins: A family of cell surface receptors. Cell 1987;48 549-54.
13. Asch AS, Barnwell J, Silverstein RL, Nachman RL. Isolation of thrombospondin membrane receptor. J Clin Invest 1987;79:1054-61.
14. Tandon NN, Kralisz U, Jamieson GA. Identification of glycoprotein IV (CD-36) as a primary receptor for platelet-collagen adhesion. J Biol Chem 1989;264:7576-83.
15. Kowalszyk AP, Tullon RH, McKeown-Longo PJ. Polarized fibronectin secretion and localized matrix assembly sites correlate with subendothelial matrix formation. Blood 1990;75:2335-43.
16. De Groot PhG, Reinders JH, Sixma JJ. Perturbation of human endothelial cells by thrombin or PMA changes the reactivity of their extracellular matrix towards platelets. J Cell Biol 1987;104:697-704.
17. Bevilacqua MP, Pober JS, Majeau GR, Cotran RS, Gimbrone MA Jr. Interleukin-1 (IL-1) induces biosynthesis and cell surface expression of procoagulant activity in human vascular endothelial cells. J Exp Med 1984;160:618-23.
18. Michelson AD, Adelman B, Barnard MR, Carroll E, Handin RL. Platelet storage results in a redistribution of glycoprotein Ib molecules. Evidence for a large intraplatelet pool of glycoprotein Ib. J Clin Invest 1988;81: 1734-40
19. Fijnheer R, Modderman PW, Veldman H, et al. Detection of platelet activation with monoclonal antibodies and flowcytometry: Changes during platelet storage. Transfusion 1990;30:20-5.

TRENDS IN THE PRODUCTION AND USE OF COAGULATION FACTOR CONCENTRATES

J.K. Smith

The major concerns today in coagulation factor production and use are virus safety, other aspects of immediate and long-term safety, and the possibility of immune modulation by repeated injection of impure factor VIII.

Virus safety

Last time I was in Groningen, in 1984, we were the first to hear the news that very mild heating, in the dry state or in solution, killed HIV-1 [1]. That announcement, unfortunately, did not quite end HIV transmission by concentrates, and of course it said little about hepatitis viruses. Some fractionators still see HCV as the main problem of the last decade, from which HIV was a tragic but brief and readily resolved diversion. We have known for five years now at least three or four standard methods of virus inactivation with very broad application, which will reliably inactivate HCV in factor VIII (FVIII), as well as HIV and probably HBV. Yet there are still FVIII concentrates on sale today which are known to be capable of transmitting HCV.

Although blood-borne viruses are not the subject of this session, I will keep stressing that secure virus inactivation must now be part and parcel of the design of all coagulation factor production processes, not just an afterthought to the elegant chemistry.

Purity

As a chemist, I can understand the naive ideal of putting a pure substance into a vial and labelling it FVIII, but that is not the proper endpoint of pharmaceutical production. The aims are to prepare homogeneous batches of an active substance, consistently the same, batch after batch, in a form which is stable during processing, storage and after preparation for i.v. injection, which is easy to prepare for injection, which does the desired job in replacing a deficient protein for a predicted time, and which carries a very low risk of side effects which might be worse than the deficiency itself.

If increased purification increases virus safety and stability of the coagulant factor activity, without loss of yield or the introduction of new problems and hazards, it should be welcomed. However, my experience shows that purification can work against the severity of virus inactivation procedures almost as often as it helps; and purification is inimical to stability at least as often as it is beneficial.

In the last few years, there has been a lot of discussion about the immune modulating effects of "junk protein" injected along with FVIII concentrates. I will make only one or two points against over-inflation of this issue. Hemophiliacs do not show abnormal mortality or morbidity usually associated with immune dysfunction, for example bacterial or viral infections, or cancer. Even when attention passes, properly, to immune modulation in HIV-negative hemophiliacs, we will still have to deal with a legacy of HCV and possibly other bloodborne infections.

Without exception all FVIII concentrates deliver, in a 1000 IU dose, approximately 250 μg of FVIII; 10-500 mg of major contaminants (fibrinogen, vWF, albumin monomer) and several mg unidentified or denatured proteins, e.g. albumin polymers, IgG. The "major" unidentified proteins are unique in each type of concentrate, and nobody knows the effect of injecting them frequently over a hemophiliac's lifetime. In vitro tests of immune modulation are of value only in showing where clinical studies might be directed, and clinical studies in patients exposed to only one kind of concentrate are in very short supply.

Other aspects of safety will include freedom from allergenic or vasoactive side-effects, no unusual incidence of inhibitor antibodies after treatment, and the absence of certain specific complications such as thrombosis following treatment with prothrombin complex concentrates.

Factor VIII concentrates (Table 1)

Among the real incentives to increase the specific activity of FVIII concentrates in the mid-80s was the need to make them more soluble and to improve the efficacy of some forms of virus inactivation. We therefore saw a number of relatively high-yielding concentrates with 2-10 IU/mg, prepared by novel precipitation methods. These concentrates usually contain von Willebrand factor (vWF) in the same proportion to FVIII coagulant activity as in plasma, but they have had most of the fibrinogen removed, and may have remarkably low concentrations of some other contaminants, like IgG.

Let me remind you that vWF, the natural carrier protein for FVIII in plasma, is the dominant partner by mass. Pure FVIII has a specific activity of about 4000 IU/mg, but purified FVIII complex (that is,

Table 1. Specific activity of factor VIII concentrates.

2-10 IU/mg:	Intermediate purity – precipitation methods
5-10 IU/mg:	Immuno-affinity purified (rVIII similar)
>50 IU/mg:	Purified by "conventional" chromatography e.g.gel filtration standard ion-exchangers "tailored' ion-exchangers; polyelectrolytes

FVIII plus vWF) would have a specific activity of not more than about 50 IU/mg. Any separation method which removes some of the vWF will have a very large effect on the numerical specific activity. It is not obvious to what extent some modern concentrates have been positively *designed* to have little or no vWF, since there seems to be no good case for removing this natural carrier and stabilizing molecule. Dissociation of the complex may have been incidental to the removal of other contaminants, or the effective recovery of FVIII by adsorption from virucidal mixtures, and the resulting high specific activity has been accepted as a bonus, however physiologically dubious.

One way to absorb FVIII complex effectively from plasma or cryo is to use an immuno-affinity reagent, i.e. an immobilized mouse monoclonal antibody to either FVIII or vWF. Both approaches result in dissociation of the adsorbed complex. One of the methods requires dissociation of the bond between FVIII and the antibody with a chaotropic reagent. Since the initial binding of FVIII to the antibody column is very strong and highly specific, copious washing can remove most other contaminants, and effect a very useful reduction in titre of some viruses. The very highly purified FVIII seems to be unstable on its own, so it is formulated in human albumin.

"Human albumin" like "FVIII concentrate" is a euphemism for a solution containing 90-95% monomeric albumin, the rest being dimerized and polymerized albumin, a collection of high molecular weight "minor" contaminants like IgG, haptoglobin and hemopexin, some of these possibly co-polymerized with albumin.

One of the immuno-affinity purified concentrates also has detectable mouse protein. These concentrates are almost universally referred to as "highly purified FVIII" but, as encountered by the hemophilic vein, might be more accurately described as intermediate-purity FVIII, in which fibrinogen and vWF have been replaced by an impure albumin preparation.

The concentrates represent a commendable industrial tour de force. They are very soluble and can be injected at very high potency, seldom cause immediate side effects and, if the manufacturers choose, can be prepared at least as virus-safe as conventional intermediate-purity

FVIII. At the moment, there is some debate about the prevalence of inhibitory antibodies in patients receiving one of these concentrates.

However, there are at least two FVIII concentrates which are of much higher specific activity than intermediate purity concentrates, as injected into the patient. These are prepared by relatively conventional chromatography on familiar DEAE anion-exchangers, and on newer charge-based ligands of very high capacity and specific activity. Again, the high specific activity is obtained largely be removal of most of the fibrinogen and vWF, but this time the FVIII is stable enough to be formulated without the addition of albumin. In our hands, this class of ion-exchanger is rarely blessed with both high capacity and complete elution of FVIII. It seems that FVIII itself binds to the exchanger rather than vWF, and one can imagine that heterogeneous binding sites on the exchanger allow multiple attachment and incomplete elution of a proportion of the FVIII, or loss of its original conformation. We should not necessarily assume that chromatography is always the gentlest of processes. One wonders whether the molecule emerges wholly in its native state after dissociation from vWF, removal of most of the vWF, and re-association with a greatly reduced portion of this carrier protein.

Dr. Pavirani will be talking about recombinant factor VIII (rVIII) later [2]. At the moment, the fractionator would have to class this along with the immuno-affinity purified concentrates, since rVIII is purified that way and is formulated with human albumin. Just to touch again on the motif of preservation of activity, I understand that at least one manufacturer prefers to co-express human vWF to stabilize FVIII activity in cell culture.

Current FVIII processing schemes include the entire range of well-proven approaches to virus inactivation. Methods such as pasteurization in solution and solvent-detergent treatment are applied at a relatively early stage, heating at controlled moisture content or in heptane are applied very late in processing, and severe dry heating at 80°C is performed in the sealed final container. Chromatography can make a very substantial contribution to reducing the titre of blood-borne viruses, but must not be relied upon as the sole safeguard.

Before leaving FVIII, I should mention progress at the other end of fractionation. The subject of FVIII stability in plasma is an old favourite at these meetings, and we should not lose sight of the extra yield that can be won by paying attention to the optimum collection of FFP. Until recently, all industrial FVIII processes have started from bulk cryoprecipitate. Large-scale cryoprecipitation, which is more Art than chemical engineering, typically yields only 350-450 IU/kg plasma, and perhaps about 200-300 IU/kg is lost. Several groups are now looking for ways of adsorbing FVIII directly from plasma, without going through cryoprecipitate, and Dr. Over's group at the Central Laboratory of the Dutch Red Cross in Amsterdam have been particularly innovative and successful. There are many implications for recovery of other coagulation factors – and many potential pitfalls.

Von Willebrand factor

In pursuing FVIII for classical hemophilia, we must not forget that people with von Willebrand's disease (vWD) need the other half of the complex, vWF. Some newer concentrates have been deliberately depleted of vWF. Even some methods of intermediate-purity processing lose most of the vWF activity, and it is possible that it is vulnerable to some methods of virus inactivation. There has therefore been much searching for high molecular weight multimers, measuring ristocetin cofactor activity, bleeding times and platelet retention times after treatment with new or modified concentrates.

There are at least two virus-safe concentrates (pasteurized and severely dry-heated) which have high ristocetin cofactor activity, approximately normal distribution of multimers, and a good record in treating all types of vWD – but they have not necessarily been successful in every bleed in every patient. Even cryoprecipitate, with an essentially full set of multimers, does not always work. Our experience is that even measurement of bleeding time is not a reliable index of successful hemostasis; you really have to stop the patients bleeding. HMW multimers are probably not the whole story; they may be necessary, but not sufficient, to stop bleeding, and we do not have a good assay for their functional activity, only their size. This is one example of not really knowing what activity we are trying to preserve. There may be unidentified cofactors adventitiously present in some concentrates and not in others.

At least one manufacturer is preparing a vWF concentrate from the side-fraction of a chromatographic FVIII process. This concentrate seems to have an excellent multimer content and is effective in correcting bleeding time and stopping bleeding in many patients. This is a rational approach to getting both FVIII and vWF from the same plasma.

Factor IX

There are now two kinds of factor IX, the traditional PCCs which have been used for 20 years as a source of factor IX, II and X but now have virus inactivation stages added, and concentrates derived from these which are intended to provide factor IX with only a low content of other factors.

This further purification of factor IX was first done by chromatography on immobilized sulphated dextran and then on heparin-Sepharose. Inevitably, immuno-affinity purification is now appearing, some methods using "smart" calcium-dependent monoclonal antibodies. Two laboratories are working on metal-chelate chromatography for separation of the vitamin K-dependent factors. All these methods increase specific activity of factor IX from about 2 IU/mg protein in PCCs to between 50 and 250 IU/mg, and they contain differing small amounts of factor X, inter-α-trypsin inhibitor, protein C and other trace proteins.

Standard virus inactivation measures cover the whole range applied to FVIII concentrates. There is also a factor IX concentrate treated with beta-propiolactone virucide. Virus inactivation has resurrected yet another 20 year old problem – should we add heparin to PCCs? Currently, we add both heparin and antithrombin III (ATIII) to our PCC, in order to neutralize, immediately and irreversibly, any activated IX_a, X_a or II_a formed during heat-inactivation of viruses. Other manufacturers arrange to leave some endogenous ATIII in the factor IX fraction.

Those who take immune modulation seriously would argue that it is worth going to further purification stages, just to get rid of "junk protein". Even more fractionators would hope that factor IX devoid of factor II may be less likely than PCC to cause thrombosis when used in high doses in patients with high risk factors. For many years we have been told that IX_a and X_a are responsible for thrombotic side effects, but there are now concentrates which do contain activated factors but are non-thrombotic in the canine DIC model, and concentrates with the reverse properties; "something else", which we do not necessarily measure routinely, makes PCCs potentially thrombogenic. Not knowing what it is, we do not know how to remove it, but I look forward to good clinical trials of several highly purified factor IX concentrates with different characteristics. Since incidents with current PCCs are already infrequent and unpredictable, it will take many years to prove a statistical improvement with any new concentrate. Of course, it will still be necessary to use PCCs in acquired deficiencies of vitamin K-dependent proteins, and we must not forget that these must also be made as safe as possible from additional risks of causing thrombosis.

Recombinant factor IX has been described, and human-sequence factor IX has also been harvested from the milk of transgenic sheep.

Some see a need for a factor X concentrate to treat the few hundred patients identified worldwide. If required, factor X is easily recovered as a byproduct of factor IX purification. However, the most seriously affected patient in the UK has done very well on treatment with alternate day infusions of traditional II, IX and X concentrate, with no signs of thrombosis.

Protein C (PC) and protein S (PS)

It may well be worthwhile to isolate PC (and possibly PS) from the crude mixture of vitamin K-dependent, heavily carboxylated proteins which are easily adsorbed on to ion-exchangers from plasma.

PC is not easy to separate clearly from coagulation factors, but it can be done using ion-exchange, immobilized sulphate polysaccharides, immuno-affinity reagents or metal-chelate chromatography. Treatment of PC deficiency has been described, using a concentrate of low purity. As more hematologists start looking for predisposing risk factors for thrombosis, and as assays become more accessible, we will see more PC concentrates reaching serious clinical trial, just as happened with ATIII.

Factor VII/VII$_a$

Factor VII is useful in congenital and acquired deficiency and has been available since the mid-70s as a minor constituent of PCCs, or as a concentrate in its own right. Factor VII is less strongly charged than factors II, IX and X at neutral pH and one can take advantage of this by using a more highly substituted ion-exchanger to adsorb factor VII from factor IX supernatant. The concentrate made in England is severely dry-heated to inactivate blood-borne viruses. Factor VII has also been prepared by adsorption of plasma on aluminium hydroxide gel, and of course there is the potential for preparation by immuno-affinity chromatography.

Recently, attention has focussed more on the activated form of factor VII, which is gathering momentum as the "inhibitor bypassing activity" of the 90s. This can be prepared from plasma-derived factor VII or by recombinant technology. There are ingenious ideas about how it might work, and impressive evidence that it stops some patients bleeding. We eargerly await the controlled trials against alternative treatments. The alternatives are the "inhibitor bypassing" concentrates of the 70s, unactivated PCCs, porcine FVIII and even that old standby, FVIII itself.

There is good evidence that VII$_a$ is not thrombogenic and it could be used in place of factor VII itself. If VII$_a$ "bypasses" FVIII inhibitors it might also work well in hemophilia, and this is being tried. Perhaps it would be cheaper to make than rVIII.

Fibrin adhesives

The coagulation factors I and II$_a$ (fibrinogen and thrombin) appear together in fibrin glues and sealants, which are much used in soft-tissue surgery. The fibrinogen need not be very highly purified but must be made virus-safe e.g. by heating or solvent-detergent treatment.

Virtually pure thrombin has been made from prothrombin complex either by ion-exchange or by affinity chromatography. Surprisingly, it withstands severe dry-heating. Human thrombin is enjoying a new lease of life, ironically because virus inactivation treatments have made it seem safer than the bovine protein.

Factor XIII

Factor XIII deficiency is probably still inadequately diagnosed, and is just as dangerous as hemophilia A or B. Fortunately, its half-life is very long, and monthly prophylaxis with factor XIII concentrate keeps patients free of bleeding. Rare factor XIII inhibitors are very difficult to treat except with potent concentrates. Some clinicians have advocated factor XIII supplementation, e.g. scleroderma, wound healing and sub-arachnoid hemorrhage, but promising initiatives have not yet been widely accepted.

Factor XIII can be made from human placentae, lacking b-subunits but apparently no less effective hemostatically than plasma-derived factor XIII possessing both a- and b-subunits. Both are pasteurized and seem to be virus-safe.

Factor XI

Factor XI deficiency is quite common in the UK and US, especially in people of Ashkenazi Jewish descent. Congenitally deficient patients do not bleed spontaneously into muscles and joints, but may bleed badly after trauma or surgery, with a severity which cannot be predicted by their resting level of factor XI. FFP is the old standby, but patients often become refractory to repeated treatment.

A few years ago, we found that our ATIII concentrate contained factor XI but that its biological activity would not withstand pasteurization. We now make an ATIII rich factor XI concentrate, severely dry-heated at 80°C. We have kept the ATIII in the factor XI concentrate because XI_a is thrombogenic and ATIII is its natural inhibitor.

Conclusion

There has been a common thread in this rapid survey – the preservation of biological activity of coagulation factors through some of the severe challengers of exposure to cell culture, proteases, harsh chromatographic media, aggressive purification, virus inactivation and loss of their natural partners.

There are some inspired friendships between plasma proteins which should not be despised automatically in the pursuit of purity. I hope to be asked back in one or two years' time when there will be a larger and more convincing body of clinical evidence from which to discuss the questions of purity, immune modulation and other immunological hazards.

Reference

1. Gerety RJ. Prevention of transmission of virus infections by blood transfusions and removal of virus infectivity from clotting factor concentrates. In: Smit Sibinga CTh, Das PC, Seidl (eds). Plasma fractionation and blood transfusion. Proceedings 9th Intern. Symp. on Blood Transfusion 1984. Boston, Dordrecht, Lancaster: Martinus Nijhoff Publ., 1985: 143-6.
2. Pavirani A, Krishnan S, Jallat S, et al. Structural and functional properties of recombinant coagulation factors. In: Smit Sibinga CTh, Das PC, Mannucci PM (eds). Coagulation and blood transfusion. Proceedings 15th Intern. Symp. on Blood Transfusion 1990. Dordrecht, Boston, London. Kluwer Academic Publ. 1991:119-24.

IMMUNOAFFINITY PURIFICATION OF FACTOR VIII/ VON WILLEBRAND FACTOR COMPLEX

K. Koops, H.S. Hoff, J.J. van Weperen, P.C. Das, C.Th. Smit Sibinga

Introduction

Over the last 20 years several procedures have been developed for purification of proteins for clinical use. Especially in the 80s chromatography has been developed as one of the main approaches for the purification of coagulation protein factor VIII (FVIII) [1].

Some of these methods are shown in Table 1. One of the several types of affinity chromatography is the immunoaffinity. This type achieves its best performance in using monoclonal antibodies (MAbs). Especially in the purification of trace amounts of protein in very heterogeneous mixtures this technique has great advantages compared to the traditional techniques, because of its rather, high specificity. This is in contrast with the other techniques which are not specific for one protein.

One of the crucial steps in the development of an immuno affinity chromatography (IAC) method is the preparation of the solid phase with the immobilized antibody [2].

The three main parts of the system are: 1) solid support; 2) coupling chemistry; 3) antibody.

These three items will determine the quality of an affinity adsorbent by affecting:

- the binding capacity of the antibody for the antigen and recovery of the antigen after binding. This will determine the yield and actually proves the functionality of the immobilized MAb.

Table 1. Chromatographic methods for the purification of FVIII.

Controlled pore glass	Based on adsorption of contaminating proteins
Ion-exchange	Based on the charge of proteins
Gelfiltration	Based on size exclusion
Ultrafiltration	Based on size exclusion
Affinity	Adsorption of protein to certain ligand

- the life cycle of the column, which has an impact on the cost-effectiveness.
- the extent of antibody leakage from the carrier material: which relates to the safety of the purified product.

An immunoaffinity system can be separated in two main subjects:

a) *the component system*. This covers the actual solid phase supports, the chemistry used for activation of coupling and blocking, the ligand itself and the physical conditions.

b) *the system performance*. This covers content of ligand per volume of support for the target molecule, the elution/regeneration solutes required, the control and measurement of leakage of the antibodies from the solid support and the sterilization and cleaning of the solid phase and functionality of MAb.

The basic principle of immunoaffinity (Figure 1) involves a monoclonal antibody which is for instance directed against the von Willebrand factor (vWF). To this immobilized antibody, FVIII derived from cryoprecipitate is bound as a complex with the vWF. Following washing, to remove the majority of unnecessary and undesirable impurities (contaminants), the FVIII/vWF complex is then eluted in a highly purified state.

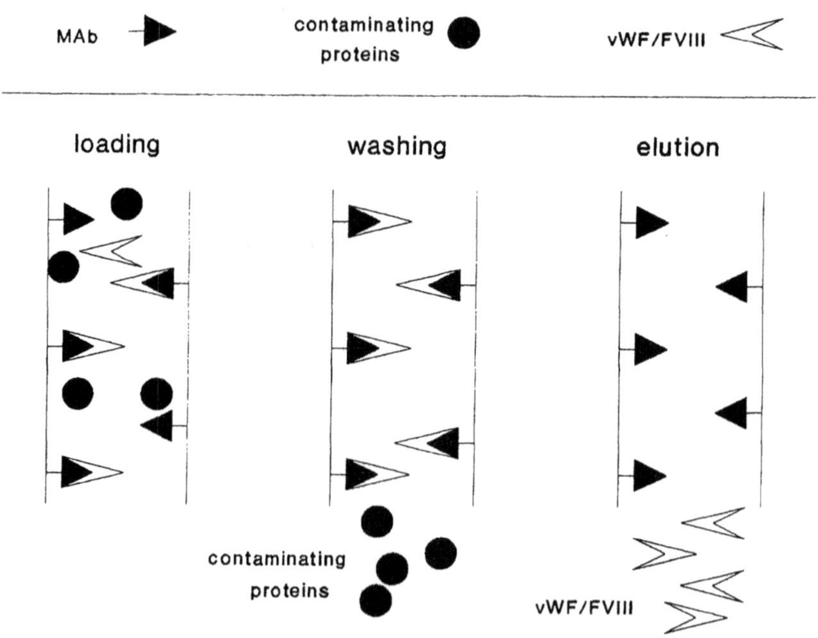

Figure 1. Principle of immuno affinity chromatography.

Except for two commercial manufactures most previous studies are limited to laboratory scales [3,5], which did not proceed to a pilot scale or the end of production schedules. In this study the development of a prototype for pilot scale when following the elution of FVIII/vWF from the immunoadsorbent column is reported.

The Red Cross Blood Bank Groningen-Drenthe and Bio-Intermediair B.V. Groningen started the development and application of this technique as a model system to purify the FVIII protein.

A model system was chosen to obtain experience and knowledge on the specific problems belonging to IAC. The difficulties are related to the items mentioned above. Once the experience and knowledge is obtained, it can be used as a principle for purification of a variety of other proteins. Additional to the knowledge, the aim for self-sufficiency and the superior characteristics of the FVIII product in purity, yield and safety compared to traditionally purified product have been the main reason to start the project, while the commercial sector has already advanced into this technology. Our approach was to use an anti-vWF antibody to purify the complex FVIII/vWF. The FVIII:C can be stabilized by the presence of vWF and such a preparation with this complex could be used for von Willebrand's disease (vWD) too. The use of an anti-vWF antibody has been applied before [6], but only the FVIII:C which was separated from vWF was purified, while anti-FVIII:C antibodies have been used by several other groups [4].

The project was started as a feasibility study. Initially a set up for purification was made with antibodies obtained from the Scottish National Blood Transfusion Service (SNBTS) and from a commercial source, followed by the development of our own antibodies with the special application of immunopurification in mind.

The first part reports a summary of the preliminary results of the design of an immunoaffinity purification of the FVIII/vWF complex on laboratory scale. The second part will be an overview of our approach

Cryoprecipitation from plasma

⇓

Prefiltration of cryoprecipitate

⇓

Immunoaffinity column chromatography

⇓

Gelfiltration column chromatography

⇓

Freeze drying

⇓

Virus inactivation

Figure 2. Flow chart of monoclonal purified FVIII.

on the development and screening for an anti-vWF antibody suitable in an immunoaffinity purification system.

The design for a purification scheme in this study comprised the steps shown in Figure 2.

Concerning the immunoaffinity purification three important items will be discussed in part 1: 1) preparation of the immunoadsorbent; 2) utility of the immunoadsorbent; 3) leakage of monoclonal antibodies.

Development of immunoaffinity chromatography

The immunoaffinity columns were produced with a concentration of approximately 1 mg antibody/ml solid support, which was Sephacryl S-1000. The CNBr-coupling method [7] as well as the periodate-oxydation (IO) coupling method [8] were used and proved to be useful techniques with at least 99% coupling of the MAbs. These two coupling methods with three different antibodies were studied for their ability to purify FVIII. An excess of FVIII was added to make use of the full capacity of the MAbs. The results of this comparative study are shown in Table 2.

The FVIII was recovered in the eluted peakfraction in concentrations of 10-20 IU/ml using MAb1 or MAb3 and 5-15 IU/ml for MAb2. According to the specific activity the purification of FVIII:C with MAb1 and MAb3 is approximately 3000-fold relative to plasma. Immunoaffinity chromatography presents a very powerfull separation because fibrinogen, fibronectin and albumin were not detectable in the purified FVIII/vWF pool. Especially the removal of fibrinogen and fibronectin is important, because these proteins may hamper efficient drying and virus inactivation of the product. Remarkable is the total release and recovery of the adsorbed FVIII for especially MAb1. When the process of loading could be optimized for this antibody the process of purification will produce almost no loss and theoretically all FVIII could be recovered. Based on these preliminary results and the availability of the different antibodies the follow-up of these experiments

Table 2. Comparative study on three antibodies and two coupling methods in their recovery, yield and purification of FVIII:C.

MAb	Coupling methods	Recovery[1] %	Yield[2] %	Specific activity IU/mg
MAb1	CNBr	98.5 ± 9.1	62.2 ± 6.9	44.6 ± 6.9
MAb1	IO4	96.7 ± 9.1	64.7 ± 6.3	38.0 ± 6.3
MAb2	CNBr	65.2 ± 19.5	42.6 ± 4.2	19.6 ± 4.2
MAb3	IO4	84.6 ± 10.2	75.2 ± 7.7	40.8 ± 20.3

1. Eluted FVIII as a percentage from adsorbed FVIII:C.
2. Eluted FVIII as a percentage of added FVIII:C.

was performed with MAb1. Besides the cryoprecipitate some other starting materials were examined. Plasma and HEP/CIG S [9] have been tested as starting material for purification. HEP/CIG S is a purified FVIII concentrate produced by the Blood Bank Groningen-Drenthe. Due to the differences in concentration of FVIII:C and contaminating proteins in these materials a better benefit for the pre-purified material was theoretically expected. But comparing these starting materials no benefit in recovery and purification for the pre-purified materials was found.

The utility of the antibody is defined as the binding capacity, which is the amount of FVIII:C activity bound per mg of MAb. The capacity of the S-1000-MAb1 column, with 1 mg/ml antibody, was determined by adding different amounts of FVIII:C to the gel and the recovered FVIII:C was measured. In Figure 3 the results of the coupling chemistry dependence for capacity is shown. This figure indicates a capacity of maximal 20 IU/mg MAb1 in case of the periodate coupling, while the CNBr coupled MAb1 has a capacity of 40 IU FVIII:C/mg. The capacity for vWF:Ag for the CNBr coupled MAb is 100 IU/mg MAb1. The ratio FVIII to vWF in the purified pool was 1:2.5.

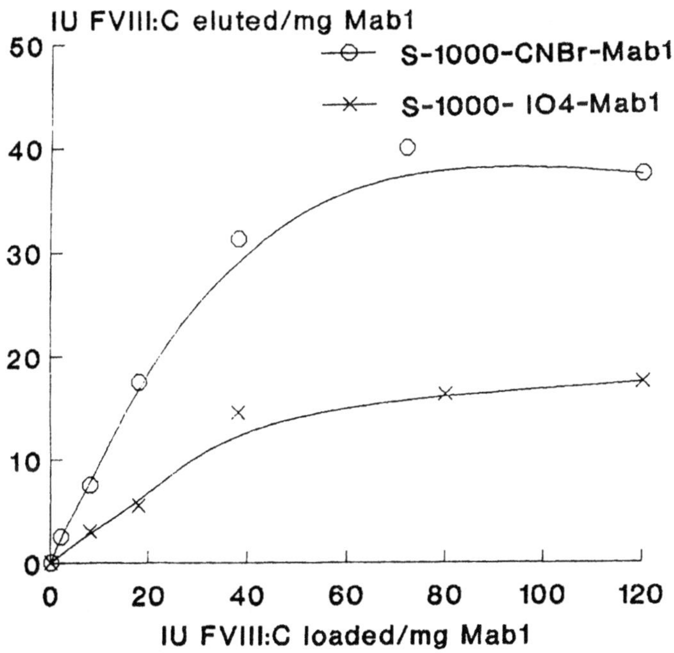

Figure 3. Influence on functionality of the MAb due to the coupling chemistry. Sephacryl S-1000 immobilized MAb1, coupled by CNBr (O) and periodate (×) method.

Theoretically there is a limit of two antigen molecules bound per antibody molecule, which means that 1 mg of MAb should bind 3 mg vWF:Ag. In the case of the CNBr-MAb1 3000 IU vWF could be bound theoretically. A utility of 100 IU vWF:Ag per mg MAb, corresponds with 3.3% of the MAb being active. This low percentage of functionality can be a result of at random coupling of Fc and Fab fragments due to binding of NH2-groups to the activated carrier material. For the periodate coupled antibodies the functionality is even half of this value. Probably the antibodies are more rigidly fixed to the carrier by this method resulting in a low binding of the antigen by the Fab fragments. Evenso the recycling of the two adsorbents shows a benefit in favour of the CNBr coupled antibody: after 30 cycles there was still a constant yield of FVIII. On the other hand the periodate coupled antibody showed a decrease in yield after only 15 runs. Comparing both methods the periodate is easier and more users' friendly, but the results with the immobilized antibody are in favour of the CNBr method for both the capacity and the reuse of the column.

For both methods we determined the release of antibody during the several phases in the immunopurification. Ionic strength, pH and composition of the buffers utilized may disrupt the binding between the

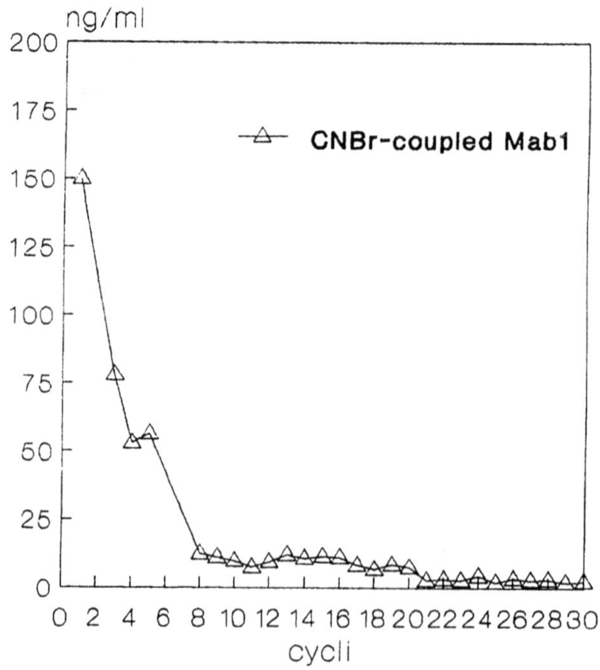

Figure 4. Leakage of murine IgG (anti-vWF antibody) in the eluted product fraction. Sephacryl S-1000 coupled with antibody by the CNBr method.

substrate matrix and the affinity ligand. In the loading and washing step there was no detectable leakage. However in the elution phase there is a certain amount of leakage. The chaotropic KI, which is a component of the elution buffer, probably will disrupt the covalent binding between carrier and antibody. After the fifth cycle the amount of IgG in the product is less than 50 ng/100 IU FVIII:C. In Figure 4 the leakage of IgG in the elution buffer and therefore in the product is shown. We measured no significant difference between the two coupling methods. In the first run there was a substantial leakage, which decreased over the first five runs and then stabilized at values of about 2-10 ng/ml.

The next phase in the purification scheme following the immunoaffinity is the gelfiltration, to exchange the buffer used to release the vWF/FVIII complex from the antibodies. KI is one of the components in the elution buffer that has to be removed. Before the filtration step, albumin was added in order to stabilize the FVIII:C. Without albumin there was 40% loss of activity when stored at –40°C. The last two steps, which are actually the freeze drying [9] and heat treatment (24 hours at 60°C) [9], were performed according to the standard operation procedure of the Blood Bank. In the freeze drying step 102 ± 3% was recovered. However, without added albumin there was a loss of 38 ± 15% of activity. During heat treatment there was no further loss of activity (103 ± 13%).

The overall recovery of the successive steps in this model are shown in Table 3.

Table 3. Recovery.

	%
Cryoprecipitation	60
Prefiltration	90
Immunoaffinity	70
Gelfiltration	85
Freeze drying and heat treatment	100
Overall recovery	32%

Thus estimated overall recovery from plasma is 32% and from cryoprecipitate is 54%. These values are the preliminary results of laboratory scale experiments.

Since these results on laboratory scale showed good prospects the follow-up of these experiments was focused on the development of MAbs (directed against vWF) and to fit the selected antibody in the purification scheme as it had been developed with MAb1.

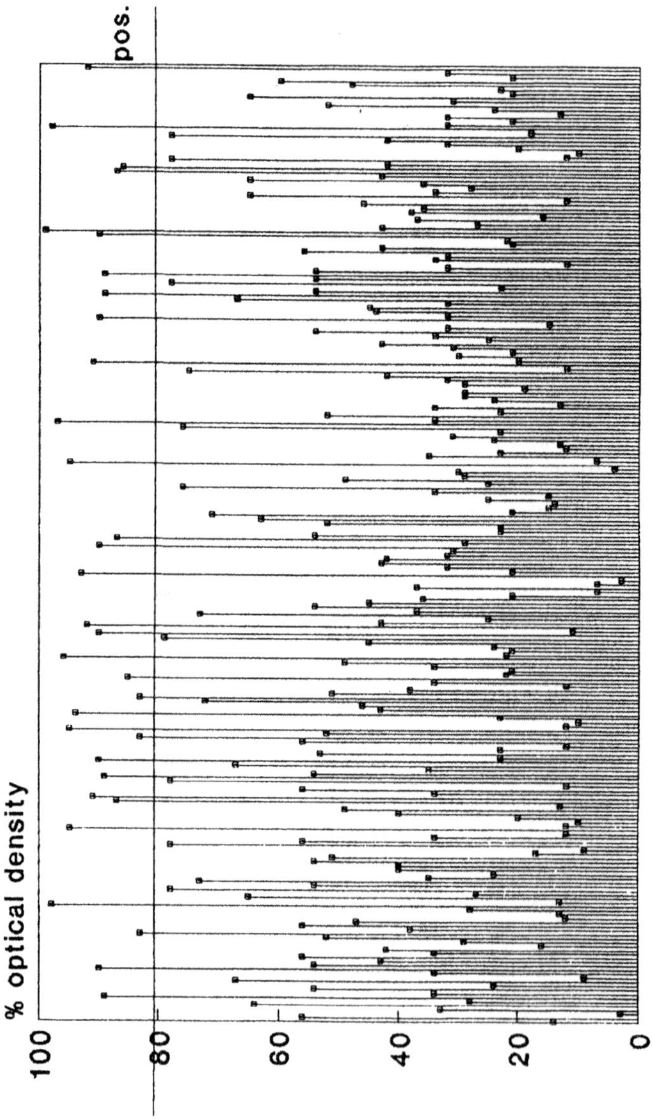

Figure 5. Primary screening on hybridomas for selection on anti-vWF antibodies.

Development of MAbs for IAC

Antibodies needed for the special application of immunoaffinity purification must bind the antigen (vWF) strongly, but on the other hand must be capable to release the antigen under mild conditions. The selection of the generated antibodies was adapted to these circumstances. The development of antibodies directed against vWF consisted of the following steps:
- purification of the antigen von Willebrand factor;
- standard immunization process of mice;
- cloning of cells with myeloma cells to generate hybridomas;
- subsquent screening of the different cell-lines producing the antibodies.

The vWF protein was purified with the antibodies mentioned in part 1. The purified vWF was used for immunization of the mice and for the screening assays. The immunization of the mice was performed by regular immunization schedules [10]. Following growing of the hybridomas the screening of the cells was performed with the specific purpose of immunoaffinity. The first screening for positive clones was carried out by a standard sandwich ELISA. Microwell plates were

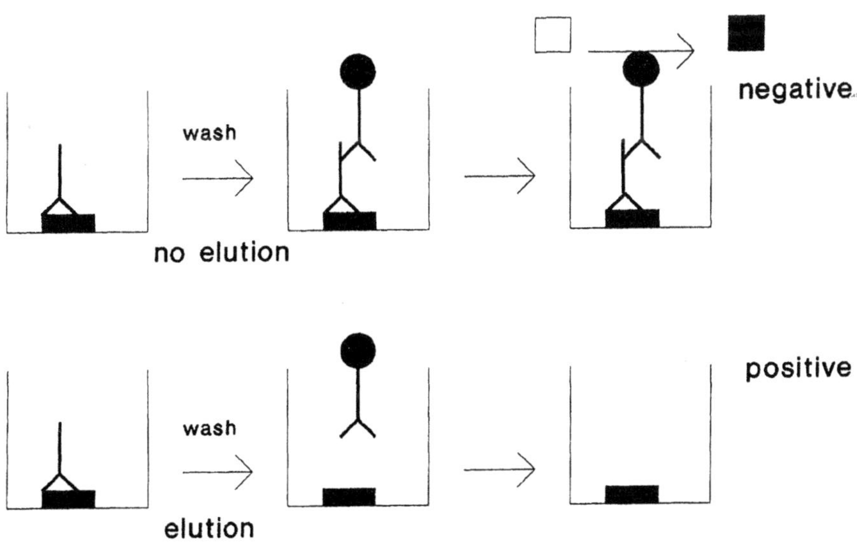

Figure 6. Principle of secondary screening of anti-vWF antibodies on functionality for immunoaffinity purification.

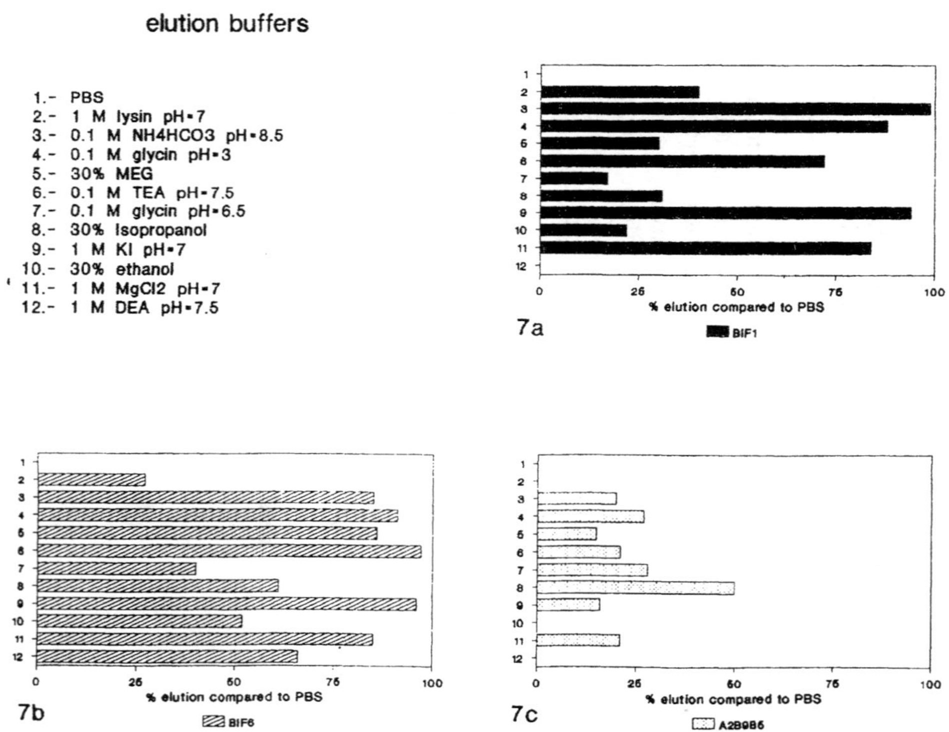

Figure 7. Results of the functionality screening of three MAbs with eleven elution buffers.

coated with the antigen vWF and after incubation with supernatant of the hybridoma, an incubation with peroxidase anti-IgG was performed. Standard colouring by adding substrate to the peroxidase could be measured at OD450. This resulted in 140 positive clones, in which a positive clone showed an optical density (OD) signal of two times the background signal, in this case about 20% of the maximal OD. A typical figure for positive and negative clones was obtained (Figure 5).

On 32 of these 140 positive clones, with the highest positive signal (actually four times the background signal), a secondary screening was performed [11]. This screening was a test on functionality to select the MAbs which were able to bind the antigen, but also were capable to release the antigen under mild elution conditions. This was also performed by an ELISA test. vWF was coated on plastic wells, the supernatant with the anti-vWF antibody was incubated and after binding of the antibody to the antigen, the wells were washed with the selected buffers. In the case of elution the antibody is released from the antigen and after incubation with the enzym-conjugated antibody no colour was detected. On the other hand when no elution took place the antibody was not removed and after incubation with peroxidase conjugated anti-IgG a colour signal was measured, indicating negative result. Each antibody was tested with eleven potential elution buffers, compared with PBS as a non-eluting control. The principle of assay is shown in Figure 6.

These experiments provide a "fingerprint" of each antibody for the capability to release the binding between antibody and antigen. The "fingerprint" has been established by expressing the optical density of each eluant as a percentage of elution in the saline control which was taken as 0% and plotting these in a histogram for each antibody with the eleven eluants. With the other buffers the binding between antigen and antibody can be released and so the percentage of elution will increase. In Figure 7 an example of three different antibodies is shown. The figure shows an antibody (7c) which is not capable to release the antigen; this is compared with the other two (7a and 7b), which show easy release of the antibody with some of the buffers. A positive antibody showed more than 50% elution with some of the buffers.

The next screening consists of an FVIII:C elution test on immobilized MAbs. The six selected antibodies were immobilized on Sephacryl S-1000 with the periodate oxydation method. They were tested on purification efficiency by the standard method described in part 1. The immunoadsorbent was mixed with cryoprecipitate, incubated and then eluted with the selected buffers. Again three examples of three different antibodies are shown in Figure 8 (a, b and c). On the horizontal axes the amount of elution of FVIII:C is shown. In this figure also the results of the secondary screening (Figure 7) are presented, which is the vWF:Ag elution. Remarkable are the differences in results between the screening on vWF:Ag or FVIII:C. In the secundary screening a

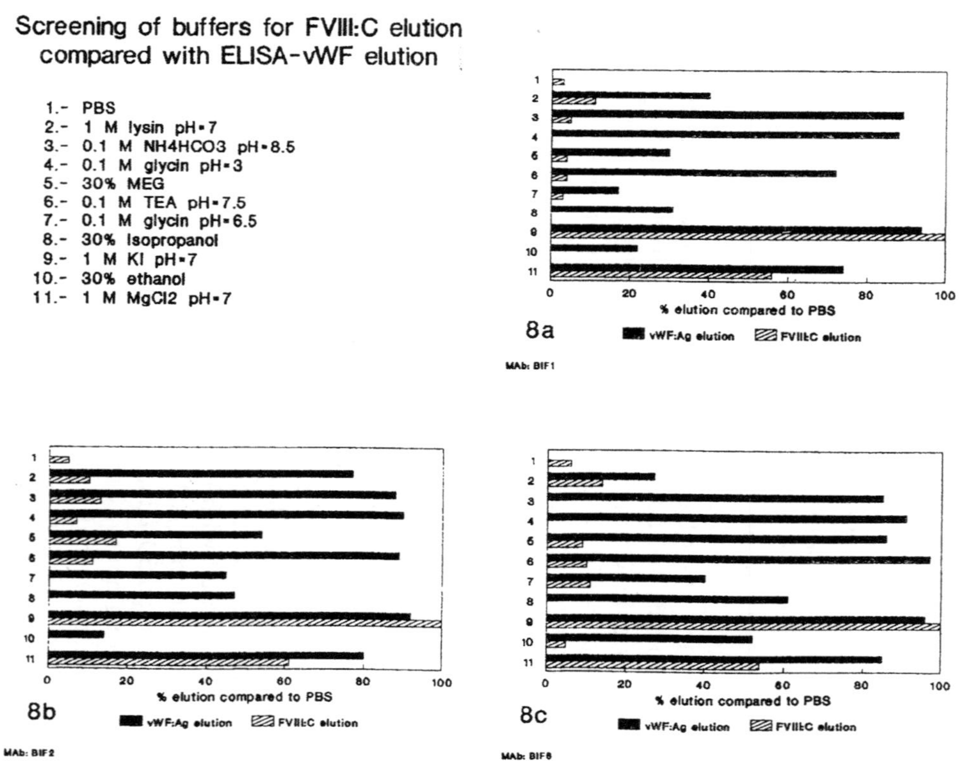

Figure 8. Screening of eleven elution buffers for elution of vWF/FVIII from immobilized MAbs.

Table 4. Summary of the results of the immunoaffinity purification experiments of six MAbs immobilized on Sephacryl S-1000 (n=5).

	Capacity IU/mg MAb	**Specific activity IU/mg**	**Recovery %[1]**	**Leakage IgG ng/ml**
BIF1	19 ± 7	47 ± 15	60 ± 7	26 ± 9
BIF2	13 ± 4	35 ± 4	62 ± 15	19 ± 6
BIF5	8 ± 3	51 ± 20	27 ± 5	19 ± 3
BIF6	15 ± 3	48 ± 13	76 ± 14	11 ± 3
BIF7	13 ± 3	36 ± 6	49 ± 14	17 ± 6
BIF8	10 ± 3	48 ± 15	48 ± 14	96 ± 35

1. Recovery in percentage from added FVIII.

number of buffers seems to be effective in eluting the antibody from the antigen. On the other hand when eluting the antigen from the antibody only the KI buffer seems to be effective.

There are some possible reasons for this phenomenon:

- the other buffers are not capable of releasing the vWF/FVIII antigen from the immobilized antibody;
- in the secondary screening the antibody was destroyed by the buffer instead of released from the antigen, after which the anti-IgG was not bound and a positive result was found;
- in the secondary screening the vWF and the antibody were eluted together from the well which showed a positive result;
- the eluted FVIII is not stable in the buffer, and is degraded before or when the assay was performed.

The last check on the selected MAbs is the real performance experiment on mini-column scale. The MAbs (immobilized on Sephacryl S-1000 with the periodate method) are screened for their capacity, yield and purification grade. These results are shown in Table 4.

From the results shown in Table 4 it can be concluded that:

1. the purification grade is good, but apparently there is no significant difference between the six MAbs. The specific activity of the purified FVIII is in the same range for all six MAbs.
2. large difference exist in capacity of the different MAbs. This can be due to different affinity for the antigen or different epitope recognition. BIF1 and BIF6 show the best results for capacity.
3. large differences in recovery, which identify the functionality of the MAb. BIF6, BIF1 and BIF2 gave more than 60% recovery of FVIII from the added FVIII.
4. leakage of mouse IgG is dependent on the type of antibody, since the coupling chemistry (periodate method) and solid support (Sephacryl S-1000) in all experiments are the same. Especially BIF8 shows

large leakage values compared to the other five MAbs, where BIF6 shows low leakage values compared to the other BIFs.

The overall conclusions on the development of antibodies directed against vWF are:

1. the structure of the antibody probably is affecting the leakage, immobilization efficiency, the capacity and recovery for vWF/FVIII.
2. the importance of a functional MAb is shown.

These results prove the importance of obtaining an excellent antibody for this technique, and that the success of the immuno affinity purification is in the first place dependent on the functionality of the MAbs.

Following these results BIF6 and BIF1 have been chosen as the antibodies to use for further experiments, and one of these two will be used in the system for purification as shown in the first part.

The investigations will be continued by modifications and improvements of immunoadsorbent, up/down stream processing and the implementation of a modified virus inactivation method based on the solvent/detergent principle. With the knowledge and experience of the aspects of immunoaffinity purification and the development of a specific MAb, the next phase will be to combine these two to a new system, which may lead to the production of a new product on Blood Bank scale.

Acknowledgement

We would like to thank Dr. D.S. Pepper and Dr. C.V. Prowse (Scottish National Blood Transfusion Service, Edinburgh, Scotland) for their support and advice in the development of the immunoadsorbent. Dr. J.K. Smith (Plasma Fractionation Laboratory, Churchill Hospital, Oxford, England) has been most helpful during this project.

References

1. Levine PH. Human factor VIII:C purified using monoclonal antibodies to von Willebrand factor. Thromb Haem Seminars in Haematology 1988;45 (Suppl.1):1-45.
2. Chase HA. Affinity separations utilizing immobilized monoclonal antibodies: A new tool for the biochemical engineer. Chem Eng Sci 1983;39:1099-125.
3. Mejan O, Fert V, Delezay M, Cheballah R, Bourgeois A. Immunopurification of human factor VIII/vWF complex from plasma. Thromb Haemostas 1988;59:364-71.
4. Griffith M, Liu S, Neslund G, Tsang I, Lettelier D, Berkebile R. Preparation of high specific activity plasma AHF by anti-FVIII:C immunoaffinity chromatography. Thromb Haemostas 1987;58:307(abstr.1123).

5. Hornsey VS, Griffin BD, Pepper DS, Micklem LR, Prowse CV. Immunoaffinity purification of FVIII complex. Thromb Haemostas 1987;57:102-5.
6. Zimmermann TS, Fulcher CA. Ultrapurification of factor VIII using monoclonal antibodies. US Patent 1982;4:361,509.
7. Kohn J, Wilchek M. A new approach (cyano-transfer) for cyanogen bromide activation of Sepharose at neutral pH which yields activated resins free of interfering nitrogen derivates. Biochem Biophys Res Comm 1982; 107:878-84.
8. Hornsey VS, Prowse CV, Pepper DS. Reductive amination for solid-phase coupling of protein. A practical alternative to cyanogen bromide. J Immun Methods 1986;93:83-8.
9. S.O.P. Component Department Red Cross Blood Bank Groningen-Drenthe, Part 3, Groningen 1990.
10. Boyd JE, Keith J. Development of monoclonal antibodies. In: Young H, McMillan A (eds). Diagnoses of sexually transmissible diseases with polyclonal and monoclonal antibodies. New York: Marcel Dekker Inc., 1987:1-56.
11. Bonde M, Frokier H, Pepper DS. Selection of monoclonal antibodies for immunoaffinity chromatography: A fingerprint of the elutibility. J Immunol Methods (submitted).

STRUCTURAL AND FUNCTIONAL PROPERTIES OF RECOMBINANT COAGULATION FACTORS[1]

A. Pavirani, S. Krishnan, S. Jallat, F. Perraud, A. Balland, W. Dalemans, D. Ali-Hadji, T. Faure, P. Meulien

Introduction

Current recombinant DNA technology enables the production of pure and safe preparations of coagulation factors destined for the treatment of the bleeding disorder hemophilia.

Production of large quantities of biologically active recombinant factor VIII (FVIII) and factor IX (FIX) has been, however, a difficult challenge for the biotechnology industry. This is mainly due to the complexity of these proteins, that is, the need of complex posttranslational modifications necessary to insure full procoagulant activity [1-3]. Such a fact has prompted the development of performant, efficient and specific heterologous expression systems capable of ensuring production of recombinant FVIII and FIX at an industrial scale.

Human recombinant FVIII preparations derived from genetically engineered chinese hamster ovary (CHO) and baby hamster kidney (BHK) cell lines are at present in clinical trials, preliminary results being very encouraging [4,5]. However, expression levels of recombinant FVIII harvested from the supernatant of these cells are relatively low when compared to the expression of other recombinant proteins [6].

In the case of recombinant human FIX the heterologous expression hosts so far employed have not been capable to ensure an adequate industrial process for the production of the recombinant molecule [7,8]. The low procoagulant activity observed may be associated with the limited choice of mammalian cell hosts which have not the capacity to ensure the posttranslational modifications required for full procoagulant activity of the recombinant protein when the latter is expressed at high levels.

1. Work on FVIII and FIX was made possible by support from TM-Innovation, France, and Institut Merieux, France, respectively.

Here we describe novel biotechnological approaches with industrial potential for the production of recombinant FVIII and FIX.

Results

Recombinant FVIII variants

In the past years our work has been focussed on the manipulations of the FVIII gene in order to construct novel FVIII derivatives. Our aim was to try to: a) investigate the functional properties of the molecule; b) simplify the complex electrophoretic profile of FVIII; c) increase expression levels in heterologous systems; d) develop molecules with new properties and with potential applications as improved pharmaceuticals. Several B-domains deleted variants of FVIII were constructed characterized biochemically and tested in vitro for procoagulant activity.

One particular variant is FVIIIΔII [9] in which the deletion extends from Pro771 to Asp1666, numbering of the amino acids (aa) being according to [10], thus including the cleavage site at aa Arg1648-Glu1649 (processed by an unknown protease). This cleavage is known to be the primary event in FVIII activation [11]. The 1436 aa polypeptide thus lacks the major part of the B-domain and the N-terminal part of the light chain. FVIIIΔII has the following characteristics: a) it retains procoagulant activity; b) it is expressed at higher levels than recombinant FVIII in comparable expression systems; c) it migrates on a SDS gel as a single band; d) it binds to von Willebrand factor (vWF); e) it is activated by thrombin to greater extent than recombinant FVIII or plasma-derived FVIII.

CHO cell lines have been engineered to produce large amounts of FVIIIΔII. After immunopurification using anti-factor VIII monoclonal antibodies the recombinant molecule has been analyzed with respect to thrombin cleavage [12]. The profile of the kinetics of thrombin activation is similar to that of plasma-derived and recombinant FVIII. The fragments generated upon thrombin activation were subjected to N-terminal aa sequencing and found to correspond to the predicted aa sequence. This demonstrates that the structural elements necessary for thrombin cleavage are present in FVIIIΔII despite the 900 aa deletion.

FVIIIΔII has been tested several times in a hemophilic dog model [13]. The novel FVIII variant displays full biological activity by correcting the bleeding time of the animal and by displaying an in vivo half-life similar to that of plasma-derived FVIII.

Recombinant FIX

In order to circumvent the problems linked to the expression of fully active recombinant human (rh)FIX in heterologous mammalian cell systems we investigated the potential use of transgenic mice as source of cell lines specifically engineered for the expression of biologically active rhFIX [14].

Transgenic technology allows the generation of novel mouse lines in which the foreign gene (the transgene) is expressed in a tissue-specific manner [for a review see 15]. This is achieved by engineering a DNA construct in which transgene expression is controlled by tissue-specific DNA regulatory sequences such as promoter/enhancers.

In the past years we have developed a procedure, we have termed transimmortalization [16], consisting of targeting the co-expression of an *onc* gene, such as c-*myc* and SV40TAg, and a gene-of-interest coding for a human recombinant protein to a tissue or cell type of choice in the transgenic mouse. Tumours develop, the neoplastic cells of which express the recombinant protein. Cell lines can be then established from tumour cells secreting the recombinant human protein in the supernatant. Hepatocytes were the candidates of choice for rhFIX expression since liver is the natural site of synthesis for the coagulation factor.

Approximately 5 kb of 5′ flanking promoter region of the FIX gene were used to direct the synthesis of several FIX genetic constructs in transgenic mouse hepatocytes, i.e.: a) the complete human gene (pTG 3960); b) the minigene (pTG3954) that is a DNA construct in which only one intron (the first intron of the FIX gene) is present; and c) the complete cDNA (pTG4915).

Table 1. Generation of double and triple transgenic mice.

	Transgene
Mouse lines	
TMTG3960	hFIX gene
TMTG2984	hα1AT[1] promoter/c-*myc*
TMTG4912	hα1AT promoter/SV40TAg[2]
	Circulating antigen levels
Double cross	
TMTG3960 × 2984	rhFIX = 25-40 μg/ml
Triple cross	
TMTG3960 × 2984 × 4912	rhFIX = 40-60 μg/ml

1. Human α1-antitrypsin.
2. Simian Virus 40 TAntigen.

Table 2. Characteristics of two trans-hepatic cell lines secreting recombinant human (rh)FIX.

	Cell line TMhepTG39	**Cell line TMhepTG48**
Productivity (rhFIX)	~0.15 $\mu g/10^6$ cells/24h	0.30-0.55 $\mu g/10^6$ cells/24h
Production (rhFIX)	~0.05 µg/ml/24h	0.37-0.55 µg/ml/24h
High level density long term production (rhFIX)	~0.3-0.4 µg/ml/24h	~0.7-0.8 µg/ml/24h
FIX activity/antigen (%)	70-124	>100

Several transgenic mouse lines were generated. The presence of one intron was found to be beneficial for high level rhFIX expression in the circulation of the animal, since transgenic mice bearing the cDNA construct had 40-200 fold lower level of FIX antigen in their plasma when compared to pTG3960 and pTG3954 mice having plasma levels ranging between 8-40 µg/ml. Expression of the transgene was restricted only to liver cells. rhFIX was characterized in terms of activity, immunorecognition and N-terminal aa processing and shown to be indistinguishable from plasma-derived FIX. Mouse lines (MTG3960) were successively crossed with transgenic mice (TMTG2984 and TMTG 4912) prone to develop hepatocellular carcinoma by hepatic tissue-specific *onc* gene expression (c-*myc* or SV40TAg, respectively) [17,18]. The resulting triple transgenic mice (Table 1) develop hepatomas after 3-14 months depending on the *onc* gene used. Providing favorable culture conditions cell lines could be established from several trans-hepatomas. rhFIX was harvested from the supernatant of these lines (Table 2) and proved to be fully active and correctly processed. At the present time, we are evaluating the industrial potential of these lines in terms of "scale-up" culturing and rhFIX production.

Discussion

The data reported show how it is possible to improve the yield and quality of complex recombinant coagulation factors using biotechnology. In the case of recombinant FVIII, FVIIIΔII could well represent a second generation molecule for the treatment of hemophilia A patients, after extensive testing relevant to potential neoantigenicity is performed. Fully active recombinant human FIX has been expressed in trans-hepatic cell lines derived from transgenic mice. These lines may have the potential for the industrial development of new preparations of FIX for the hemophilia B community.

Acknowledgements

We are sincerely grateful to J.P. Lecocq for encouragement and advice, to P. Chambon, P. Kourilsky and E. Eisenmann for support, to M. Courtney, C. Roitsch, H.V.J. Kolbe, C. Mazurier, D. Meyer, N. Bihoreau, G. Mignot, P. Paolantonacci, A. Sauger, V. Toully for helpful discussion, to all the technicians in Transgene involved in this work and to S. Perinel for excellent secretarial assistance.

References

1. Furie B, Furie BC. The molecular basis of blood coagulation. Cell 1988;53: 505-18.
2. Pavirani A, Meulien P. Advances in biotechnology of factor VIII. In: Seghatchian, Savidge GF (eds). Factor VIII von Willebrand factor. Volume 1. Biochemical, methodological and functional aspects. Boca Raton, Florida: CRC Press Inc, 1989:25-39.
3. Pittman DD, Kaufman RJ. Structure-function relationship of factor VIII elucidated through recombinant DNA technology. Thromb Haemostas 1989;61:161-5.
4. White GC, McMillan CW, Kingdon HS, Shoemaker CB. Use of recombinant antihemophilic factor in the treatment of two patients with classic hemophilia. N Engl J Med 1989;320:166-70.
5. Schwartz RS, Abildgaard C, Aledort L, et al. Preliminary report of phase I and II clinical investigation of human FVIII derived from recombinant DNA. Thromb Haemostas 1989;62:548a.
6. Kaufman RJ, Pittman DD, Marquette KA, Wasley LC, Dorner AJ. Factors limiting biosynthesis and secretion of factor VIII in mammalian cells. In: Alitalo KK, Huhtala ML, Knowles J, Vaheri A (eds). Recombinant systems in protein expression. Amsterdam: Elsevier Science Publishers B.V., 1990: 63-74.
7. Kaufman RJ, Wasley LC, Furie BC, Furie B, Shoemaker CB. Expression, purification, and characterization of recombinant γ-carboxylated factor IX synthesized in Chinese hamster ovary cells. J Biol Chem 1986;261:9622-8.
8. Balland A, Faure T, Carvallo D, et al. Characterization of two differently processed forms of human recombinant factor IX synthesized in CHO cells transformed with a polycistronic vector. Eur J Biochem 1988;172:565-72.
9. Meulien P, Faure T, Mischler F, et al. A new recombinant procoagulant protein derived from the cDNA encoding human factor VIII. Protein Eng 1988;2:301-6.
10. Wood WI, Capon DJ, Simonsen CC, et al. Expression of active human factor VIII from recombinant DNA clones. Nature 1984;312:330-7.
11. Eaton D, Rodriguez H, Vehar GA. Proteolytic processing of human factor VIII. Correlation of specific cleavages by thrombin, factor Xa, and activated protein C with activation and inactivation of factor VIII coagulant activity. Biochemistry 1986;25:505-12.
12. Krishman S, Kolbe HVJ, Lepage P, et al. Thrombin cleavage analysis of a novel antihemophilic factor variant: Factor VIIIΔII. Eur J Biochem 1991; 195:637-44.

13. Van de Pol H, Mignot G, Bihoreau N, et al. In-vitro and in-vivo studies of a biologically active genetically engineered factor VIII molecule. Thromb Haemostas 1989;62:623a.
14. Jallat S, Perraud F, Dalemans W, et al. Characterization of recombinant human factor IX expressed in transgenic mice and in derived trans-immortalized hepatic cell lines. EMBO J 1990;9:3295-301.
15. Jaenisch R. Transgenic animals. Science 1988;240:1468-74.
16. Pavirani A, Skern T, Le Meur M, et al. Recombinant proteins of therapeutic interest expressed by lymphoid cell lines derived from transgenic mice. Bio/Technology 1989;7:1049-53.
17. Dalemans W, Perraud F, Ali-Hadji D, et al. New cell lines for the production of recombinant human proteins derived by *onc* gene induced tumours in transgenic mice. In: Alitalo KK, Huhtala ML, Knowles J, Vaheri A (eds). Recombinant systems in protein expression. Amsterdam: Elsevier Science Publishers B.V., 1990:187-8.
18. Dalemans W, Perraud F, Le Meur M, Gerlinger P, Courtney M, Pavirani A. Heterologous protein expression by transimmortalized differentiated liver cell lines derived from transgenic mice. Biologicals 1990;18:191-8.

DISCUSSION

L.W. Hoyer, P.C. Das

H.J.C. de Wit (Leeuwarden, NL): Prof. Sixma, you did excellent work on the role of fibronectin in platelet adhesion, but blood bankers are interested in situations where a deficiency can be important. Can you tell us in what patients fibronectin deficiency could play a role in hemostasis, whether fibronectin suppletion could be useful and in what pharmaceutical form fibronectin could be administered.

J.J. Sixma (Utrecht, NL): For fibronectin the situation is different than for von Willebrand factor (vWF). The reason for this is that there is so much fibronectin present in connective tissue and the vessel wall that there is no need for fibronectin in plasma or in platelets. There has been a report on a family described with fibronectin deficiency in plasma and a deficient platelet aggregation. This is possible because fibronectin not only works in adhesion. Eva Bastida together with us showed that thrombus formation and aggregation in shear also requires fibronectin.[1] So, if fibronectin deficiency exists, you would expect some abnormality in platelet aggregation. There are also data from various other groups that have shown that fibronectin/GP-IIb/IIIa interaction plays a role in aggregation. But as an adhesive surface the vessel wall and connective tissue in general has so much fibronectin, that there will be no local deficiency.

R.L. McShine (Groningen, NL): Dr. Holme, do you have an explanation for the difference in mean platelet volume between filtered platelets and unfiltered platelets. Secondly, have you or do you know anybody who has done platelet function tests on filtered platelets and unfiltered platelets in vitro and in vivo.

1. Bastida E, Escolar G, Ordinas A, Sixma JJ. Fibronectin is required for platelet adhesion and for thrombus formation on subendothelium and collagen surfaces. Blood 1987;70:1437-43.

S. Holme (Norfolk, VA, USA): With regard to the first question whether we have an explanation for the differences in size, we also see with filtration that there is approximately 15-20% loss in platelet count, which suggests to us that probably the large platelets are selectively removed during the filtration process. The second question whether there is any difference in function before or after filtration. We have done quite a lot of testing like aggregation, hypotonic shock response and shape change, and so forth. We have not found any effect of filtration with regard to these in vitro parameters. We never tested in vivo or ex vivo function of filtered platelets.

J.J. Sixma: In our laboratory Dr. van Marwijk Kooy[2] looked at the in vivo effects of filtration and he found that filtered platelets had a good survival, but also corrected the bleeding time well. In the perfusion system that I described we also compared the effects of removing leukocytes by filtration or by centrifugation and found no difference. The concentrates behaved similar in the perfusion system.

R.L. McShine: Dr. Holme, another question. There is evidence in the literature that there is probably good correlation between platelet size and biological activity.[3,4,5] How could you explain the fact that, although you find a lower MPV after filtration, that there is still no difference in biological activity in vitro.

S. Holme: Well, first of all I do not think it is very well documented that large platelets are functionally better than small platelets. On the other hand, the differences that we see in mean platelet sizes are so small that you are probably not able to detect any effect at all. So, I really do not have any answer to that question.

M. Harvey (Leiden, NL): I understood that large platelets are generally younger. Is this so?

J.J. Sixma: The large platelets are usually the younger platelets.

2. Van Marwijk Kooy M, van Prooijen HC, Moes M, Bosma-Stants I, Akkerman JWN. Use of leukocyte-depleted platelet concentrates for the prevention of refractoriness and primary HLA alloimmunization: A prospective, randomized trial. Blood 1991;77:201-5.
3. Karpatkin S. Heterogenicity of human platelets VI. Correlation of platelet function with platelet volume. Blood 1978;51:307-16.
4. Thompsom CB, Eaton KA, Princiotta SM, Rushin CA, Valeri CR. Size-dependent platelet subpopulation relationships of platelet volume to ultrastructure, enzymatic activity and function. Br J Haematol 1982;50:509-19.
5. Wong T, Pedvis L, Frojmovic M. Platelet size affects both micro- and macro-aggregation: Contribution of platelet number, volume fraction and cell surface. Thromb Haemost 1989;62:733-41.

S. Holme: I think that is also disputed whether the large platelets are young platelets. I have not seen any good evidence for it.

M. Harvey: Well, I understand that if you do survival studies on platelets which have been taken over a gradient, you will find that the large platelets generally have the longest survival. This would correlate with your data that filtered platelets have a generally shorter survival time than unfiltered.

S. Holme: Yes, this probably could explain if it is so that large platelets have longer survival time. That could explain the findings of the shorter survival time with filtered platelets.

M. Harvey: We also see a slight decrease in platelet size on filtering. I think it is a point of attention for the manufacturers, because we have just switched over from day fresh platelets to filtered stored platelets and we are having to transfuse more often to keep the same hemostatic level in patients. One thing which is a great problem is the lowered initial hemostatic potential of stored platelets, what you beautifully showed in the first 24 hour-recovery period. If you are transfusing patients which are i.e. infected, you have a shortened recovery from other origin and maybe the platelets are destroyed by toxins before they get a chance to recover. Have you any idea what the most essential fact is in recovery of platelet function after storage?

S. Holme: No, but that is something that is worth investigating. I do not know what is causing the loss of function during storage. It appears that the loss of function of platelets during storage is not that all related to loss of viability. The loss of function has not been found to be related to energy metabolism, and is not related to any apparent changes in glycoproteins. Furthermore, there are no changes in respiration, hypotonic shock response or anything we have measured that correlates with this loss of the in vitro function. So at present, it is uncertain what is causing the loss of in vitro function.

M. Harvey: Prof. Sixma, I wonder have you tried something like recalcifying before you transfuse platelets.

J.J. Sixma: With Dr. Fijnheer from the Central Laboratory we recently have started to look at platelet concentrates, that have been stored for a while and that had lost their ability to aggregate with ADP. We have added that mixture to red blood cells, perfused them in the perfusion chamber and found to our surprise that platelets that could not aggregate well within the test tube formed nice thrombi on the vessel wall. It may well be that when you are testing with ADP, you may be underestimating in some respect the potential of the platelets to give a hemostatic reaction.

H. Storch (Suhl, FRG formerly DDR): Dr. Holme, what is your opinion about UV-irradiation of platelets to reduce the immunogenicity. Do you foresee clinical application in the near future?

S. Holme: I have no experiments, but I know that people in the audience are familiar with this.

C. Coffe (Besançon, F): We are at present trying a machine to UV-irradiatiate platelet concentrate. In France a multicentre protocol has started to irradiate by UVB platelet concentrate and to transfuse patients. In vitro, in the mixed lymphocyte culture system, lymphocyte activity is affected. But in vivo we are not yet able at the present time to provide information, since we began the protocol recently and hope to have approximately 200 patients in the study, by the end of 1991.

C.Th. Smit Sibinga (Groningen, NL): Adding to that information, of course, Dr. van Prooijen in Utrecht has done already some work on UV-irradiation. We should not forget about the messages which we go last year about the platelets as well.[6] Dr. Slichter from Seattle reported at the WAA meeting in Amsterdam[7] promising in vitro work with dogs. I want to come back to the opening remark of Prof. Sixma. He was wondering why he was invited and what his work has to do with blood transfusion. Well, it is quite evident because what he has illustrated is actually what we need to preserve in blood transfusion. When we store platelets for transfusion purposes, we want them to function, to survive and to act when transfused. Sofar, we have never actually developed any usable test system to really measure in vitro and predict the in vivo function of platelets. What you have shown is extremely important and you focused nicely and precisely on the role of cell receptors in the first phenomenon of adhesion. What Dr. Holme is pondering about, why is it that platelet viability does not really relate to function loss when storing, might very well be related to an effect on the receptors on the membrane in ageing of platelets. It might very well deal with the different storage media. Probably you both could comment, because here might be something in our hands to develop for the next few years as a test system in

6. Holme S. Storage of platelet concentrates in plasma-free synthetic media. In: Smit Sibinga CTh, Das PC, Meryman HT (eds). Cryopreservation and low temperature biology in blood transfusion. Dordrecht: Kluwer Academic Publ., 1990:119-27.
7. Slichter SJ. UV-irradiation: Effects on the immune system and on platelet function, viability, and alloimmunization. In: Smit Sibinga CTh, Kater L (eds). Advances in haemapheresis. Dordrecht: Kluwer Academic Publ., 1991:(in press).

vitro to predict a little more accurately how platelets are going to actually function in vivo.

J.J. Sixma: Thank you, the point is well taken. I think that the perfusion system could be used very well for this purpose. However, I should warn you. It was a very time consuming technique and there are still many tricks and pitfalls. But if you have it working I think it is the system that probably comes closest to the in vivo situation. I think though that you still have to prove that platelets that do well in the perfusion chamber also shorten the bleeding time.

J. Over (Amsterdam, NL): Mr. Koops, I was wondering whether you had a look into the contaminants in the vWF/FVIII preparations that you got in purifying them with monoclonal antibodies. Because when the FVIII/vWF complexes are essentially native and non-denatured, the specific activity will be about 100 units of vWF per mg protein. I noticed that you have only about 40 to 50. So, are there any other contaminants present?

K. Koops (Groningen, NL): They were not detectable. But maybe that is due to the amount of vWF compared to the FVIII:C. We could not detect fibrinogen, albumin or other proteins.

J. Over: So, the specific activity of vWF antigen, so to say, is 100 units/mg.

K. Koops: Yes, but the differences between our data presented and the theoretical value could be due to the protein assays, or FVIII assay. There are always some discrepancies in the literature about that.

P.M. Mannucci (Milan, I): A comment related to the presentation of Dr. Smith, on the interest of developing pure vWF concentrates. I think that such concentrates are interesting, but perhaps a word of caution should be made. Because there is a tendency on the basis of these new developments to ignore that probably 90% of the patients with von Willebrand disease (vWD) can be treated without blood derivatives, but with DDAVP, which is safer than any concentrate. I think that even if these concentrates are probably safer in terms of viruses than first generation concentrates, there is still considerable risk while DDAVP does not carry any risk. Hearing at various meetings presentations on the use of these concentrates in patients with vWD I am appalled to notice that these concentrates are given to patients that definitely could be treated with DDAVP. In my opinion the only patients for whom vWF concentrates could be considered are patients with severe type 3 vWD, type 2A and type 2B. These patients are extremely rare, they probably represent no more than 10% of all the patients with vWD in whom plasma derived von Willebrand concentrates in gneeral are needed, one has to remind that these patients are deficient in FVIII. They do bleed probably more frequently, because they are deficient in FVIII than because they are deficient in vWF. So, these pure vWF concentrates are interesting because FVIII is probably raised in an alternative way. I do agree with you that one should not ingore that in FVIII concentrate there is a lot of vWF. One should not ignore that in vWD type 3 FVIII is needed as much as vWF for the treatment of these patients.

M. Mikaelsson (Stockholm, S): Dr. Smith, I am not happy with the way you handle the question of purity. Are you stressed yourself, the major concern in the production of therapeutic concentrates is the virus safety. However, the degree of purification is the most important character of the purification process, not the final specific activity which depends on the added albumin. If you take the immunoaffinity purified products, the overall degree of purification is about 200,000 times over plasma. But for ordinary, high purity concentrates it is about 1000 to 2000-fold purification. That has importance when you look at the removal or inactivation of viruses, removal of different types of impurities, aggregated proteins etc.

J.K. Smith (Oxford, UK): I would certainly agree with out if a) it was shown that the proteins which have traditionally been present in FVIII concentrates are caousing immunosuppression or immunomodulation and b) if in fact such a highly purified FVIII was being delivered and infused into the hemophiliac. That is not so at the moment. The most highly purified concentrates transfused into the hemophiliacs are, in fact, the moderately purified ones, which contain vWF. The specific activity of the two monoclonally purified concentrates represent perhaps, addition of different amounts of albumin.

L.W. Hoyer: Does not this really come down to the question of which proteins you would prefer to have with the FVIII as the contaminant, since some other protein is necessary for FVIII stability, in other words, which set of proteins have the most potential for harm; the vWF, fibronectin and fibrinogen in intermediate purity products; or the albumin ant the small number of contaminants found with the albumin preparations in the monoclonal purified products. I do not know of any data that really address this question. It is a very important clinical issue whether or not there are either safety or efficacy differences between these products that end up with the same specific activity.

C.R.M. Hay (Liverpool, UK): I did find Dr. Smith's comments on the relative importance of immune disfunction in HIV negative hemophilic patients a little biased. I believe that there is some evidence that there may be an excess mortality from carcinoma and an increased risk of infection in this group and that this might be attributable to immunomodulation caused by intermediate purity FVIII. To get back to Dr. Hoyer's comments; it is true that after albumin has been added to monoclonally immunopurified concentrates, their specific activity compares with some of the chromatographically prepared concentrates. But certainly in vitro the immunopurified concentrates inhibit lymphocyte function and monocyte function very much less than chromatographically prepared concentrates, suggesting that not all impurities are the same in the eyes of the immune system and that products with albumin added are very much less likely to cause adverse immunological effects. Finally, if this immune disfunction is such a minor concern perhaps Dr. Smith could tell us why it is that the Blood Products Laboratory has decided to start to make immunopurified FVIII concentrate.

J.K. Smith: To take the question first, we recognize that there are many different views within one country on the preference for contaminants one has along with one's FVIII. So it is BPL policy that we are making the existing concentrate. To go back to your earlier comments, I would like to see any publication on an increased risk of cancer or infections in HIV negative hemophiliacs, compared with unaffected individuals. I knew of only one very indirect piece of evidence that is Frank Hill's case of tuberculosis[8] in Birmingham many years ago, which could have other explanations and was, of course, before the HIV era. All other clinical evidence suggests to me that there is no difference between different concentrates in their tendency to produce immunomodulation as presently denoted by T4, T8 and IgG levels in HIV-negative hemophiliacs.

T.W. Barrowcliffe (Potters Bar, UK): Dr. Smith, you mentioned the possibility of improvements in the problem of thrombogenicity of factor IX (FIX) concentrates by going to more purified FIX preparations. I wonder if you can comment about the possible role of activated FIX, which at least in some animal models is extremely thrombogenic. Do you think this is going to be a problem with the new types of FIX concentrates that we have to test for limited amounts of activated FIX.

J.K. Smith: I believe that with some of the chromatographic methods IX_a does tend to travel along with IX and it is difficult to separate. I do not know at what levels we should be getting worried about IX_a. I simply point to a current concentrate which contains so much ATIII

8. Beddall AC. Unusually high incidence of tuberculosis among boys with haemophilia during an outbreak of the disease in a hospital. J Clin Pathol 1985;38:1163-5.

and heparin that IX_a should not be a problem. Yet it still gives a slight response, when given to dogs in the DIC model. I wonder whether only IX_a is involved here or whether there are still some unidentified thrombogenic factors or cofactors.

T.W. Barrowcliffe: Dr. Pavirani, I was very interested in your data on thrombin activation with the modified FVIIIΔII. You said you got something like a 40-fold increase in activity. We have looked at thrombin activation in regular concentrates and we find it very difficult to measure. Maybe it is just our incompetence, but we find it very difficult to reproduce these sort of activities. I think one of the problems is on the assay systems where thrombin activated and non-activated material is not parallel. So, I just wonder, if you are really convinced that there is a real big difference between your modified FVIII and ordinary FVIII.

A. Pavirani (Strasbourg, F): We have done the experiment a number of times and we are very well convinced that what I have shown is essentially an average profile of activation for the molecule called FVIIIΔII. Usually we find between 30 and 50-fold activation. We found at least three fold more activation with respect to recombinant FVIII (rVIII) or for instance, plasma derived FVIII. So, we are definitely convinced about that. I cannot tell you why that is. I would be very pleased to know the functional background about the observed phenomenon.

T.W. Barrowcliffe: We have some evidence that ordinary rVIII is at least partially activated. So, it maybe that the difference is because the regular rVIII has already been partially activated.

L.W. Hoyer: So, does it mean that the FVIIIΔII in this case is not activated?

T.W. Barrowcliffe: Well, there is a possibility, I think we could look at this in another system and that would be very interesting to see.

A. Pavirani: I have a comment, which could be of interest in this discussion. We found that neither fibronectin nor fibrinogen had a possitive effect on stabilizing the activity of rVIII preparations.

L.W. Hoyer: In contrast to vWF.

C.Th. Smit Sibinga: To follow-up to the question of Dr. Barrowcliffe, I was wondering what is it actually that in the changed molecules provides the tremendous increase in expression of FVIII. In other words what is it precisely in the ΔII that gives that so much better effect.

A. Pavirani: We have seen these activation profiles with thrombin only for ΔII. Probably I was not clear in my presentation. ΔI has a profile similar to rVIII as well as what we call ΔVI. So, actually only ΔII has this strange feature. We think that we have hit an important portion of the molecule by extending the deletion to just that particular aminoacid. Definitely, it has profound consequences in the conformation of the new analogue, but if you ask me more in detail, I really do not know why.

S. Stienstra (Nijmegen, NL): Mr. Koops, as Dr. Smith presented Heimburger uses a method in extracting the surplus of vWF from his FVIII preparations,[9] and helping two patients with one preparation. Do you think that in your preparation, which is fairly von Willebrand enriched, also this procedure can be used to make a FVIII product which has a higher FVIII concentration and to get in the same time a FVIII product. Does it make any sense?

K. Koops: It is of course possible to bind von Willebrand, elute FVIII:C, collect separately and afterwards release the von Willebrand from the antibody. But, probably the stabilization of the FVIII:C will be a problem. Of course, it is possible, but the question is if it is effective!

J. Over: A comment, which is touching upon a few points that Dr. Smith was mentioning. I am referring to a project in the Central Laboratory which is aiming for directly isolating FVIII from plasma by affinity chromatography. The fundamental work for it has been done by the Technical University in Twente a few years ago[10], but it has been our task up till now to further develop this procedure and to scale it up.[11] The ligand that has been chosen finally after the fundamental work had been done, turns out to be a multipurpose ligand. It has shown an affinity for both FVIII, vWF, factor V (FV) and the prothrombin complex factors. So, in the pilot scale in which about ten batches of 150 kg plasma were run, we succeeded to get a preparation with a final recovery of 300 units per kg of plasma. This ligand is also showing an

9. Heimburger N, Kumpe G, Wormsbacher W. A new pasteurized high purity factor VIII concentrate: FVIII:C P. 17th International Congress of the World Federation of Hemophilia. Madrid, 26-31 May 1988. Abstract book:25.
10. Te Booy MPWM, Riethorst W, Faber A, Over J, König BW. Affinity purification of plasma proteins: Characterization of six affinity matrices and their application for the isolation of human FVIII. Thromb Haemost 1989;61:234-7.
11. Te Booy MPWM, Faber A, de Jonge E, et al. Large-scale purification of factor VIII by affinity chromatography: Optimization of process parameters. J Chromat 1990;503:103-14.

affinity to FV. The FV level is pretty high in this concentrate. In the same time vWF is present in normal multimeric composition. It might turn out that this preparation would also be suitable for treating vWD patients. We are wondering at the moment whether it is acceptable to have preparation which is containing both FVIII and FV in high concentrations. But we could solve this problem by first isolating FVIII by, for instance, cryoprecipitation and then apply this affinity matrix to the plasma for isolating FV. So, I think that would be a good possibility to produce a FV concentrate.

III. LABORATORY ASPECTS

PLATELET COUNTING AND FUNCTION TESTING

B. Brozovic, R.L. McShine

During the last two decades the demand for platelet concentrates (PC) required for treatment of thrombocytopenic patients receiving multiple transfusions of PC has been steadily growing. This demand has been met by increasing rate of preparation of PC using conventional methods as well as by developing novel techniques. As a consequence there has been a need to improve our understanding on functional changes of the platelet during processing and storage of PC and to develop methods suitable for quality monitoring of critical stages in that process.

The quality of PC can be qualified in terms of conformance to product specification based on the requirements set by the users (clinicians) and those set by the producers (blood bankers). The users require evidence for a satisfactory outcome of a platelet transfusion, as measured by the survival, recovery and hemostatic capacity of the transfused platelets, the subject which is discussed in detail elsewhere [1]. The users have a wide range of in vitro tests of varying complexity to choose from for assessing the quality of PC. In this presentation only the in vitro tests considered to be essential for quality control of PC are reviewed. In addition, results of recent studies on novel methods applicable to quality control of PC are presented.

Essential tests for the quality control of platelet concentrates

Essential tests for the quality control of PC are: determination of volume, enumeration of platelets, evaluation of platelet function using at least one of the many tests available for that purpose, and determination of leukocyte count.

Volume

Volume of PC can be easily determined and it provides an indication of the consistency of the operator's performance or the reproducibility of the automated processor when the latter is used in the manufacturing process. As a measure of quality it should always be used in conjunction with the platelet count.

Platelet count

Platelet count can be calculated from the platelet concentration, determined with an automated hematology cell counter, and the volume of PC. The accuracy and precision of the platelet count in blood samples depend on many factors [2] and in particular on the care applied for obtaining a representative sample from PC, the type of anticoagulant used, and the lapsed time from the collection of sample to the counting of platelets. The influence of the anticoagulants and the effect of the elapsed time on the accuracy of platelet counting has been recently investigated by McShine and collegues [3]. These authors have reported that the platelet count in samples of blood taken from healthy individuals into sodium citrate, ACD(A), CPDA-1 or EDTA anticoagulants[1] decreased by up to 30% within the period of six hours after collection of blood (Figure 1). The decrease of the platelet count in the blood samples was essentially the same with any of the three citrate containing anticoagulants, but it was almost negligible (invariably less than 10%) in samples anticoagulated with EDTA. The effect of EDTA on the platelet count was also seen when EDTA was added to blood samples already anticoagulated with a citrate containing anticoagulant. It is of interest to note that the platelet count in citrated samples of blood spontaneously rose after 24 hours but did not reach either the initial value or that obtained by counting platelets in the sample with EDTA. The mechanism by which EDTA is capable of affecting the platelet count is discussed below. The study of McShine and collegues [3] has highlighted the necessity to add EDTA to all samples of blood and blood components taken for platelet counting even when they already contain one of the citrate anticoagulants.

Determination of platelet function

It has been now generally accepted that the structure and function of platelets are subject to change during the period from blood collection to administration of PC to the patient. These changes are characterized by the diminished platelet metabolism, function and viability, and they are collectively named the platelet storage lesion. The extent of the platelet storage lesion is determined by the action of many diverse factors of which the main ones are: the type and shape of the platelet pack, the composition of anticoagulant, the concentration of platelets (and leukocytes), and conditions of storage such as temperature, oxygenation and agitation of the pack.

1. ACD(A), acid-citrate-dextrose (NIH formula A); CPDA-1, citrate-phosphate-dextrose-adenine formula 1; EDTA, trisodium or tripotassium salt of ethylenediamine tetraacetic acid.

Tests which can be used in vitro to measure the degree of the storage lesion can be conveniently grouped into those which a) demonstrate changes in the membrane structure, as for example loss of glycoproteins GP-Ib and GP-IIb/IIIa or emergence of membrane glycoprotein MGP140, b) measure rates of various metabolic processes and concentrations of end products as well as the ability of platelets to respond to stimulation by agonists, and c) estimate changes of the platelet morphology (Table 1). One can demonstrate some degree of storage lesion using any one of these tests. However, the magnitude of the storage lesion revealed by the chosen test may vary from almost negligible, e.g. loss of GP-IIb/IIIa, to near complete, e.g. absence of platelet aggregation on stimulation with a low dose of ADP. Because of this there is almost invariably a good correlation between the results obtained by any of the two tests selected for demonstrating the platelet storage lesion. For details on conventional measurements of platelet function the reader should consult reference [4].

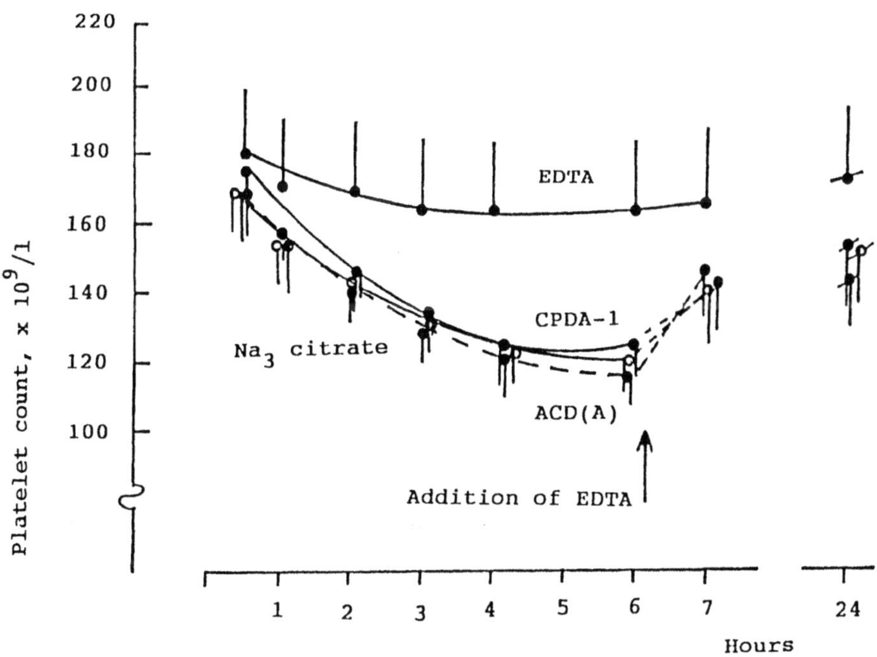

Figure 1. Changes of platelet counts in blood samples anticoagulated with Na3citrate, ACD(A), CPDA-1 or EDTA, and the effect of EDTA on platelet countof citrated samples (n=12). In samples with citrate anticoagulants the blood count was carried out at six hours after collection and prior to addition of EDTA and again one hour later. Vertical bars represent 1 SD (modified from: McShine et al [3]).

Table 1. Methods available for investigating the storage lesion of the platelet.

Platelet structure	Membrane glycoproteins Granules (alpha granules, dense granules and lysosomes)
Platelet function	Adhesion Aggregation Metabolic changes Release reaction
Platelet morphology	Morphology score (light and electron microscopy) Shape change in stirred suspensions Hypotonic shock response

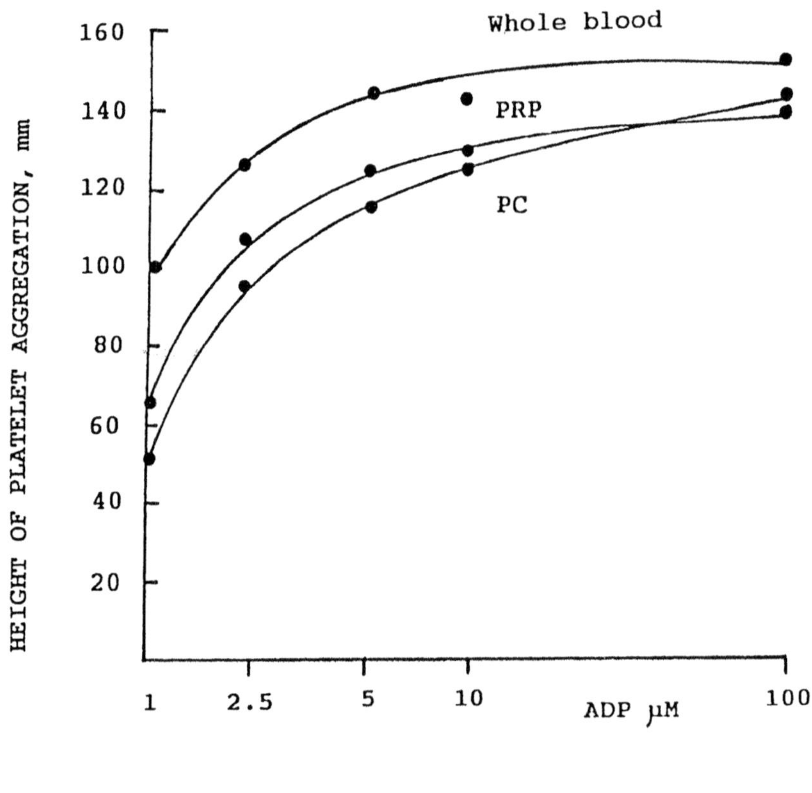

Figure 2. The aggregation response of platelets tested during the stages of preparation of platelet concentrates (PC). Each point represents the mean height of platelet aggregation response in six PC. PRP: platelet rich plasma. The difference between the platelet aggregation response in whole blood and in PRP and PC was significant ($p<0.05$) for concentrations of ADP up and including 10 µM (modified from: Bateson [6]).

Determination of leukocyte content

The presence of leukocytes in PC is undesirable because of their propensity to release proteolytic enzymes, their potential to sensitize the recipient against HLA alloantigens and their capacity to shelter dormant viruses (CMV, EBV and HTLV-I). Therefore, the determination of leukocyte content in PC is an essential test for the quality control of the production of PC. The role of leukocytes in blood transfusion has been reviewed elsewhere [5].

New approaches in the quality control of platelet concentrates

In vitro tests available for evaluating platelet function and storage lesion of the platelets in PC have come into blood transfusion from the hospital or research environment. We have therefore explored the possibility to modify two of the tests, the platelet aggregation and the

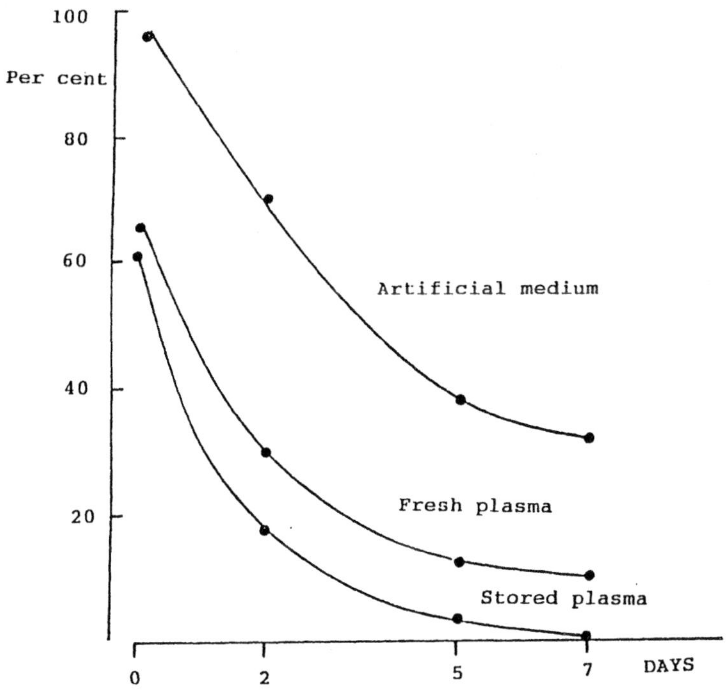

Figure 3. Enhancement of platelet aggregation in stored CPDA-1 platelet concentrates (PC) using fresh allogeneic plasma and artificial medium. The values represent the mean of 12 measurements [8].

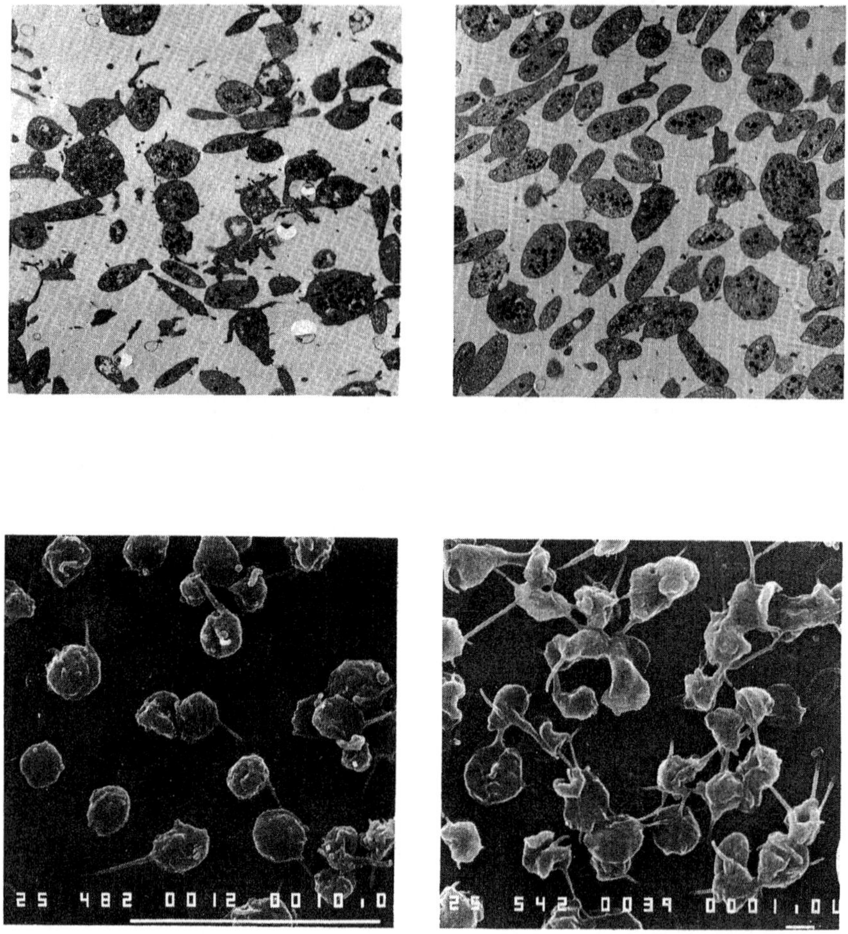

Figure 4. Transmission (a,b) and scanning (c,d) electron microscopy of fresh platelet concentrates (PC) in CPDA-1 before (a,c) and after addition of EDTA (b,d); magnification for a and b is × 2250 and c and d × 1350.

platelet response to EDTA, and thus make them more relevant to use in blood transfusion practice.

Platelet aggregation

Platelet aggregation induced by ADP has been used as a yardstick for measuring platelet function in the authors' laboratories. The test has been found sufficiently sensitive to demonstrate a diminished response of platelets to stimulation with low concentrations of ADP even in freshly prepared PC (Figure 2) [6].

Earlier observations made in the author's laboratory by J. Bateson that fresh plasma carries a beneficial effect when added to stored platelets and that the "rejuvenated" platelets increase the residual capacity to aggregate on stimulation with ADP [6] led us to explore further that phenomenon as well as to extend the study to the use of a balanced salt solution, similar in composition to the one described by Rock et al [7]. The results of this study carried out on PC collected from 12 healthy donors and stored for seven days are illustrated in Figure 3. The highest aggregation response to stimulation with 10 μM ADP was obtained in fresh PRP and assigned the value of 100%. The aggregation of platelets after addition of fresh plasma was better than that in the control PC, but was far exceeded by aggregation of platelets after addition of the balanced salt solution [8].

These findings have indicated that it is possible to rejuvenate platelets in stored ADP, and probably to increase their clinical efficacy by incubation with an artificial medium before transfusion. Furthermore, these findings have provided a way to assess the residual function of stored platelets. Finally, this study has provided an explanation for the lack of correlation between the results of in vitro and in vivo tests used for assessment of platelet function.

Platelet shape change

The degradation of the platelet function during storage is associated with the platelet shape change from discoid to spherical [9]. The transformation can be seen using light microscopy and can be quantitated either by scoring the transformed cells or by using electronic systems [10,11]. The ability of platelets to maintain their shape can be also deduced using hypotonic shock response test [12]. It has been recognized for quite some time that the platelet shape change and the change of platelet volume are closely associated and bear relationship to platelet aggregation and adhesion [13-15]. It has also been recognized that subpopulations of platelets of different volume and density have different functional properties, as well as different viability in vivo (for a review of the heterogeneity of platelets see [16]). We have exploited the information previously published to extend our studies in two directions: firstly, to investigate separation of platelet subpopulations from whole

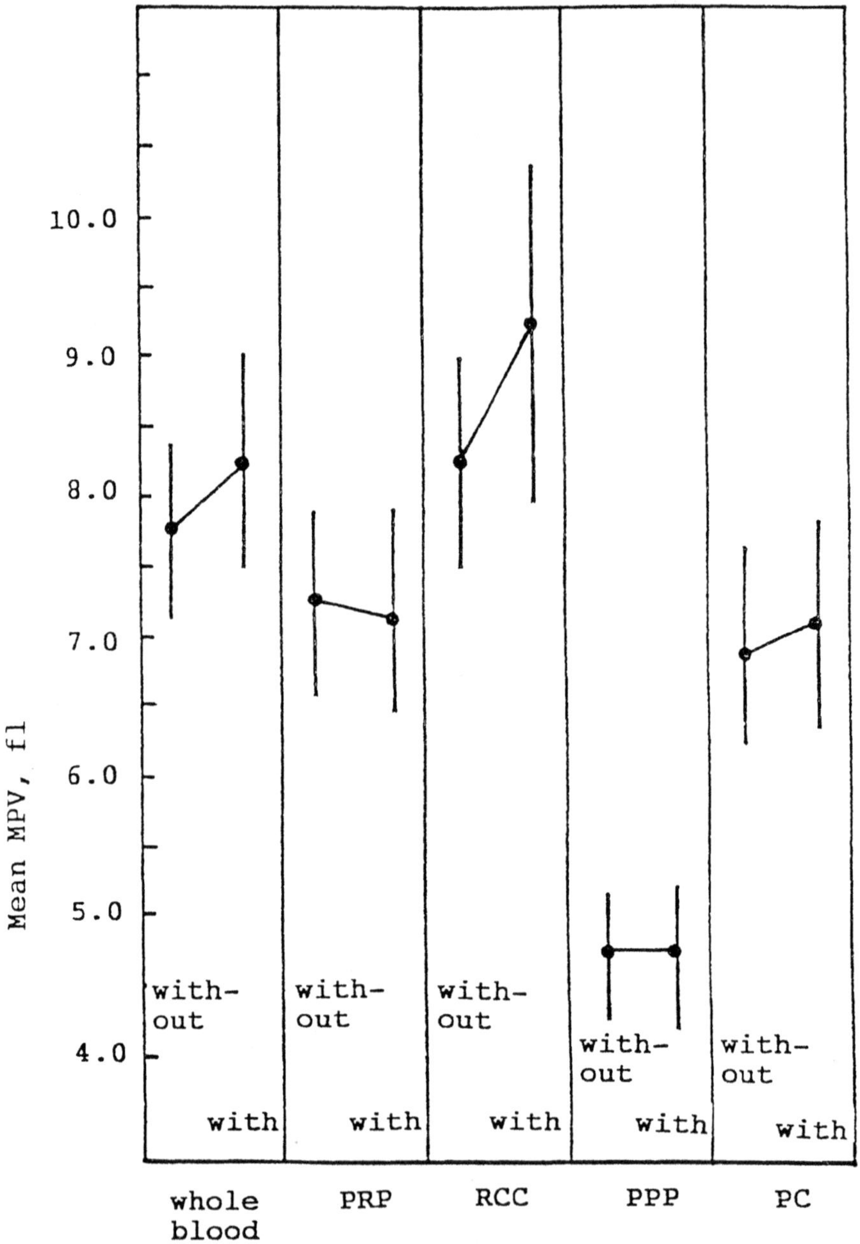

Figure 5. Mean platelet volume (MPV) in whole blood collected in CPDA-1, platelet rich plasma (PRP), red cell concentrate (RCC), platelet poor plasma (PPP) and platelet concentrate (PC). On the left of each column are values - obtained in samples without EDTA and on the right in samples with EDTA(n=12).Vertical bars represent 1 SD [19].

blood into blood components, concentrated red cells, platelet poor plasma (PPP) and PC, and secondly, to follow the changes of the platelet volume during storage of PC. In addition, in both studies, carried out concurrently in London and Groningen, we have measured the response of platelets suspended in citrate solutions to addition of EDTA using automated hematology cell counters. Following addition of EDTA platelets become spherical and increase their size, the phenomenon previously described [17] and illustrated in Figure 4. We have measured the extent of the EDTA effect on platelets in suspension by the difference between the mean platelet volume (MPV) of platelets in citrate solution and MPV after addition of EDTA. This difference which we have called dMPV has proved to be of great interest in estimating the platelet storage lesion as explained below.

In the first set of experiments McShine has shown that during preparation of PC subpopulations of platelets of different size were separated and were found in different components, concentrated red cells, PPP and PC [18,19]. The ability of platelets of different sizes to change their volume after addition of EDTA was also different (Figure 5). The subpopulation of the largest platelets with the greatest response to EDTA was separated with the red cells, while subpopulation of the smallest platelets unable to respond to EDTA was found in PPP. It is of interest that in all the components the change of the platelet distribution width (PDW) of each separated subpopulation of platelets on addition of EDTA was inversely proportional to the change of MPV.

In the second set of studies Seghatchian, Vickers and Ip in London followed the changes in MPV in stored PC collected by Autopheresis C cell separator (Baxter Healthcare Ltd.) as a part of a multicentre trial [20]. These investigations also measured the change of MPV induced by addition of EDTA using Technicon H*1 hematology cell counter (Technicon Ltd.) and Sysmex 2000 hematology cell counter (TOA Medical Electronics Ltd.). Several important observations ensued from these studies.

In the studies it has been shown, firstly, that MPV (as well as PDW) of the platelets in PC changes substantially during the 7-day period of storage under conventional conditions. It has been further demonstrated that MPV increased when measured by Sysmex 2000 cell counter, which employs the aperture-impedance sizing, but it decreased when measured by Technicon H*1 cell counter which is an optical flow cytometre and utilizes the principle of measuring the diffraction of a scattered light beam. It is therefore important in an analysis of data to relate changes of absolute values for MPV to the type of instrument used for platelet sizing. These findings confirmed previous observations on the measurement of MPV in blood samples [21].

Seghatchian and collegues have also shown that the ability of platelets to change the size on addition of EDTA, as measured by dMPV is related to the length of storage (Figure 6). The importance of that in-

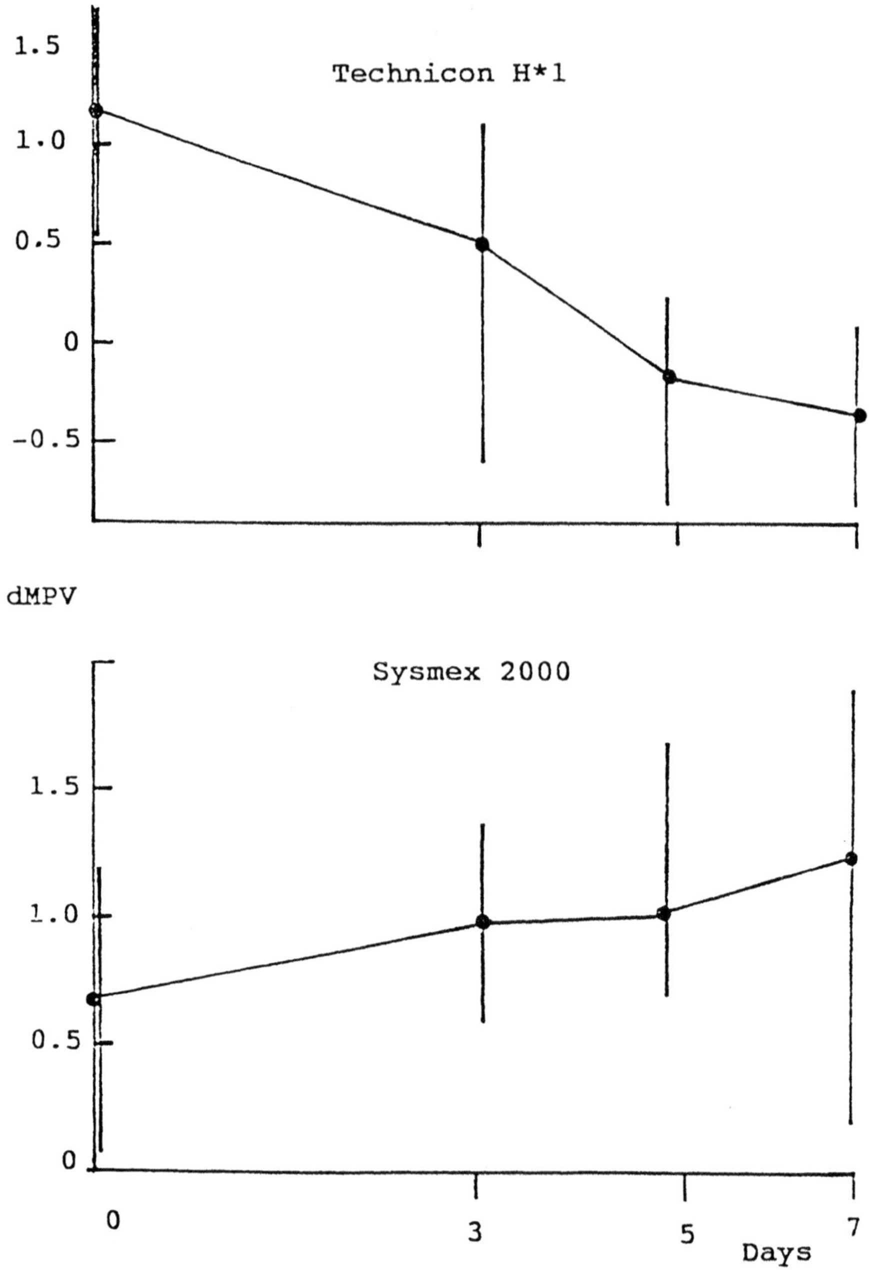

Figure 6. Effect of EDTA on mean platelet volume MPV during storage of platelet concentrates (PC) collected in ACD(A) using Autopheresis C cell separator. Values represent the mean difference between MPV measured before and after addition of EDTA (dMPV) expressed in fl, and vertical bars represent the range; n=6 for measurements with Technicon H*1 cell counter, and n=11 for measurements with Sysmex 2000 cell counter [20].

formation has become apparent when dMPV of platelets in stored PC was correlated with the results of platelet aggregation induced by ADP or ADP and collagen (Table 2). A good correlation between dMPV and the platelet response to agonists was further supported by a good correlation between dMPV and a number of tests used for measuring platelet metabolism and function: glucose consumption, lactate production and release of vWF antigen by platelets during storage of PC [22]. At present the values of MPV indicate the degree of platelet function retained by platelets during storage as well, if not better, than values obtained by any other in vitro test available.

The mechanism by which EDTA induces changes in the volume of platelets is not quite clear. Suvarov and Markosyan have suggested that EDTA increases the intracellular cyclic AMP concentration, which in turn alters the permeability of the plasma membrane of platelets [23]. Increase in intracellular fluid associated with changes in membrane permeability would cause the cell to swell. We have extended this concept to platelets in storage affected by the storage lesion: platelets with higher residual function undergo a greater shape change and have a larger increment in size – measured in the total population of platelets as dMPV. Platelets without residual function are unlikely to change the shape and size in response to addition of EDTA.

The way forward

The observation that EDTA has a capacity not only to abolish permamently aggregation but also to induce shape change of platelets suspended in citrate solutions has provided an exciting new approach for quality control of PC during storage. The complementary studies of McShine and co-workers in Groningen and Seghatchian, Vickers and Ip in London have shown how the understanding of the EDTA effect on platelets and the use of automated cell counters can be combined in developing a single test – "the system for enumeration of platelets,

Table 2. Correlation between dMPV and other variables in stored platelet concentrates (from: Seghatchian et al, 1990).

Variable correlated	**Technicon H*1 (n=6)**		**Sysmex 2000 (n=11)**	
	r	**p**	**r**	**p**
dMPV: days stored	–0.98	0.0020	0.97	0.001
dMPV: platelet count	0.96	0.0016	–0.97	0.0053
dMPV: 20 μM ADP	0.81	0.0436	–0.91	0.0091
dMPV: 10 μM ADP and 50 μM collagen	0.81	0.0414	–0.90	0.0104

pH and HSR were not significantly correlated.

measurement of platelet activity and determination of leukocyte count" (SEAL). SEAL generates accurate platelet count (and leukocyte count) and the difference between the MPV before and after addition of EDTA (dMPV) which indicate the degree of residual function of the platelet in fresh or stored PC. The replacement of plasma in PC with an artificial salt solution may provide added advantage to the use of SEAL by providing better correlation with in vivo tests used for assessing platelet viability.

SEAL has proved to be a simple, reproducible and reliable test which has already been successfully used in the authors' laboratories for a variety of purposes such as the evaluation of the procedures for preparation of PC, investigation of the platelet storage lesion and assessment of the quality of PC collected from units of blood and by cell separators. The use of SEAL to achieve high quality applications at a fast rate will become critical to success of research and development on platelet preparations in the 1990s.

References

1. De Wolf JThM. Clinical efficacy of platelet concentrates: Survival, recovery and hemostatic capacity. In: Smit Sibinga CTh, Das PC, Mannucci PM (eds). Coagulation and blood transfusion. Dordrecht: Kluwer Academic Publ., 1991:159-63.
2. Dacie JV, Lewis SM. Practical haematology. Edinburgh: Churchill Livingstone, 1991:57-8.
3. McShine RL, Das PC, Smit Sibinga CTh, Brozovic B. Differences between the effects of EDTA and citrate anticoagulants on platelet count and mean platelet volume. Clin Lab Haematol 1990;12:227-85.
4. Harker LA, Zimmerman TS (eds). Measurement of platelet function. Edinburgh: Churchill Livingstone 1983.
5. Brozovic B (ed). The role of leukocyte depletion in blood transfusion practice. Oxford: Blackwell Scientific Publications, 1989.
6. Bateson EAJ. Cryopreservation of platelets: Investigation of factors affecting recovery and function of frozen and thawed platelets. PhD thesis. London, 1988.
7. Rock G, Swenson SD, Adams GA. Platelet storage in plasma free medium. Transfusion 1985;25:551-6.
8. McShine RL, Das PC, Smit Sibinga CTh, Brozovic B. Enhancement of aggregation response in stored platelets using artificial medium. Abstract. ISBT/AABB Joint Congress, Los Angeles 1990:S545.
9. Kunicki TJ, Tucelli M, Becker GA, Aster RG. A study of variables affecting the quality of platelets stored at room temperature. Transfusion 1975;15: 414-21.
10. Holme S, Murphy S. Quantitative measurements of platelet shape by light transmission studies; application to storage of platelets for transfusion. J Lab Clin Med 1978;92:53-63.

11. Bellhouse MA, Ross I, Entwistle CC, Bellhouse BJ. Optical measurement of the viability of stored human platelets. Optics and Laser Technology 1985;Febr:27-30.
12. Kim BK, Baldini MG. The platelet response to hypotonic shock. Its value as an indicator of platelet viability after storage. Transfusion 1974;14:130-8.
13. Mannucci PM, Sharp AA. Platelet volume and shape in relation to aggregation and adhesion. Br J Haematol 1967;13:604-17.
14. Karpatkin S. Heterogeneity of human platelets. VI. Correlation of platelet function with platelet volume. Blood 1978;51:307-16.
15. Frojmovic MM, Milton JG. Human platelet size, shape, and related functions in health and disease. Physiol Rev 1982;62:185-261.
16. Martin J, Trowbridge A (eds). Platelet heterogeneity. Biology and pathology. Heidelberg: Springer-Verlag, 1990.
17. Holme S, Murphy S. Coulter counter and light transmission studies of platelets exposed to low temperature, ADP, EDTA and storage at 22°C. J Lab Clin Med 1980;96:481-93.
18. McShine RL. The organisation of techniques used for quality control of platelet concentrates within the blood transfusion service. MPhil thesis. London, 1990.
19. McShine RL, Das PC, Smit Sibinga CTh, Brozovic B. The effect of EDTA on platelet count and other platelet parameters in blood and blood components collected with CPDA-1. Vox Sang 1991;(in press).
20. Seghatchian MJ, Vickers M, Ip AHL, et al. Changes in the mean platelet volume and the quality control of platelet concentrates. Abstract. ISBT/AABB Joint Congress, Los Angeles 1990:S523.
21. Trowbridge EA, Reardon DM, Hutchinson D, Pickering C. The routine measurement of platelet volume: A comparison of light-scattering and aperture-impedance technologies. Clin Phys Physiol Meas 1985;6:221-38.
22. Tandy N, Cutts M, Brooker V, et al. Evaluation of storage characteristics of platelets collected using the Autopheresis C Plateletcell™. Abstract. ISBT/AABB Joint Congress, Los Angeles 1990:S536.
23. Suvarov AV, Markosyan RA. Some mechanisms of the effect of EDTA on platelet aggregation. Bul Exp Biol Med 1981;91:651-3.

THE PREDICTIVE VALUE OF ELISA PLATELET CROSSMATCHING FOR THE SELECTION OF PLATELET DONORS FOR ALLOIMMUNIZED PATIENTS

K. Sintnicolaas[1], W. Sizoo[2], R.L.H. Bolhuis[3]

Introduction

The development of platelet alloantibodies in multitransfused patients represents a major problem in platelet supportive therapy as 40-100% of patients with acute leukemia become alloimmunized during treatment [1,2]. Therefore, the provision of compatible platelets for alloimmunized patients is an important task for the blood transfusion service. Compatible platelet donors are usually selected based on HLA-matching between donor and recipient. Drawbacks of this approach are that 1) a large HLA-typed donor panel is required that needs continuous updating and is therefore very expensive; and 2) a significant percentage (13-31%) of HLA-matched platelet transfusions does not result in satisfactory post-transfusion platelet increments [3-6]. Another approach is to select platelet donors from the random donor population only using a platelet crossmatch test. This requires the availability of an assay for the detection of antiplatelet alloantibodies that is senstive, rapid and can be performed on preserved donor cells. The microplate platelet-ELISA meets these criteria [7]. Preliminary studies have indicated that the ELISA crossmatch allowed successful selection of compatible platelet donors from the random donor population [8]. Here, we describe our further experiences with platelet transfusions of ELISA crossmatch negative platelets into alloimmunized patients, comparing the results with those obtained from HLA-matched transfusions.

1. Blood Transfusion Service, The Dr. Daniel den Hoed Center, Rotterdam, The Netherlands
2. Department of Hematology, The Dr. Daniel den Hoed Center, Rotterdam, The Netherlands
3. Department of Immunology, The Dr. Daniel den Hoed Center, Rotterdam, The Netherlands

Materials and methods

Patients

Eighteen patients with hematological neoplasia (15 with acute leukemia and three with myelodysplastic syndrome) were studied. The sex ratio F:M was 14:4. The median age was 62 years (range 30-74). All patients were refractory to random donor platelets due to alloimmunization as indicated by the presence of antiplatelet alloantibodies in the serum. At the time the platelet transfusion there were no other factors present known to interfere with platelet increments (fever, sepsis, splenomegaly, massive bleeding, disseminated intravascular coagulation).

Platelet ELISA

For compatibility testing a microplate ELISA was used with platelets coated onto the plastic to form a solid phase as detailed elsewhere [7]. In brief, platelets were isolated from donor blood and resuspended in EDTA-PBS at 100×10^9/l. Platelets (5×10^6) were coated onto the wells of microtiter plates or strips. After washing with PBS-Tween (0.05% v/v), 50 µl of serum was added and incubated for 60 min at 37°C. After washing, 100 µl of $F(ab')_2$-fragments of goat-anti-human IgG conjugated to horseradish peroxidase diluted in PBS-Tween-BSA (4%) was added and incubated for 30 min at 37°C. Tween was added since it reduced non-specific binding of serum-IgG to the plastic. Enzymatic activity was measured using orthophenylenediamine as substrate. The reaction was stopped by adding 50 µl 4N H_2SO_4. Optical densities (O.D.) of the wells were read by an automated micro-ELISA-reader (Titertek, Multiscan MC) at 492 nm (against 620 nm, dual wavelength).

Donor selection by ELISA platelet crossmatch

Platelets from regular platelet apheresis-donors were coated onto microtiter strips. Following the addition of 200 µl of PBS-DMSO 10% the strips were frozen and stored at –70°C. When a patient developed serum alloantibodies, the patient serum was tested against a number of ABO compatible donors. Usually 15-50 donors were tested. Donors with a negative crossmatch test were used for plateletapheresis using the Haemonetics V50 I autosurge cell separator.

Donor selection by HLA-matching

HLA-matched donors were recruited either from family members, usually brothers or sisters, or from a large unrelated HLA-typed donor pool (Red Cross Blood Bank, Leiden; Department of Immunohematology, University Hospital, Leiden).

Random multiple donor platelet concentrates

Random multiple donor platelet concentrates were prepared from 6-12 units of whole blood by standard centrifugation techniques (Red Cross Blood Bank, Rotterdam).

Evaluation of platelet collection and transfusions

For evaluation of the transfusion results, a blood platelet count was done in triplicate just prior to, at one hour and at 16 hour following transfusion and the in vivo recovery of the platelets was calculated by use of the following formula:

$$\text{Recovery (\%)} = 100 \times \frac{\text{platelet increment} \times \text{blood volume}}{\text{number of platelets transfused}}$$

Blood volume (liters) was estimated to be 2.5 times body surface area (m^2) [9].

Results

Platelet crossmatching (Xm)

Platelet donors were selected from the random donor population for 18 alloimmunized patients by the ELISA platelet crossmatch. The frequency of ELISA negative donors varied from 0-50% (median 18) per patient. For two patients no donors were found. Fifty-three transfusions obtained from donors with a negative ELISA crossmatch were studied. In Figures 1 and 2 the post-transfusion platelet recoveries are shown. A satisfactory one-hour post-transfusion recovery (>20%) [8] was obtained in 40 out of 53 (75%) transfusions. In nine out of these 40 transfusions the survival of the transfused platelets was greatly reduced as indicated by a 16-hour post-transfusion platelet recovery of less than 10%. Thus, 31 out of 53 (58%) platelet transfusions with ELISA crossmatch-negative (Xm-neg) platelets into alloimmunized patients were associated with a fully successful transfusion response.

HLA-matched transfusion (Xm)

HLA-matched transfusions were administered into the same patient population, both from related (n=31) and unrelated (n=34) donors. Satisfactory one-hour post-transfusion recoveries were obtained in 28/31 (90%) and 26/34 (76%) transfusions respectively. A significant reduction in the survival of transfused platelets was observed in 1/27 (3%) and 3/32 (9%) respectively. Thus, 27/31 (87%) and 23/34 (66%) of the transfusions from HLA-matched related and unrelated donors were associated with a fully successful transfusion response.

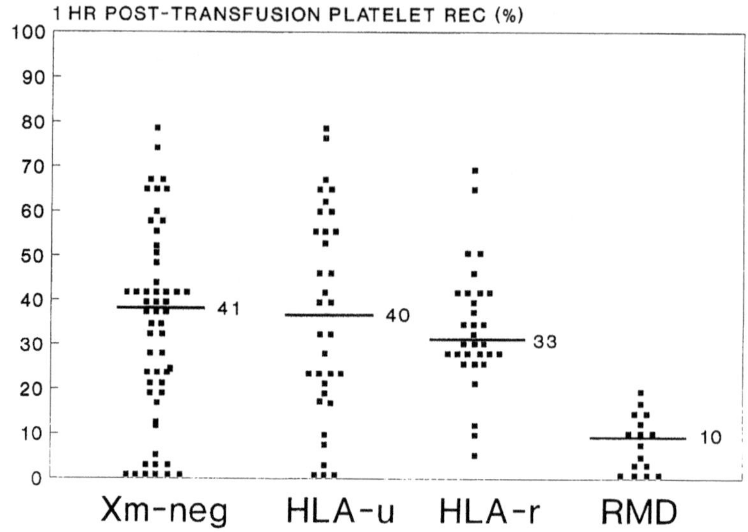

Figure 1. One hour post-transfusion platelet recoveries following the transfusion of ELISA-crossmatch negative platelets (Xm-neg), HLA-matched platelets from related donors (HLA-r), HLA-matched platelets from unrelated donors (HLA-u) and random multiple donor platelets (RMD) into alloimmunizedrecipients. Horizontal lines indicate medians.

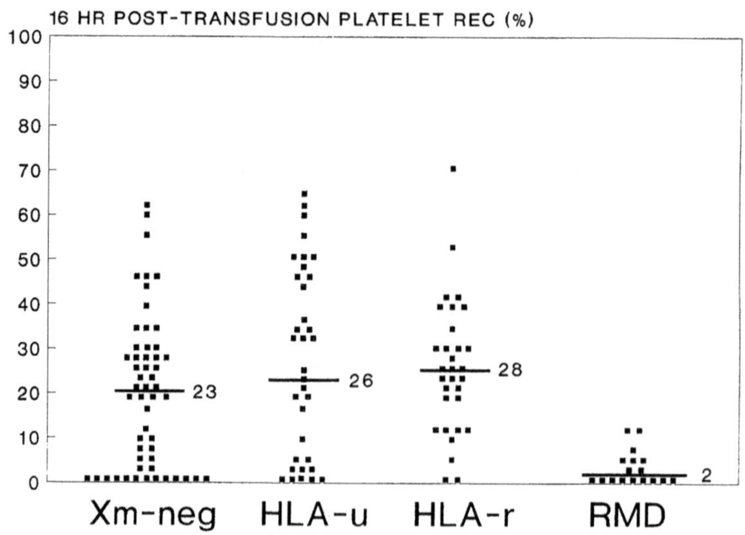

Figure 2. Sixteen hour post-transfusion platelet recoveries following the transfusion of ELISA-crossmatch negative platelets (Xm-neg), HLA-matched platelets from related donors (HLA-r), HLA-matched platelets from unrelated donors (HLA-u) and random multiple donor platelets (RMD) into alloimmunized recipients. Horizontal lines indicate medians.

Random multiple donor (RMD) platelet transfusion

Random multiple donor platelets were transfused on 15 occasions. Fourteen of the 15 (93%) transfusions were unsuccessful, confirming the refractory state of the patients.

Comparison of donor selection by ELISA platelet crossmatch and HLA-matching

There was no significant difference in both the one-hour and 16-hour post-transfusion platelet recoveries between Xm-neg and HLA-matched transfusions (Xm-neg vs HLA-related: $p=0.07$ and 0.10 for one-hour and 16-hour recoveries respectively; Xm-neg vs HLA-unrelated: $p=0.62$ and 0.16 respectively). Also, the differences between related and unrelated HLA-matched transfusions were not significantly different ($p=0.67$ and 0.76 for one-hour and 16-hour recoveries respectively). However, as expected, each donor selection method was significantly better than no selection i.e. random multiple donor platelet transfusions ($p<0.005$). P-values were calculated using the Wilcoxon ranksum test.

Analysis of transfusion failures

ELISA platelet crossmatches were repeated in 15 transfusion failures using fresh test cells. Nine corssmatches, corresponding with poor platelet recoveries at both one-hour and 16-hour post-transfusion, were all positive when repeated with fresh cells. Six crossmatches associated with platelet transfusions with initial good one-hour platelet recovery but reduced survival, were repeatedly negative.

When extrapolated, these data suggest that 13 of the 20 crossmatch failures might be prevented by improving the storage technique for the test platelets. In the group of HLA-matched transfusions, the frequency of unsuccessful transfusions was clearly related to the HLA-matching degree. The combined data for related and unrelated HLA-matched donors showed 5/55 (9%) transfusion failures when donors had no major antigen mismatches; however, when one or two major antigen mismatches existed, 7/7 (100%) of the transfusions were failures.

Discussion

Using the microplate ELISA platelet crossmatch assay [7] it was possible to screen large numbers of frozen test cells (50-100) within half a day. This makes prospective donor selection by platelet crossmatch feasible. In this study we used only the ELISA platelet crossmatch to select donors from our pool of platelet apheresis donors for alloimmunized patients. Therefore, we did not use HLA-typing as a selection criterion. A surprising finding was that for almost all (16/18 i.e. 89%) alloimmunized patients negative crossmatches were obtained.

This means that even with a small donor pool we were able to find crossmatch-negative donors. A similar observation has been made in a study where a platelet radioactive antiglobulin platelet crossmatch assay was used [11]. For optimal evaluation of the value of any platelet crossmatch assay it is essential to directly compare the test result with the transfusion outcome. Therefore we used platelets from the same donor for both test and transfusion. Thirty-one of the 53 (58%) transfusions with ELISA crossmatch negative platelets into alloimmunized patients proved fully successful. This was significantly better than transfusion results obtained with random donor platelets. Using HLA-matched donors, successful transfusions were obtained in 50/65 (77%) occasions. This also was significantly better than transfusing random donor platelets. However, still 23% of these transfusions were failures. It appeared that the degree of HLA-matching was of major importance to the transfusion outcome (Figure 3). In the absence of major HLA-antigen mismatches, only 5/55 (9%) of the transfusions failed. However, in the presence of one or two HLA-antigen mismatches all transfusions (n=7) proved failures. Thus the best platelet transfusion results were obtained using HLA-matched platelets (91% success), whereas ELISA-crossmatch negative platelets showed a 58% success

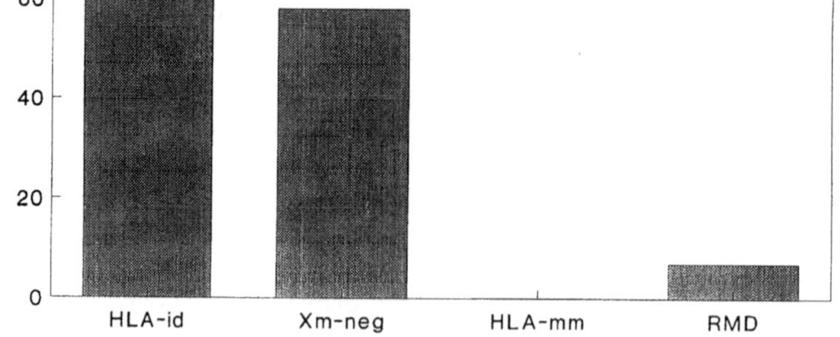

Figure 3. Percentage of successful platelet transfusions into alloimmunized patients obtained using different donor selection methods: HLA-id = HLA-matched, no major antigen mismatches; HLA-mm = HLA-mismatched, one or two major antigen mismatches; Xm-neg = negative ELISA platelet cross match; RMD = random multiple donor transfusion.

rate. The use of HLA-mismatched platelets proved no better than not selecting at all.

In order to improve donor selection by ELISA platelet crossmatch, the cryopreservation procedure of the test platelets has to be optimized. When stored cells would retain full test reactivity, it might be assumed that 13 of the 20 transfusion failures could be prevented, theoretically increasing the success rate from the actual 62% to 87%. A drawback of platelet crossmatching is that this is not applicable to alloimmunized patients without demonstrable antibodies. In this situation, HLA-matched donors remain necessary. A drawback of HLA-matching is that HLA-matched donors are not always available. In this study 9% of the transfusions could not be fully HLA-matched and resulted in transfusion failures. Here, platelet crossmatching could be advantageous over HLA-matching.

We conclude that for alloimmunized patients HLA-matched platelet donors without major HLA-antigen mismatches, are the first choice. When such donors cannot be found, platelet crossmatching is the best alternative. The use of HLA-mismatched donors did not have any advantage over random donors. As both HLA-matching and platelet crossmatching have their own advantages and disadvantages, both methods ideally should be available for optimal platelet supportive therapy.

Acknowledgements

We gratefully acknowledge Gertie Bokken and Dew Doekharan for their invaluable technical assistance and Johanna Dumon Tak-Garschagen for typing the manuscript. This work was supported by a grant from the "Josephine Nefkens Foundation".

References

1. Tejada F, Bias WB, Santos GW, Zieve PD. Immunologic response of patients with acute leukemia to platelet transfusions. Blood 1973;42:405-12.
2. Dutcher JP, Schiffer CA, Aisner J, Wiernik PH. Alloimmunization following platelet transfusion: The absence of a dose-response relationship. Blood 1981;57:395-8.
3. Duquesnoy RJ, Filip DJ, Rodey GE, Rimm AA, Aster RH. Successful transfusion of platelets "mismatched" for HLA-antigens to alloimmunized thrombocytopenic patients. Am J Hemat 1977;2:219-26.
4. Brand A, van Leeuwen A, Eernisse JG, van Rood JJ. Platelet transfusion therapy: Optimal donor selection with a combination of lymphocytotoxicity and platelet fluorescence tests. Blood 1978;51:781-8.
5. Pegels J, Bruynes E, Engelfriet C, von dem Borne AEGKr. Serological studies in patients on platelet- and granulocyte-substitution therapy. Br J Haematol 1982;52:59-68.

6. Bonacossa IA, Perchotte M-RY, Olchowecki JK, Schroeder ML. Role of lymphocytotoxicity and Staph-Protein A assays in platelet donor selection. Curr Stud Haematol Blood Transf 1986;52:58-64.
7. Sintnicolaas K, van der Steuyt KJB, van Putten WLJ, Bolhuis RLH. A microplate ELISA for the detection of platelet alloantibodies: Comparison with the platelet immunofluorescence test. Br J Haematol 1987;66:363-7.
8. Sintnicolaas K, Sizoo W, Bolhuis RLH. Prospective selection of compatible platelet donors for alloimmunized patients by an ELISA platelet crossmatch only. In: Smit Sibinga CTh, Das PC, Engelfriet CP (eds). White cells and platelets in blood transfusion. Boston, Dordrecht: Martinus Nijhoff Publishers 1987:53-7.
9. Brassine A. Le volume sanguin de l'homme normale: Recherche de formule de prediction. Rev Hémat 1949;4:481-501.
10. Van der Velden KJ, Sintnicolaas K, Löwenberg B. The value of a ^{51}Cr platelet lysis assay as crossmatch test in patients with leukemia on platelet transfusion therapy. Br J Haematol 1986;62:635-40.
11. Freedman J, Hooi C, Garvey MB. Prospective platelet crossmatching for selection of compatible random donors. Br J Haematol 1984;56:9-18.

CLINICAL EFFICACY OF PLATELET CONCENTRATES

J.Th.M. de Wolf

Clinical efficacy of platelet concentrates is related to the ability of platelet concentrates (PC) to control or prevent bleeding in thrombocytopenic patients. It has to be separated from quality.

The *quality* of PC can be evaluated by viability. measurements and platelet function tests. It is clear that good quality is a prerequisite for effectiveness.

Appropriate use refers to the use of PC in situations in which its use has been demonstrated to be effective. For instance: a patient with bone marrow failure, platelet count 50×10^9/l, template bleeding time slightly prolonged but within two times the upper limit of normal and without bleeding diathesis received a platelet transfusion. Platelet count increased from 50 to 100×10^9/l and the bleeding time was corrected completely to normal. Although the recovery was excellent and the function of the transfused platelets good, the transfusion was not effective as in this situation there was no bleeding to control or to be expected.

Quality

Accepted indicators of viability are platelet increments, the recovery, and survival after transfusion. To allow comparison between patients the recovery can be expressed in a way in which the increment of platelet count is related to the patient's size (using surface area or blood volume) and to the number of platelets given.

Platelet recovery

Corrected count increment (CCI) =

$$\frac{\text{Post-, minus pre-transfusion counts}}{\text{platelets given} \times 10^{11}} \times \text{surface area (m}^2\text{)}$$

Corrected increment (CI) =

$$\frac{\text{Post-, minus pre-transfusion counts}}{\text{units of platelets given}} \times \text{ surface area } (m^2)$$

Percentage recovery =

$$\frac{\text{Post-, minus pre-transfusion counts}}{\text{platelets given} \times 10^{11}} \times \text{ blood volume}$$

A CCI of 10; a CI of 7.5 and a percentage recovery of 30 are considered acceptable one hour post-transfusion recoveries. Although a good recovery is an indicator of viability, an unsatisfactory recovery could be related to preparation and storage but also to patient factors like sepsis, splenomegaly, bleeding or alloimmunization.

Survival

In order to be able to compare platelet survival results from different laboratories a standardized protocol was developed by the Platelet Radiolabeling Study Group [1]. Rock et al [2] compared this protocol with their previous chromium-51 method of determining platelet survival and recovery following storage in a variety of conditions.

Platelet function

In addition to viability measurements like recovery and survival, hemostatic function is also important in clinical response. The most acceptable in vivo platelet function test is the template bleeding time. Harker and Slichter [3] not only showed a direct inverse relation between the bleeding time and the platelet count, but also a predictable shortening in bleeding time when the platelet count is increased by transfusion of fresh PC.

Let us go back to clinical efficacy, the ability of PC to control or prevent bleeding.

The quantitative relation between the degree of thrombocytopenia and the risk of hemorrhage was studied by Gaydos et al [4] in patients with acute leukemia; 92 patients with acute leukemia had been followed throughout the entire clinical course of their disease (85 till death; six were still alive at the end of the study; one was lost to follow-up study). The days that a given patient spent in a certain platelet category were recorded (platelet categories: <0.5, 1-3, 3-5, 5-10, 10-20, 20-50, 50-100 and >100 × 10^9/l), as well as all hemorrhagic manifestations. A progressive increase in frequency of all kinds of hemorrhage was observed as the platelet count decreased. If only major bleedings as gross hematuria, melena and hematemesis were considered, gross hemorrhage rarely occurred at levels over 20×10^9/l. Especially a platelet count below 5×10^9/l was associated with an increase in serious bleeding episodes. In 16 of the 92 patients fatal intracranial hemorrhage occurred; eight of these 16 were associated with blast crisis, where at autopsy intracerebral leukostasis and leukemic nodules were found. In the remaining eight patients only one patient had a platelet level over 5.0×10^9/l and non exceeded 10×10^9/l.

Slichter and Harker [5] studied the relation between the degree of thrombocytopenia and bleeding by measuring faecal blood loss in aplastic thrombocytopenic patients. Their red cells were labeled with ^{51}Cr and stools were collected for 1-2 weeks. In patients with platelet counts greater than 10×10^9/l stool blood loss was less than 5 ml/day, not different from normals. At levels between 5 and 10×10^9/l blood loss was slightly increased: 9 ± 7 ml/day. Platelet counts less than 5×10^9/l were associated with markedly elevated blood loss (50 ± 20 ml/day). Prednisone and penicillines could markedly increase gastrointestinal blood loss.

These studies showed the relation between the degree of thrombocytopenia and the risk of bleeding; but, are platelet transfusions capable of controlling bleeding in these thrombocytopenic patients?

Most of the studies concerning this subject used the same criteria for evaluation of the hemostatic effects of platelet transfusion, namely: arrest of hematuria was considered due to the transfusion if clearing of the urine occurred not later than two consecutive urine specimens after the transfusion; effects on epistaxis and gum bleeding within 60 minutes after transfusion; arrest of hematemesis was associated with the transfusion when bleeding did not recur at least within 24 hours; melena was considered arrested when normal stools were passed within 48 hours. In 1959 Freireich et al [6] conducted a randomized double blind trial. Bleeding thrombocytopenic acute leukemia patients were treated either with socalled bank blood, stored for 2-9 days before being used, or with fresh whole blood anticoagulated with EDTA; nine patients were treated for 28 bleeding periods. Each pateint was his own control. In 9/14 bleeding episodes fresh blood transfusions were effective in controlling hemorrhage compared to 2/14 treated with stored bank blood. In 1963 Freireich et al [7] published the results of the treatment of 28 thrombocytopenic acute leukemia patients; 51 out of 57 hemorrhagic episodes were arrested by the transfusion of single donor platelet rich plasma. Alvarado et al [8] treated 19 thrombocytopenic acute leukemia patients with fresh PC from multiple donors. In 15 cases the hemorrhages, including epistaxis, hematuria, melena and hematemesis were arrested by the transfusions. Furthermore it was noticed that the likelyhood of controlling bleeding was related to the post transfusion platelet increment. The higher the increment the higher the number of arrested bleedings. Van Eys et al [9] reported only 40% control of thrombocytopenic bleeding episodes by transfusion of PC. The primary factor precluding good recovery and control of bleeding was the number of previously administered platelet transfusions, which probably determined the occurence of alloimmunization: more prior transfusions, less adequate recovery and control of bleeding.

In summary we can conclude that platelets are effective in controlling bleeding in the thrombocytopenic patient.

Are prophylactic platelet transfusions effective?

Indications for the succesful use of prophylactic platelet transfusions in the prevention of bleeding episodes and thereby of mortality comes from retrospective studies. For instance Roy et al [10] compared the incidence of bleeding episodes during the prophylactic use of PC with the incidence in periods in which patients were not prophylactically transfused. The differences were highly significant.

However there are only a few prospective randomized trials which evaluated the effectiveness of prophylactic platelet transfusion [11-13]. Most of these studies showed a significant decrease in the occurrence of bleeding episodes in the patients with prophylactic platelet transfusions, but no study has shown that death can be prevented. The largest and most extensively published study is the one from Murphy et al [13] which shall be discussed in more detail; 66 patients with acute lymphoblastic and nonlymphoblastic leukemia entered the study. The prophylactic group received platelets when the platelet count dropped below 20; the therapeutic group received platelets when thrombocytopenia was associated with uncontrolled epistaxis, gross gastrointestinal or genitourinary bleeding, central nervous system or any other life-threatening bleeding episode.

Prophylactic platelet transfusion delayed the time to the first episode of bleeding, as well as the number of bleeding episodes, especially in the first year of randomization. During the entire study period there were significantly fewer bleeds per 100 patients months in the prophylactic group: 1.9 compared to 7.9 in the therapeutic group. Separate analysis of the ALL and AnonLL groups gives the same results. During the last month of life bleeding episodes were significantly longer and often unresponsive to random platelet transfusion in the prophylactic group probably caused by immunologic refractoriness. It must be noticed that HLA-matched platelets were not available for these patients at that time. This is probably the reason why in the entire study period, despite a significantly reduced number of bleeds in the prophylactic group, the total number of days of bleeding did not differ in the two groups. There was no difference in survival between the two groups, suggesting that bleeding episodes in patients who do not receiveplatelets prophylactically can be treated very well with PC without influencing survival.

Summary

If the purpose of prophylactic platelet transfusion is reduction of bleeding, we can conclude that prophylactic platelet transfusion is effective. However if we try to lower mortality with prophylactic platelet transfusion, effectiveness has not been shown.

References

1. Snijder EL, Morroff G, Heaton A, and members of the Ad Hoc Platelet Radiolabeling Study Group. Recommended methods for conducting radiolabeled platelet survival studies. Transfusion;1986:26.37-42
2. Rock G, Tittley P. A comparison of results obtained by two different chromium-51 methods of determining platelet survival and recovery. Transfusion 1990;30:407-10.
3. Harker LA, Slichter SJ. The bleeding time as a screening test for evaluation of platelet function. N Engl J Med 1972;287:155-9.
4. Gaydos LA, Freireich EJ, Mantel N. The quantitative relation between platelet count and hemorrhage in patients with acute leukemia. N Engl J Med 1962;266:905-9.
5. Slichter SJ, Harker LA. Thrombocytopenia: Mechanism and management of defects in platelet production. Clin Haematol 1978;7:523-39.
6. Freireich EJ, Schmidt PJ, Schneiderman MA, Frei E. A comparative study of the effect of transfusion of fresh and preserved whole blood on bleeding in patients with acute leukemia. N Engl J Med 1959;260:6-11.
7. Freireich EJ, Kliman A, Gaydos LA, Mantel N, Frei EA. Response to repeated platelet transfusion from the same donor. Ann Int Med 1963;59: 277-87.
8. Alvarado J, Djerassi I, Farber S. Transfusion of fresh concentrated platelets to children with acute leukemia. J Pediatr 1965;67:13-22.
9. Van Eys J, Thomas D, Olivos B. Platelet use in pediatric oncology: A review of 393 transfusions. Transfusion 1978;18:169-73.
10. Roy AJ, Jaffe N, Djerassi I. Prophylactic platelet transfusion in children with acute leukemia: A dose response study. Transfusion 1973;13:283-90.
11. Higby DJ, Cohen E, Holland JF, Sinks L. The prophylactic treatment of thrombocytopenic leukemic patients with platelets: A double blind study. Transfusion 1974;14:440-6.
12. Solomon J, Bofenkamp T, Fahey JL, Chillar RK, Beutler E. Platelet profylaxis in acute non-lymphoblastic leukemia. Lancet 1978;i:267.
13. Murphy S, Litwin S, Herring LM, et al. Indications for platelet transfusion in children with acute leukemia. Am J Hematol 1982;12:347-56.

PRINCIPLES OF COAGULATION FACTOR ASSAYS

A.M.H.P. van den Besselaar

Introduction

Coagulation factor assays are most commonly performed by a one-stage procedure, using a modified tissue thromboplastin time (extrinsic coagulation pathway) or activated partial thromboplastin time (intrinsic pathway). In these bio-assays, the concentration of the factor to be assayed is made rate limiting in an otherwise competent system utilizing clot formation as its end point. The determination of factor VIII coagulation activity (FVIII:C) is one of the most common specific coagulation factor assays performed in Europe and in the United States [1]. Although both one-stage and two-stage coagulation assays are used, the one-stage procedure seems more popular. The methodology of the two-stage assay of FVIII:C has been treated in detail elsewhere [2]. In the present paper, the basic principles of the one-stage coagulation factor assays will be illustrated by the FVIII:C assay.

Statistical methods have been developed to enable the assessment of the validity of the bio-assay, as well as an estimation of the relative potencies of the preparations with some indication of the precision of each estimate [3,4]. Design of a bio-assay is essential for a reliable result. Furthermore, reproducibility can be enhanced through appropriate choice of reagents and instruments.

For many coagulation factors and inhibitors specific chromogenic or fluorogenic substrate methods are commercially available or are being developed. The advantage of this type of assay is that it does not require deficient plasmas and can be easily automated.

Basic principles

A coagulation factor assay is based on the determination of the relationship between the concentration of the factor and the resultant clotting time, other reagent concentrations being kept constant. The fundamental requirement for two preparations to be comparable is that they should behave as if one (the weaker) were a simple dilution of the

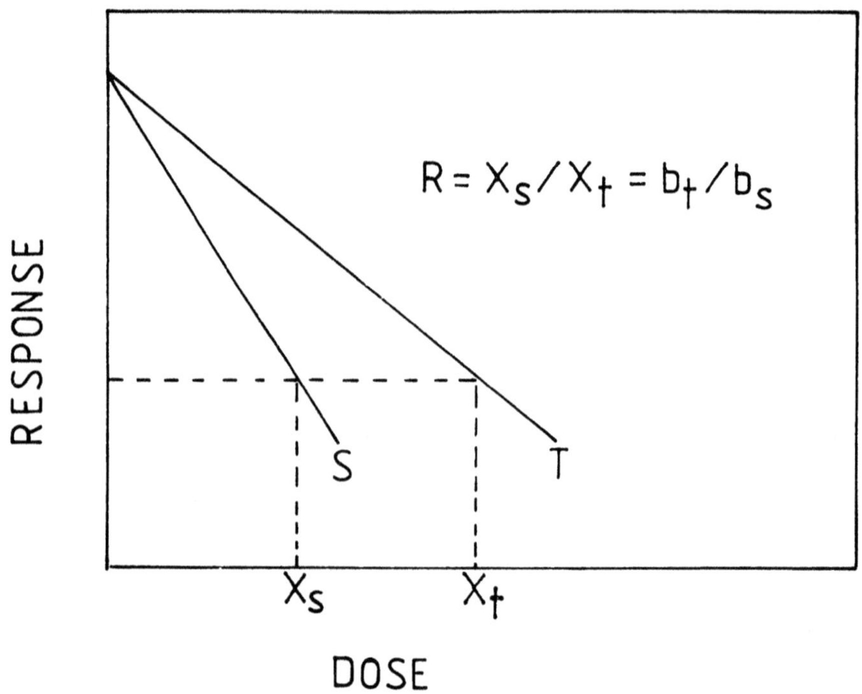

Figure 1. Slope ratio assay. Response (Y) is plotted as a function of dose (X) for both standard (S) and test (T) preparation. The potency ratio (R) can be obtained from the slopes b_t and b_s of the lines for test and standard preparation, respectively.

other (the stronger). If this is the case, then the concentration-clotting time relationships should be identical apart from an adjustment for the concentration ratio, or potency ratio, between them.

Estimation of the potency ratio is simplified if the relationships in a dose-response plot are linear. There are two established models for analyzing the data: the slope ratio assay and the parallel line assay.

In the slope ratio assay (Figure 1), the potency ratio (R) is estimated from the ratio of equivalent doses (X_s/X_t) which equals the ratio of the slopes (b_t/b_s) of the dose-response relations. The slope ratio assay requires linear dose-response relations and is useful for evaluation of chromogenic substrate assays.

In the parallel line assay (Figure 2), the potency ratio (R) is estimated from the horizontal distance (M) between the parallel log dose – (log) response relations of test (T) and standard (S) preparations. The parallel line assay requires linear dose-response relation after log/lin or log/log transformation. It is useful for evaluation of coagulation assays and for many chromogenic substrate assays.

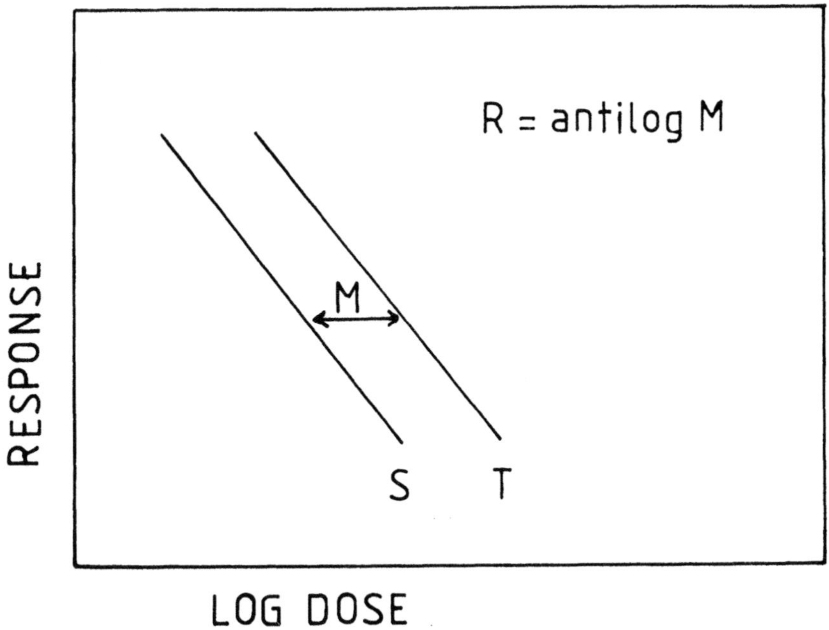

Figure 2. Parallel line assay. Response is plotted as a function of log dose for both standard (S) and test (T) preparation. The potency ratio (R) can be obtained from the horiontal distance (M) between the lines for test and standard preparation.

For both the slope ratio and parallel line assay, an analysis of variance provides a check of validity and confidence limits of the potency estimate.

Assay design

Many components of coagulation assay systems are labile and no preparation can be relied upon to give the same mean response or assay slope from one assay to another. It is, therefore, essential that each assay includes a fresh sample of a suitable standard preparation. In this way, the potency estimate for the test preparation will be largely independent of variation in reagents and instruments between assays.

The linearity of the dose-response relationship can only be checked if there are at least three dose levels (dilutions).

In all cases it is important that the responses of each test sample are in the same range as those of the standard to avoid the need for extrapolation. For a proper analysis of variance (see next section) we need some measure of the extent of deviations which could reasonably be attributable to random variation. This can be achieved by independently replicating the doses of at least one of the preparations tested (usually the standard). The differences between the replicate responses represent the magnitude of the cumulative error from all of the experimental steps which are independently replicated.

If replicate samples of one of the preparations are tested at the beginning and at the end of each assay, then any consistent difference between replicate responses is an indication of temporal drift. In order to eliminate the effect of a linear time trend, for the purpose of potency estimation, replicate samples should be tested in balanced temporal order. Table 1 shows the raw data from an assay, carried out in the author's laboratory, following a design incorporating most of the points outlined above. A graphical representation of the data is given in Figure 3.

An alternative way of minimizing the effect of temporal drift is to perform all clotting time assessments more or less at the same time. This requires the availability of an instrument (or an array of instruments) with multiple measuring chambers [5].

Table 1. Example of a balanced one-stage factor VIII:C assay design of one test preparation (T) against a standard (S). Order of testing runs from top to bottom. The test preparation was a cryoprecipitate and the standard was a pooled normal plasma.

Preparation	Dilution	Clotting time (s)
S	1/5	46.4
	1/10	51.7
	1/20	61.2
	1/40	70.5
	1/80	78.4
	1/160	87.8
T	1/5	36.3
	1/10	39.3
	1/20	46.9
	1/40	53.9
	1/80	62.7
	1/160	71.1
T	1/5	37.8
	1/10	42.3
	1/20	49.2
	1/40	57.5
	1/80	65.4
	1/160	72.0
T	1/5	46.4
	1/10	54.5
	1/20	64.0
	1/40	73.6
	1/80	84.2
	1/160	91.8

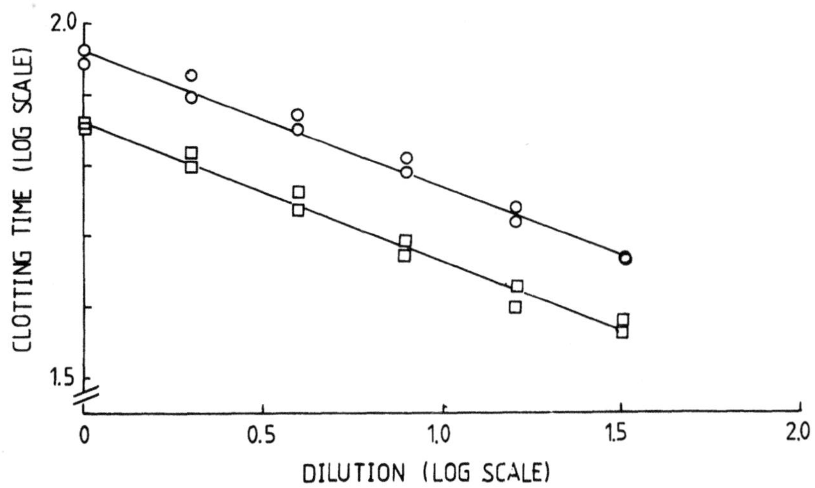

Figure 3. Parallel line assay of factor VIII:C activity. The data in Table 1 are plotted, using $\log_{10}$ clotting time as the response metameter. The lines were calculated with linear regression analysis.

Analysis of variance

The standard procedure for assessing the statistical significance of deviations from parallelism or linearity is analysis of variance [3,4], in which these deviations are expressed as variance ratios relative to the estimated random error. Table 2 shows an analysis of variance of the parallel line assay data in Table 1. In brief, the analysis of variance partitions the total variation or sum of squares (S.S. total), calculated among all clotting times, into distinct and independent components,

Table 2. Analysis of variance table for the data in Table 1, using $\log_{10}$ clotting time as the response metameter.

Source of variation	**S.S.**	**D.F.**	**M.S.**	**F-ratio**	**P**
Preparations	0.06839	1	0.06839	302	<0.001
Regression	0.24356	1	0.24356	1077	<0.001
Non-parallelism	0.00001	1	0.00001	0.06	N.S.
Non-linearity (S)	0.00072	4	0.00018	0.80	N.S.
Non-linearity (T)	0.00050	4	0.00012	0.55	N.S.
Residual error	0.00271	12	0.00023		
Total	0.31588	23			

S.S. = Sum of squares
D.F. = Degrees of freedom
M.S. = Mean square

each of which is attributable to one of the sources listed at the left. Associated with each source is a number of degrees of freedom (D.F.). The fourth column of mean squares (M.S.) is the amount of variation per degree of freedom, i.e. S.S. divided by D.F. If there were no true effect to a particular source, the mean square for that source would be roughly the same as that for the residual error, M.S. (error). Otherwise, the mean square would be greater than M.S. (error).

The fifth column, headed F-ratio, gives the value obtained by dividing the mean square for each non-error source by M.S. (error). An F-ratio around unity implies no effect due to that source, while a large F-ratio implies a large effect. Due to chance, a certain amount of randomness is to be expected in each of the F-ratios, so the statistical significance of any particular value may only be determined by reference to statistical tables.

The important determinants of assay validity are the F-ratios for "non-parallelism" and "curvature", which should not be significant. Also important is the F-ratio for "regression", which must be significant, and preferably highly so; otherwise, the assay is useless since the clotting time does not change significantly with dilution and, therefore, cannot provide a basis for relating the potency of one preparation to another. The F-ratio for "preparations" is a useful indicator of the quality of choice of relative dilution ranges for the different preparations, though its level of statistical significance is unimportant. In a well-planned assay, the "preparations" F-ratio should be small, indicating good overlap of the ranges of clotting times.

As described in a previous section (basic principles), the potency ratio of a test preparation T relative to a standard S, is estimated from the horizontal distance between the two fitted regression lines. The estimated horizontal distance M is given by the equation

$$M = X_s - X_t - (Y_s - Y_t)/b$$

in which X_s and X_t are the mean log doses for S and T, respectively, Y_s and Y_t the mean responses for S and T, respectively, and b is the common slope of the fitted parallel regression lines. The potency ratio R is calculated as R = antilog M (Figure 2).

The confidence limits of M are derived from the residual error mean square in the analysis of variance table, and are essentially a conversion of the errors in the response into a corresponding uncertainty in the potency estimate [3,4].

Variables in coagulation factor assays

Substrate plasma

The substrate plasma is usually obtained from a patient with a hereditary deficiency of the factor being measured. Although such plasmas are now generally available from commercial sources, there may be problems with plasma obtained from patients with hereditary deficiencies of the various coagulation factors. These problems include poor availability due to frequent transfusion or rarity of the disorder, risk of infectious disease, poor characterization of the hereditary defect, and variable performance in factor assays.

It is possible to prepare deficient plasmas by specific removal of the relevant coagulation factor with immuno-affinity procedures. A clear advantage of the use of immune-depleted plasmas as substrate plasmas, is that these, in general, ar better defined than the congenital-deficiency plasma. It has been well established that many patients with a hereditary coagulation defect have a functionally defective molecule rather than a true molecular deficiency. This seems to be true especially for factor VIII and factor IX deficiencies [6,7]. For most of the commercially available congenital-deficiency plasmas it is not known whether there is an abnormal molecule present or not and, if so, to what extent this abnormal molecule might interfere with the assay of the normal coagulation factor due to competition between normal and abnormal proteins, as for instance described for factor IX-Bm and factor X in the ox-brain thromboplastin time [8]. Finally it is important to check whether the selected deficient plasma is sufficiently stable (especially after reconstitution) for efficient use in daily practice, and whether batch-to-batch variation is acceptably low.

Dilution medium

Dilutions of standard and test samples are made with buffer solutions that do not bind Ca^{2+}-ions, like barbital, barbital-acetate, imidazole, Tris, etc. NaCl may be added for providing physiological ionic strength. Since both the standard and test samples usually contain similar citrate concentrations, and the clotting assay is started with an excess of Ca^{2+}-ions, the final citrate concentration in the diluted samples is not expected to affect the results of the assay to a great extent.

Concentrated standards and test materials are usually diluted to concentrations similar to those present in 1:10 or more diluted plasma [9]. Non-parallelism is frequently observed when the unknown sample and the calibration plasma are unlike materials. In such a situation one can either use a different standard or make an initial dilution of the concentrate in a plasma deficient of the relevant factor [10,11].

Reagents

For the assays of intrinsic coagulation factors (XII, XI, IX, VIII, V, X, II, prekallikrein and high molecular weight kininogen) a modified activated partial thromboplastin time (APTT) is used. An APTT reagent consists of an activator of factor XII such as kaolin, ellagic acid or micronized silica, and a phospholipid component. A wide variety of commercial APTT reagents with different sensitivity and responsiveness are available. The responsiveness (slope of the dose-response curve) and precision are influenced by the reagent [1]. Furthermore, differences in assay precision were noted between various instrument-reagent combinations [1].

For the assay of the extrinsic coagulation factors (factors II, V, VII and X) a large number of thromboplastin preparations are commercially available. Some of these thromboplastins contain $CaCl_2$ and therefore it should be checked whether such a thromboplastin will comply with the assay design (especially important for automated instruments). Secondly, it should be checked whether the thromboplastin preparation is sufficiently stable for practical use (especially lyophilized preparations requiring reconstitution). Finally, special attention should be given to its application in the factor VII assay. As the thromboplastin-factor VII complex is the rate-limiting factor in determining the actual clotting time in this assay, it is important that the thromboplastin itself does not contain factor VII, as this will result in low sensitivity and less steep calibration curves. Further, it is important to check the interaction between the thromboplastin and the factor VII-deficient plasma, especially if a congenital deficiency plasma has been selected. Brandt et al [12] demonstrated that the residual factor VII activity in this type of plasma largely varies with the type of thromboplastin used. On one hand this is due to the specificity of the thromboplastin-factor VII interaction, on the other hand this might be related to abnormalities in the variant factor VII of the patient, which are only detected with certain types of thromboplastin.

The different types of thromboplastin also differ in their ability to measure native and activated factor VII. This may result in apparently discrepant results when changing from one type of thromboplastin to another.

Chromogenic methods

For many of the coagulation factors and inhibitors specific chromogenic methods are commercially available or are being developed. The advantage of this type of assay is that it does not require deficient plasmas and can be easily automated. In most cases these assays are offered to the laboratory as complete kits; this has the obvious advantage of constant quality of the reagents. On the other hand, it is not always easy to modify the complicated design of the assay for use in a particular instrument. Moreover, different results might be obtained for the same patient samples when using kits from different manufacturers. This might be due to different sources and/or concentrations of the specific activators or enzymes used, but it also might be related to the use of different chromogenic substrates (different specificities). In conclusion, it is important to introduce chromogenic coagulation factor assays in the laboratory only after careful analysis of both the specificity and sensitivity of the various methods available [13].

Acknowledgements

The author is indebted to Mrs. J. Meeuwisse-Braun for skilfull technical assistance, and to Mrs. E.W.H. Vletter-Imanse for careful preparation of the typescript.

References

1. Brandt JT, Triplett DA, Musgrave K, et al. Factor VIII assays. Assessment of variables. Arch Pathol Lab Med 1988;112:7-12.
2. Barrowcliffe TW. Methodology of the two-stage assay of factor VIII (VIII:C). Scand J Haematol 1984;33(Suppl.41):25-38.
3. Kirkwood TBL, Snape TJ. Biometric principles in clotting and clot lysis assays. Clin Lab Haemat 1980;2:155-167.
4. Curtis AD. The statistical evaluation of factor VIII clotting assays. Scand J Haematol 1984;33(Suppl.41):55-68.
5. Veltkamp JJ, Drion EF, Loeliger EA. Detection of the carrier state in hereditary coagulation disorders. I. Thrombos Diathes Haemorrh 1968;19:279-303.
6. Bertina RM, Veltkamp JJ. The abnormal factor IX of hemophilia B^+ variants. Thromb Haemostas 1978;40:335-49.
7. Triplett DA, Brandt JT, Fair DS, et al. Factor VII deficiency: Heterogeneity defined by combined functional and immunochemical analysis. Blood 1985;66:1284-7.
8. Østerud B, Kasper CK, Lavine KK, et al. Purification and properties of an abnormal blood coagulation factor IX (factor IX-Bm)/kinetics of its inhibition of factor X activation by factor VII and bovine tissue factor. Thromb Haemostas 1981;45:55-9.
9. Over J. Quality control of the one-stage factor VIII (VIII:C) assay in the coagulation laboratory. Scand J Haematol 1984;33(Suppl.41):89-100.
10. Barrowcliffe TW, Tydeman MS, Kirkwood TBL. Major effect of prediluent in factor IX clotting assay. Lancet 1979;ii:192.
11. Over J. Methodology of the one-stage assay of factor VIII (VIII:C). Scand J Haematol 1984;33(Suppl.41):13-24.
12. Brandt JT, Triplett DA, Fair DS. Characterization and comparison of immunodepleted and hereditary factor VII deficient plasmas as substrate plasmas for factor VII assays. Am J Clin Pathol 1986;85:583-9.

13. Pabinger I, Kyrle PA, Speiser W, et al. Diagnosis of protein C deficiency in patients on oral anticoagulant treatment: Comparison of three different functional protein C assays. Thromb Haemostas 1990;63:407-12.

STANDARDIZATION OF CLOTTING FACTOR ASSAYS

T.W. Barrowcliffe

Introduction

In the blood transfusion field, assays of clotting factors are carried out for three main purposes:

1. to measure the clotting factor content of plasma used either directly for transfusion or as source material for fractionation;
2. for assay of therapeutic concentrates;
3. For assessment of the results of transfusion of concentrates in recipients' plasma.

The development of therapeutic concentrates as worldwide articles of commerce in the 1970's emphasized the need for standardization of these assays, particularly of factor VIII, which is priced by the unit. Standardization is also important for clinical purposes, so that a statement such as "a hemostatic effect was associated with a rise in factor VIII of 30%" can have the same meaning in different laboratories, perhaps performing different assay methods.

Standardization of assays should not be interpreted, as it sometimes is, to mean that all laboratories should follow exactly the same assay procedure with the same reagents. Even with such a simple test as the prothrombin time this has proved impossible on a worldwide basis. The aim of standardization is to define the minimum procedures necessary to achieve good agreement between different laboratories and different methods, with the emphasis on the use of appropriate reference standards.

In this article the progress made in international standardization of clotting factor assays in the last 20 years will be reviewed, and some recent problems associated with the development of high-purity concentrates described.

General principles of biological standardization

Standardization of clotting factor assays in the last 20 years has followed certain basic precepts which were established for other biological substances such as insulin some years before. Three of the most important principles are as follows:

1. *Establishment of stable reference standards.* The almost universal practice of defining the unit of activity for each clotting factor as the amount in "fresh normal plasma" has proved quite inadequate in practice to effect standardization, particularly in assays of therapeutic concentrates. International standards provide stable reference preparations against which local and commercial standards can be calibrated, and have now been established for all the major clotting factors.
2. *Live vs like.* This is an important principle in choosing the appropriate standard for any particular test sample. In practice the samples assayed fall into two main types; plasma and concentrates, and it has been found necessary to establish separate plasma and concentrate standards for most of the clotting factors. However differences in composition, e.g. between different types of concentrates, may give rise to discrepancies because of the non-specificity of some assay methods.
3. *Potency should be independent of the method used.* This ideal is not always easy to achieve in practice. As already mentioned, assay methods may respond differently to differences in composition between standard and test preparations, and a difficult choice may then have to be made as to the clinical relevance of the various methods.

International standards for factor VIII and factor IX

The original definition of the unit of biological activity for both factor VIII and factor IX was the activity present in 1 ml of fresh normal plasma. The main difficulty with this definition is the large variation of factor VIII and factor IX in the normal population. Table 1 shows the range of values of these factors in normal pools of at least 15 donors.

Table 1. Factor VIII and factor IX content of normal pools.

	Number of laboratories	Range of values iu/ml
Factor VIII	21	0.73–1.35
Factor IX	23	0.82–1.37

Data from international collaborative studies [1,2]. Pools in each laboratory are from at least 15 donors.

The development of factor VIII concentrates as articles of commerce in the late 1960's accelerated the need for a stable reference preparation against which these products could be compared, and the 1st International Standard for factor VIII concentrate was established in 1971 [1,2]. Since then the standard has been replaced at regular intervals, and all manufacturers of factor VIII concentrates around the world have used these standards directly or indirectly to calibrate their materials.

Similarly, a factor IX concentrate international standard (IS) was established in 1976 [3,4], and was replaced by the 2nd IS in 1987 [5,6].

For assays of plasma samples laboratories use either national plasma standards where available, commercial plasma standards, or local plasma pools. Calibration of these plasma standards against the IS for factor VIII concentrate was found to give large discrepancies between laboratories and between assay methods [7,8]. Therefore it was decided to establish a plasma standard for factor VIII to co-exist with the concentrate standard. This reference plasma was established in 1982, and calibrated for the other factor VIII-related activities as well as factor VIII:C (FVIII:C), i.e. factor VIII:Ag, and von Willebrand factor (vWF) activity and antigen [9]; it has recently been replaced by the 2nd IS for factor VIII and vWF in plasma. Similar considerations led to the establishment in 1987 of a plasma IS for factor IX; this plasma was also calibrated for the other prothrombin complex factors, II, VII, and X.

Table 2 summarizes the various plasma and concentrate international standards which have been established for factor VIII and factor IX.

Table 2. International standards for factor VIII and factor IX.

	Factor VIII		**Factor IX**	
Concentrates	1st IS	1971	1st IS	1974
	2nd IS	1978	2nd IS	1987
	3rd IS	1983		
	4th IS	1989		
Plasmas	1st IRP	1983	1st IS	1987
	2nd IS	1989		

International standards for other clotting factors

The availability of international standards for other clotting factors is summarized in Table 3. As for factor VIII and factor IX, it has been found useful to establish separate plasma and concentrate standards where therapeutic concentrates exist.

Table 3. Plasma and concentrate international standards.

	Standards available	
Factor VIII	plasma	concentrate
Von Willebrand factor	plasma	–
Factor IX	plasma	concentrate
Factor II	plasma	concentrate
Factor VII	plasma	–
Factor X	plasma	concentrate
Protein C	plasma	–
ATIII	plasma	concentrate

Prothrombin complex factors

When the IS for factor IX concentrate was replaced, opportunity was taken to calibrate the new concentrate, 84/681, for its content of factor II and factor X. This concentrate has low content of factor VII activity, and a separate factor VII concentrate was investigated, but found unsuitable as a standard because of extremely high variability of assays. Activated factor VII is now being used for treatment of hemophiliacs with factor VIII antibodies, and a standard for this material is currently under development.

In the collaborative study on factor II, factor VII, factor IX and factor X, a freeze-dried plasma was used to check laboratories' normal pools. The differences between pools, though less than those for factor VIII, were still considerable, and therefore this plasma, 84/665, was established as the international standard for factor II, factor VII, factor IX and factor X in plasma [5,6].

Protein C

Protein C measurements are mainly carried out on patients and family members with a history of thrombosis, and an international standard was established to overcome the variability of local pools [10]. When this plasma standard, 86/622, was calibrated against fresh normal plasma, there was good agreement between four types of biological activity methods, and between activity and antigen assays [10]. Since protein C concentrates are not available for therapeutic use, a separate concentrate standard has not been established.

Antithrombin III

In addition to assays of patients' plasma, assays are also done on concentrates which are available as replacement therapy. The 1st International Reference Preparation, plasma 72/1 was established in 1980 [11], and at this time concentrates were unsuitable as standards because of high assay variability and poor stability. Since then there have been improvements in production methods for ATIII concentrates, and

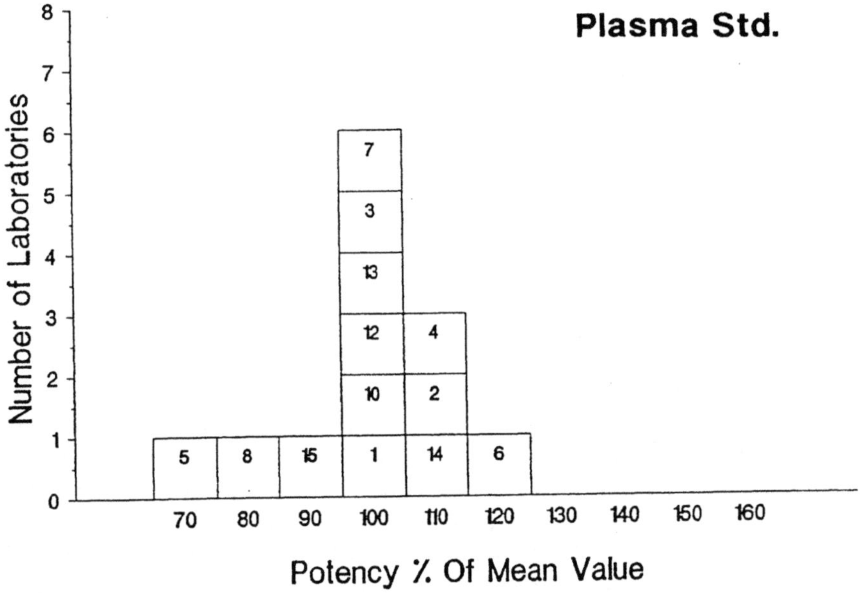

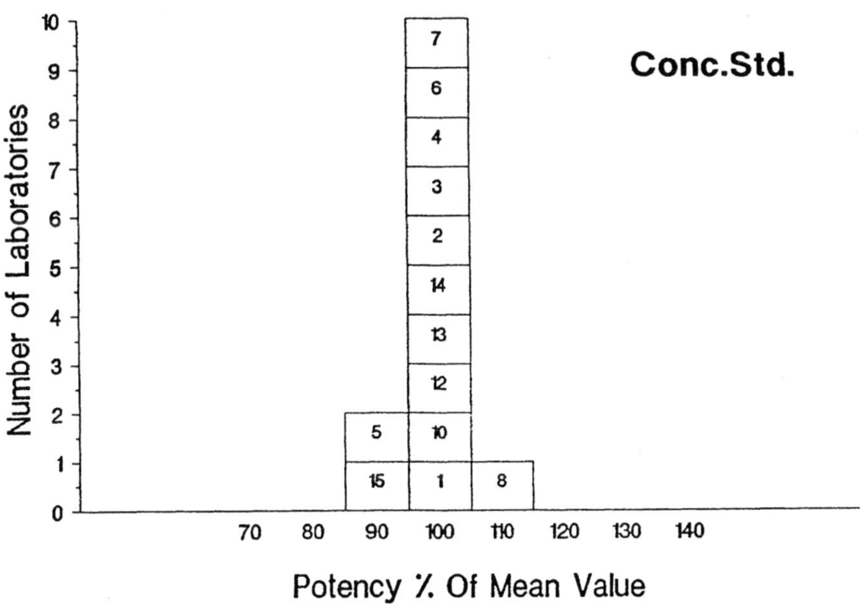

Figure 1. Comparison of inter-laboratory variability of ATIII assays (heparin co-factor activity) on concentrate C with plasma P or concentrate A as standards. Data from international collaborative study (NIBSC unpublished report).

a collaborative study was recently organized with the aim of establishing a separate concentrate standard. In this study there was good agreement between the various assay methods when the concentrates were assayed against the existing plasma standard, but, as illustrated in Figure 1, a clear improvement in inter-laboratory agreement when the plasma standard was replaced by a concentrate standard. This is another demonstration of the importance of the "like vs like" principle. Concentrate 88/548 has now been established by WHO as the international standard for ATIII concentrate.

Variability between laboratories

It must be stressed that the degree of variability between laboratories depends very much on the type of sample being assayed and its similarity to the standard being used. Thus for concentrates it has been established in many studies that variability is less when compared to a concentrate standard than when a plasma standard is used [5,11,12] – this is illustrated in Table 4 for factor VIII, factor IX and ATIII. The development of new purification methods for concentrates, including monoclonal antibody purification from both plasma and rDNA sources, has meant that some concentrates may differ in composition from the concentrate standards used. In this case, inter-laboratory variability may be considerably greater than that shown in Table 4, as discussed in a subsequent section.

Table 4. Inter-laboratory variability in collaborative studies of factor VIII, factor IX and ATIII.

	Variability, gcv%	
	C vs P	**C vs C**
Factor VIII	17.1	3.5
Factor IX	22.7	8.9
ATIII	16.0	4.1

gcv = geometric coefficient of variation

Pre-dilution of concentrates

Another factor which may affect variability between laboratories is the method of pre-dilution. It was shown by Lee et al. [13] that pre-dilution of intermediate purity factor VIII concentrates in hemophilic plasma increased their potency by approximately 25%, compared to the same concentrate pre-diluted in buffer only. A similar phenomenon was found for factor IX in the international collaborate study [5]. Therefore if concentrates are assayed in clinical laboratories against plasma standards, it is essential to pre-dilute the concentrates in the appropriate deficient plasma in order to obtain the correct potency.

Since both plasma and concentrate international standards are available for factor VIII and factor IX, it was necessary to standardize the method of pre-dilution in order to get equivalence between plasma and concentrate units. When the 3rd IS for factor VIII concentrate was established it was assayed against both the concentrate and plasma standards, using pre-dilution in hemophilic plasma for comparison against the plasma standard. In one-stage assays there was no significant difference between these two values, though a 20% difference remained in two-stage assays [12].

For factor IX the situation was somewhat more complicated, since calibration of the 2nd IS against the plasma standard, using factor IX deficient plasma as pre-diluent, yielded a value some 20% higher than that against the 1st IS concentrate [5,14]. The higher potency was chosen for the 2nd IS, to achieve comparability between plasma and concentrate units, and consistency with the factor VIII situation, and this effectively meant a re-evaluation of the unit of factor IX.

For routine assays of concentrates against a concentrate standard in our laboratory, we have not found it necessary to pre-dilute in deficient plasma. However, this policy may have to be revised when new high-purity concentrates become available, as discussed in a subsequent section.

Comparison of methods

Comparisons between one-stage and two-stage assays of factor VIII have been extensively reviewed elsewhere [15,16], and will only be mentioned briefly here. The two-stage method has given better precision in most studies than the one-stage method, both within and between laboratories, although in recent studies the differences have been small. In most collaborative studies normal plasmas have given identical results with the two methods, though somewhat surprisingly a significant difference was found in the most recent collaborative study, as shown in Table 5. It is well-known that concentrates when

Table 5. Comparison of one-stage and two-stage factor IX assays on plasma samples.

Date of study	Potency IU/ampoule one-stage	two stage
1979	0.57	0.57
1981	0.60	0.62
1982	0.70	0.69
1984	0.73	0.74
1988	0.60	0.66

assayed against a plasma standard give higher potencies by two-stage than by one-stage assays [8,12]. In previous surveys most concentrates when assayed against a concentrate standard gave similar potencies by the two methods, but some products have consistently given significant differences, with one-stage potencies usually higher than two-stage [15,16]. In a more recent survey [17], the majority of concentrates tested gave higher potencies by one-stage than by two-stage assays. This was linked to the possible presence of activated factor VIII in some concentrates [17,18], particularly the VHP plasma derived and recombinant materials.

The introduction of a chromogenic method for factor VIII, which uses purified clotting factors and an amidolytic substrate for factor X_a, could eventually lead to improved standardization. the method is the same in principle as that of the two-stage method, and in comparative assays in our laboratory the chromogenic and two-stage methods gave very similar results on most concentrates [19]. A collaborative study involving four clinical laboratories also found on significant differences in assays of clinical plasma samples by one-stage and chromogenic assays [20]. In the most recent international collaborative study of concentrates, the chromogenic method gave identical results to the one-stage and two-stage methods on a monoclonal antibody purified concentrate, but slightly higher results on an intermediate purity concentrate [21]. The 8% difference between chromogenic and one-stage assays on the latter concentrate was statistically significant (Table 6).

Table 6. Potencies of intermediate purity (IP) and very high purity (VHP) concentrates in 4th IS study.

Number of labs	Method	IP concentrates potency IU/ml	IP concentrates gvc%	VHP concentrates potency IU/ml	VHP concentrates gvc%
26	one-stage	6.10	5.6	4.97	13.8
11	two stage	6.36	5.9	4.88	7.6
15	chromogenic	6.63	9.2	4.89	14.3
28	overall	6.30	7.7	4.93	12.7

Very high purity concentrates of factor VIII

The advent of monoclonal antibody technology has led to the preparation for clinical use of concentrates of very high purity (VHP) from both plasma and rDNA sources. These concentrates, though formulated with albumin as a stabilizer, are different in both protein composition and methods of production from the concentrate standards used up to now, and our results on two monoclonal plasma-derived products indicated that these concentrates might be subject to more assay variability than conventional products [24].

A collaborative study was therefore carried out to investigate variability between laboratories and between assay methods, and to examine the need for a possible very high purity standard. Seven laboratories took part and five concentrates, i.e. two monoclonal, one recombinant and two intermediate purity (IP), were assayed against existing WHO and US concentrate standards. The results showed that for all three methods, variability between laboratories was much higher for VHP concentrates than for IP materials [25]. Of the three methods the chromogenic gave the most variability and the two-stage the least.

One aspect of VHP concentrates is that, though formulated with albumin, they tend to be less stable than IP concentrates, particularly when diluted in the assays. Although 0.1% albumin was used in the assay buffers during the above study, this may not be adequate to stabilize dilutions of some VHP concentrates. Accordingly, in the recently completed large-scale international collaborative study, organized to replace the 3rd IS for factor VIII concentrate, 1% albumin was included in all assay buffers for both candidate preparations, an IP and a VHP (monoclonal plasma-derived) concentrate. This may be responsible for the fact that inter-laboratory variability on the VHP concentrate, though greater than on the IP concentrate (see Table 6) was much less than in the previous study [21].

Two other aspects which may contribute towards variability in assays of these concentrates are the possible presence of activated factor VIII, as already mentioned, and the use of immunodepleted plasmas in one-stage assays. Preliminary studies in our laboratory indicated that some immunodepleted plasmas gave lower potencies for VHP concentrates than hemophilic plasma [24], and these results were confirmed in a recent UK collaborative study. Hemophilic plasma is therefore recommended as substrate for assay of VHP concentrates, i.e. those prepared by monoclonal antibody and recombinant techniques.

The results of these two studies emphasize the need for attention to methodological details in assessment of potency of these VHP concentrates, but indicate that at least one VHP product can be assayed satisfactorily against an IP standard. In view of this, and the fact that IP concentrates still form the bulk of the therapeutic products used around the world, the IP concentrate was chosen as the 4th IS for factor VIII concentrate. The possible need for a VHP standard will be carefully assessed in the future.

References

1. World Health Organization. Tech Rep Ser 1971;463:14.
2. Bangham DR, Biggs R, Brozovic M, Denson KWE, Skegg JL. A biological standard for measurement of blood coagulation factor VIII activity. Bull WHO 1971;45:337-51.
3. World Health Organization. Tech Rep Ser 1977;610:13.
4. Brozovic M, Kirkwood TBL, Robertson I. Study of a proposed international standard for blood coagulation factor IX. Thromb Haemostas 1976;35:222-36.
5. Barrowcliffe TW, Curtis AD. An international collaborative study of factors II, VII, IX and X. NIBSC, unpublished report, 1986.
6. World Health Organization. Tech Rep Ser 1988;771:23-4.
7. Kirkwood TBL, Barrowcliffe TW. Discrepancy between 1-stage and 2-stage assay of factor VIII:C. Br J Haematol 1978;40:333-8.
8. Barrowcliffe TW, Kirkwood TBL. Standardization of factor VIII. I. Calibration of British standards for factor VIII clotting activity. Br J Haematol 1980;46:471-81.
9. Barrowcliffe TW, Tydeman MS, Kirkwood TBL, Thomas DP. Standardization of factor VIII-III. Establishment of a stable reference plasma for factor VIII-related activities. Thromb Haemostas 1983;50:690-6.
10. Hubbard AR. Standardisation of protein C in plasma: Establishment of an International Standard. Thromb Haemostas 1988;59:464-7.
11. Kirkwood TBL, Barrowcliffe TW, Thomas DP. An international collaborative study establishing a reference preparation for antithrombin III. Thromb Haemostas 1980;43:10-5.
12. Barrowcliffe TW, Curtis AD, Thomas DP. Standardisation of factor VIII-IV. Establishment of the 3rd International Standard for factor VIII:C concentrate. Thromb Haemostas 1983;50:697-702.
13. Lee ML, Magalang EA, Kingdon HS. An effect of predilution on potency assays of factor VIII concentrates. Thromb Res 1983;30:511-9.
14. Standardization of factors II, VII, IX and X in plasma and concentrates. Report of the ICTH sub-committee on factors VIII and IX. Thromb Haemostas 1988;59:334.
15. Barrowcliffe TW. Comparisons of 1-stage and 2-stage assays of factor VIII:C. Scand J Haematol 1984;33:39-54.
16. Barrowcliffe TW. The 1-stage versus the 2-stage factor VIII assay. In: Triplett DA (ed). Advances in coagulation testing. Skokie IL, College of American Pathologists 1986:47-62.
17. Barrowcliffe TW, Edwards SJ, Kemball-Cook G, Thomas DP. Factor VIII degradation products in heated concentrates. Lancet 1986;i:1448-9 (letter).
18. Barrowcliffe TW, Dawson NJ, Kemball-Cook G. Activated factor VIII in concentrates prepared by monoclonal antibody and recombinant technology. Thromb Haemostas 1989;62(suppl.1):198(abstract).
19. Hubbard AR, Curtis AD, Barrowcliffe TW, Edwards SJ, Jennings CA, Kemball-Cook G. Assay of factor VIII concentrates: Comparison of chromogenic and 2-stage clotting assays. Thrombosis Res 1986;44:887-91.
20. Rosén S, Anderson M, Blombäck M, et al. Clinical application of a chromogenic substrate method for determination of factor VIII activity. Thromb Haemostas 1985;54:818-23.

21. Barrowcliffe TW, Heath AB. Establishment of the 4th international standard for factor VIII concentrate. NIBSC, unpublished report, 1989.
22. Mikaelsson M, Oswaldsson U. Standardization of VIII:C assays: A manufacturer's view. Scand J Haematol 1984;33:79-86.
23. Blombäck M. Synthetic chromogenic substrate assay for factor VIII. In: Triplett DA (ed). Advances in coagulation testing. Skokie IL, College of American Pathologists, 1986:21-32.
24. Dawson NJ, Kemball-Cook G, Barrowcliffe TW. Assay discrepancies with highly purified factor VIII concentrates. Haemostas 1989;19:131-7.
25. Barrowcliffe TW, Kemball-Cook G, Heath AB. A collaborative study of intermediate and very high purity factor VIII concentrates. NIBSC, unpublished report, 1989.

PROTEIN C AND S IN SWISS BLOOD DONORS

R. Pflugshaupt, P. Baillod, W. Etter, G. Kurt

Introduction

Protein C, which is produced by the liver, is a vitamin K-dependent two-chain glycoprotein with a molecular weight of 62 kd [1]. It has a short half-life of six hours [2,3] and is found in plasma in an inactive form with a concentration of 4.8 ± 1.0 µg/ml. Activated protein C is a potent inhibitor of factors V_a and VIII_a; in this way it functions as a regulator of coagulation. In addition, protein C stimulates fibrinolysis by inhibiting plasminogen activator-inhibitor (PAI). Protein S is also synthesized by the liver and vitamin K-dependent. It has no enzymatic activity by itself, but enhances as a cofactor protein C activity by forming a complex which promotes the inhibition of factors V_a and VIII_a. Approximately 40% of circulating protein S is in the free form; the rest is inactive, being bound to the C4b-binding protein.

Congenital deficiency of protein C is inherited as an autosomal dominant disease and occurs in two variants: type 1 shows a decreased level of protein C antigen; type 2 has a normal protein C antigen level but reduced protein C functional activity, suggesting that this may be due to the presence of an abnormal protein C molecule [4]. The homozygous form is characterized by severe thromboembolic manifestations early in life [5,6,7]. The heterozygous form shows a protein C-level of 25 to 50% of normal; patients may show a tendency to thrombotic disorders.

Congenital deficiency of protein S is inherited as an autosomal dominant disease; it occurs in a few variants which are not yet completely understood. The description of deficient persons should include total and free protein S, C4b-binding protein and functional protein S measurement [8].

The aim of the study was to measure the protein C and protein S distribution in the Swiss population and to establish a normal range for our laboratory.

Methods and material

The following methods have been used:

The micro-method protocols were applied.

- Protein C, immunological, ELISA, Boehringer-Mannheim Kit
- Protein C, functional, chromogenic, Baxter Kit
- Protein S (total), immunological, ELISA, Boehringer-Mannheim Kit
- Protein S (free), immunological after precipitation with polyethyleneglycol, ELISA, Boehringer-Mannheim Kit

Two hundred plasma samples were obtained during blood collection by mobile teams in various locations in the Swiss midlands.

Results

All samples were tested for protein C-antigen, total protein S-antigen and free protein S-antigen. The results are shown in a number of tables and figures. Table 1 contains the overall results. In Table 2 the results of men and women are presented separately. The values of protein S

Table 1. Results of protein C, protein S (total) and protein S (free) in all samples. The mean values and the range seem to be lower than those stated by the producer of the kits.

	N	$\bar{x}$ %	SD	$\bar{x}$ + 2 SD	Normal range % (Boehringer)
Protein C immunological	197	85.52	18.29	48.9–132.1	70–140
Protein S (total) immunological	197	90.00	19.51	50.9–129.0	70–140
Protein S (free) immunological	915	81.05	19.39	42.3–119.8	70–140

Table 2. Protein C shows no sex-related differences, while the values for protein S (total and free) differ significantly between men and women.

	Sex	N	$\bar{x}$ %	SD	Difference
Protein C immunological	men	115	86.75	19.24	not significant
	women	82	83.79	16.83	
Protein S (total) immunological	men	115	93.89	19.71	significant t test
	women	82	84.55	17.98	p=<0.001
Protein S (free) immunological	men	114	87.14	16.70	significant t test
	women	78	70.56	16.70	p=<0.001

(total and free) found in women are significantly lower than those found in men, while protein C shows no difference between men and women. In Figure 1 the values of total protein S are plotted against those of free protein S. Figure 2 and 3 show mean values and standard deviation of protein S (total) and protein S (free) according to sex and age. Some samples with low protein C levels have also been examined with a functional test; the results are presented in Table 3.

Table 3. In ten samples with low protein C levels, no difference between immunological and functional determination was found.

Samples with low level of protein C	N	$\overline{X}$ %	SD	$\overline{X}$ + 2 SD	Normal range %
Protein C functional	11	64.09	4.48	55.13–73.06	70–130 (Baxter)
Protein C immunological	11	62.14	322	55.70–68.57	70–140 (Boehringer)

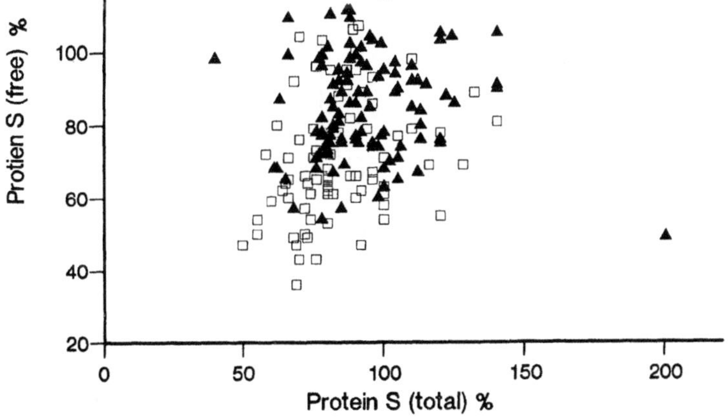

Figure 1. Results of protein S (all donors). Total protein S plotted against free protein S; men and women identified by different marks. The two groups differ significantly.

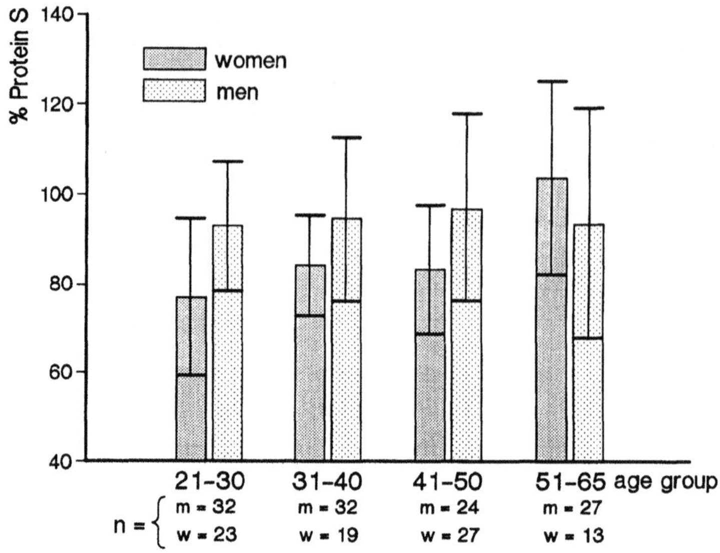

Figure 2. Means and standard deviations of total protein S according to age and sex.

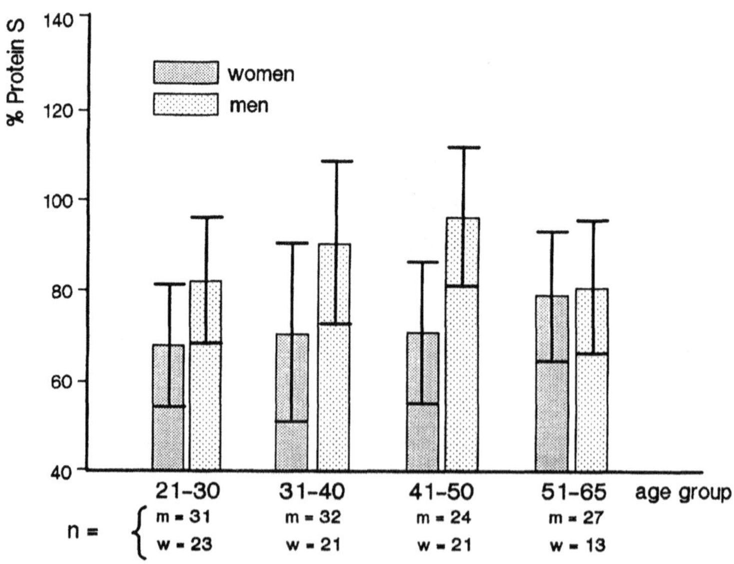

Figure 3. Means and standard deviations of free protein S according to age and sex.

Discussion

Our results show that total protein S and free protein S have different normal values in men and women. This is mainly seen in women from twenty to fifty years of age. Women above fifty years show no differences in total or in free protein S compared with men of the same age group. This observation could support Huisveld et al.'s hypothesis that protein S-levels could be influenced by oral contraceptives [9]. However, we did not find a difference between total and free protein S, as reported by Huisveld. Unfortunately, we have no information on the contraceptive use by our female donors.

The normal values stated by the producer of these kits seem to be too high. It might therefore be important to establish normal values with a sufficient number of subjects for each laboratory using a standard pool of normal plasmas as references. An international reference plasma is urgently needed.

Acknowledgement

Some of the protein C and protein S kits have been donated by Boehringer-Mannheim (Schweiz) AG, Switerland.

References

1. Kisiel W. Human plasma protein C: Isolation, characterization and mechanisms of activation by (alpha)-thrombin. J Clin Invest 1979;64:761-9.
2. Epstein DJ, Bergum PW, Bajaj SP, et al. Radio-immunoassays for protein C and factor X: Plasma antigen levels in abnormal hemostatic states. Am J Clin Pathol 1984;82:573-81.
3. Comp PC, Nixon RR, Esmon CT. Determination of functional levels of protein C, an antithrombin protein, using thrombin-thrombomodulin complex. Blood 1984;63:15-21.
4. D'Angelo SV, Comp PC, Esmon CT, et al. Relationship between protein C antigen and anticoagulant activity during oral anticoagulation and in selected disease states. J Clin Invest 1986;77:416-25.
5. Brockmans AW, Veltkamp JJ, Bertina RM. Congenital protein C deficiency and venous thromboembolism. N Engl J Med 1983;309:340-4.
6. Seligson U, Berger A, Abend M, et al. Homozygous protein C deficiency manifested by massive venous thrombosis in the newborn. N Engl J Med 1984;310:559-62.
7. Marciniak E, Wilson HD, Marlar RA. Neonatal purpura fulminans. A genetic disorder related to the absence of protein C in blood. Blood 1985; 65:15-20.
8. Comp PC. Laboratory evaluation of protein S status. Seminars in Thrombosis and Haemostasis, 1990;16:177-81.
9. Huisveld IA, Hospers JEH, Meijers JCM. Oral contraceptives reduce total protein S, but not free protein S. Thromb Res 1987;45:109-14.

CLINICAL EFFICACY OF CLOTTING FACTOR CONCENTRATES: SURVIVAL, RECOVERY AND HEMOSTATIC CAPACITY[1]

I.M. Nilsson, E. Berntorp

Factor VIII concentrates are necessary for the treatment not only of patients with hemophilia A but also for those with severe von Willebrand's disease (vWD), especially the type III or the type II variants. Earlier, above all cryoprecipitate, and low and intermediate purity concentrates were used. The intermediate purity concentrates contained 1-3 units of factor VIII clotting activity (FVIII:C) per mg protein, factor VIII itself being only a trace protein. Since 1984, all commercial factor VIII concentrates have been subjected to some form of virus inactivation. In the last years several plasma-derived, superpure factor VIII concentrates have been developed to eliminate the risk of viral transmission, and to reduce other side effects caused by the multiplicity of foreign proteins and alloantigens the concentrates of intermediate purity contain. Clinical trials of recombinant factor VIII have also been started. Correction of the bleeding defect in vWD requires a concentrate containing almost native von Willebrand factor (vWF).

Here we shall be reporting on the biochemical properties of six plasma-derived, superpure factor VIII concentrates, one recombinant preparation and for comparison two other concentrates, one of high purity, the other of intermediate purity. The in vivo properties of the superpure factor VIII concentrates and one conventional high purity concentrate have also been studied.

Materials and methods

Factor VIII concentrates

Table 1 shows the various concentrates studied, their preparation procedures, and forms of virus inactivation.

1. The study was supported by grants from the Swedish Medical Research Council (00087).

Table 1. Factor VIII concentrates; data given by manufacturers, and virus inactivation.

Preparation	Preparation procedure	Virus inactivation
Monoclate (Armour)	Affinity purification by vWF MAb[1]	Dry heat 60°C 30 h
Monoclate P (Armour)	Affinity purification by vWF MAb[1]	Pasteurization
Hemofil M (Baxter)	Affinity purification by FVIII:C MAb[1]	SDI
Octonativ M (Kabi)	Affinity purification by FVIII:C MAb[1]	SDI
Otavi (Octapharma)	Chromatographic purification	SDI
Factor VIII VHP (Bio-Transfusion)	Chromatographic purification	SDI
Recombinant factor VIII (Baxter)	DNA technology[1]	
Profilate SD (Alpha)	Cryoprec + $Al(OH)_3$ ads + PEG + glycine prec	SDI
Kryobulin TIM3 (Immuno)	Cryoprec + further purification	Steam treatment 60°C 10 h

SDI = solvent detergent inactivation
MAb = monoclonal antibodies

1. Dissolved in albumin.

Factor VIII assays

One-stage assay. FVIII:C activity was assessed from the normalizing effect on recalcification time of platelet-rich hemophilia A plasma containing less than 1% of the normal FVIII:C concentration [1]. Clotting time was measured with a Photocoagulator (Kabi).

Chromogenic assay. This was performed using the microtitre version of the Coatest kit from Kabi, Sweden, as described previously [2].

The concentrates were diluted with a) 0.05 mol/l Tris-HCl, 0.1 mol/l NaCl, 1% BSA buffer, and b) plasma from a patient with severe hemophilia A with less than 0.1 IU/dl of FVIII:C, until the activity values corresponded to those of standard plasma. Further dilutions were made in Tris buffer, 1% BSA. All assays incorporated two replicate sets of three dilutions of standard and test preparations, in a balanced design to allow for the possibility of temporal drift.

In the in vivo studies, plasma samples were assayed at three different dilutions according to the balanced design previously described by Nilsson et al [1].

As concentrate standard was used the 3rd International Standard (NIBSC 80/556) for FVIII:C concentrate, which was calibrated against our house standard (Octonativ M, Kabi). Pooled citrated plasma from 20 healthy individuals, calibrated against the 13th British Standard plasma for factor VIII (85/573), was used as the standard for FVIII:C in plasma. Results were expressed in IU/ml for the concentrates and in IU/dl for plasma.

Factor VIII coagulant antigen (FVIII:Ag) was assayed by an ELISA based on three different monoclonal antibodies against the light chain of factor VIII [3]. The concentrates were diluted both in 0.05 mol/l Tris-HCl, 0.1 mol/l NaCl, 4% BSA, 0.05 Tween 20, pH 7.5, and in plasma from patients with severe hemophilia A.

Von Willebrand factor antigen (vWF:Ag) was measured both with a quantitative electroimmunoassay (EIA) [4] and by ELISA [5].

Ristocetin cofactor activity (vWF:Rcof) was assessed with a method using formalin-fixed platelets [6].

As the standard for FVIII:Ag, vWF:Ag and vWF:Rcof was used, the same plasma as described above, calibrated against the 1st IRP for factor VIII-related activities in plasma (80/511) and expressed in IU.

Multimeric distribution of vWF:Ag in the preparations was analyzed with low-resolution SDS agarose electropheresis as described earlier [7].

Binding of vWF:Ag to collagen was measured with an ELISA method described by Brown and Bosak [8].

Fibrinogen, fibronectin, IgA and IgG were measured with ELISA methods using polyclonal antibodies from Dakopatts AB, Copenhagen (fibrinogen A080, fibronectin A245, IgA A262, IgG A423) the procedure being that recommended by the manufacturer. Protein standard plasma from the Behring Institute was used in measuring fibrinogen and fibronectin, and standard human serum, also from the Behring Institute, in the measurement of IgA and IgG.

Protein concentration was determined with the method of Bradford [9] using bovine serum albumin as the standard (Protein Standard II, Bio-Rad) for the preparations dissolved in albumin and for Profilate SD and Kryobulin. Bovine gammaglobulin (Protein Standard I, Bio-Rad) was used for the superpure concentrates prepared by conventional protein purification methods (Octavi, factor VIII VHP).

In vivo studies

The in vivo properties of six different concentrates (Table 4) were evaluated after intravenous injection in 14 patients with severe hemophilia A (referred to here as patients A, B, C, D, E, F, G, H, J, K, L, M, N, O). The patients received between one and four different concentrates. An interval of at least one week was allowed to elapse between treatments, and there were no bleeding episodes at the time of injec-

Table 2. Factor VIII assays of the various concentrates (mean values).

Preparation	1	2	3	4	5	6	7	8	9
Monoclate	3	102	123	119	118	120	157	121	9.4
Monoclate P	4	98	136	137	122	122	108	80	10.7
Hemofil M	3	115	96	97	93	97	58	47	10.8
Octonativ M	6	100	131	131	85	96	92	79	36.8
Octavi	7	27	23	23	20	22	22	17	42.6 *
Factor VIII VHP	2	21	18	19	17	19	16	14	45.2 **
Recombinant factor VIII	1	33	40	47	45	50	55	42	5.0
Profilate SD	3	42	52	46	42	45	41	44	12.4
Kryobulin TIM3	3	30	38	36	32	33	54	49	1.8

1 = Number of batches
2 = Labelled potency IU/ml

3 = FVIII:C one-stage IU/ml 1% BSA
4 = FVIII:C one-stage IU/ml hemophilia A plasma
5 = FVIII:C Coatest IU/ml 1% BSA
6 = FVIII:C Coatest IU/ml hemophilia A plasma

7 = FVIII:Ag ELISA IU/ml 1% BSA
8 = FVIII:Ag ELISA IU/ml hemophilia A plasma

9 = Specific activity IU FVIII:C/mg protein

* With albumin as standard 105.
** With albumin as standard 126.

Table 3. In vitro studies of the concentrates (mean values) (the same concentrate as in Table 2).

Preparation	**1**	**2**	**3**	**4**	**5**	**6**	**7**	**8**	**9**
Monoclate	13	14	3	5	9	739	577	8	30
Monoclate P	15	18	5	5	7	92	646	17	95
Hemofil M	1	1.2	1.6	2	79	0	0	1	8
Octonativ M	1	1.6	1.3	1	65	4	1	1	1
Octavi	7	14	6	19	2	2,335	3,304	72	495
Factor VIII VHP	3	7	4	6	3	1,425	123	35	55
Recombinant factor VIII	<1	<0.1	0	0	–	0	0	2	6
Profilate S	68	120	160	460	0.2	36,000	83,000	7,000	8,500
Kryobulin TIM3	185	157	130	76	0.4	865,000	90,000	2,400	7,200

1 = Von Willebrand factor EIA IU/ml
2 = Von Willebrand factor ELISA IU/ml
3 = Von Willebrand factor Rcof IU/ml
4 = Von Willebrand factor collagen binding IU/ml

5 = FVIII:C/vWF:Ag

6 = Fibrinogen ELISA ng/IU FVIII:C
7 = Fibronectin ELISA ng/IU FVIII:C
8 = IgA ELISA ng/IU FVIII:C
9 = IgG ELISA ng/IU FVIII:C

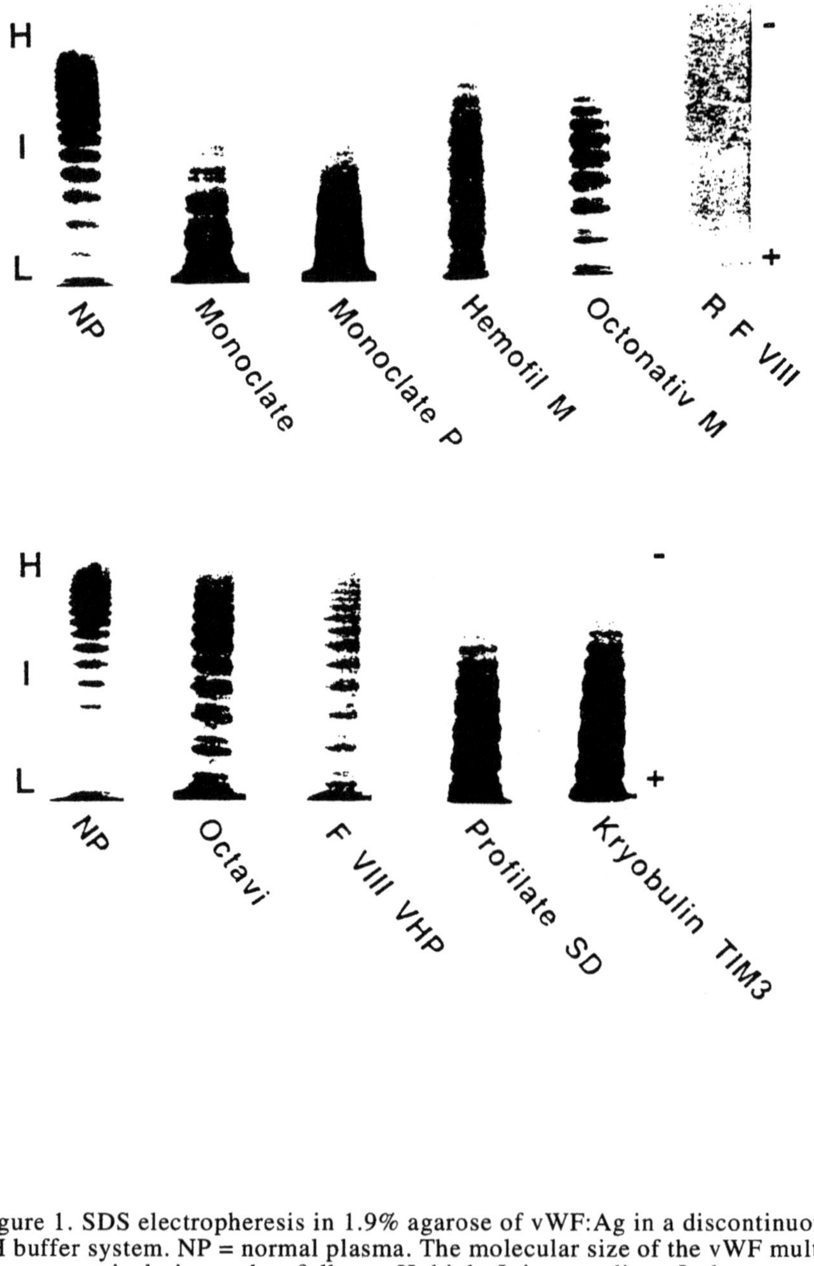

Figure 1. SDS electropheresis in 1.9% agarose of vWF:Ag in a discontinuous pH buffer system. NP = normal plasma. The molecular size of the vWF multimers is designated as follows: H, high; I, intermediate; L, low.

tion. In all cases the dose of FVIII:C was 25 IU/kg body weight (labeled activity). Venous blood was collected into evacuated tubes containing 0.129 M sodium citrate 1:9 (Becton Dickinson, Meylan, France) before and five and 30 minutes, 1, 2, 4, 6, 9, 11, 24, 36 and 48 hours after injection. Platelet-poor plasma was obtained after centrifugation at 2000 g for ten minutes, and was then immediately frozen and stored at –70°C until tested. Haemotacrit was determined before treatment. In assessing of in vivo recovery, the plasma volume was calculated according to Allain et al [10] and in vivo recovery in per cent, thus:

$$100 \times \frac{\text{plasma volume (ml)} \times \text{ observed rise in FVIII:C (IU/ml)(peak level)}}{\text{injected volume (ml)} \times \text{ labelled potency (IU/ML)}}$$

For determination of the half-life of injected FVIII:C, the plasma concentrations of FVIII:C (log) were plotted against time elapsed since injection, and disappearance rate then being determined by least-squares regression analysis using natural log values of plasma concentrations.

Results and comments

In vitro studies

The analytical data for the various factor VIII concentrates are given in Tables 2 and 3. Dilution of the recombinant factor VIII preparation in hemophilia A plasma gave higher values for FVIII:C than when the preparation was diluted in BSA buffer. This has been observed earlier and has been shown to be due to the absence of vWF in the preparations [11]. All the other preparations yielded about the same FVIII:C values whether assayed after dilution in hemophilia A plasma or in buffer. Dawson et al [12] found that one-stage assays performed with immunodepleted plasma lacking vWF yielded lower values for potency than those performed with hemophilic plasma, this was so for all concentrates tested, though the discrepancy was most marked in the case of superpure concentrates purified by monoclonal antibodies. As we use hemophilia A plasma as the test base in our one-stage assay, no such discrepancy has been observed by us, except in the case of the recombinant preparation. In two of the concentrates affinity purified by monoclonal antibodies (Monoclate P, Octonativ M), higher values were observed with the one-stage assay than with the chromogenic assay, while for the remaining preparations, the two methods yielded comparative values. Dawson et al [12] also obtained higher potency values for a superpure factor VIII concentrate by one-stage assay than by chromogenic assay. Barrowcliffe et al [13] have suggested that these results might indicate the preparations analyzed to contain activated factor VIII. It is also possible that there is variation from batch to batch. Although our FVIII:C estimates were largely in agreement with values given by the manufacturers, there were some exceptions. Our assays yielded potency values for Monoclate, Monoclate P, and the recombinant preparations that were clearly higher than the label values.

FVIII:Ag in the preparations was also determined both after dilution in buffer and in hemophilia A plasma. Some preparations (Monoclate P, Octonativ M, Octavi, FVIII VHP, Profilate SD) showed about the same values for FVIII:Ag (buffer diluent) as for FVIII:C by the chromogenic method, while the recombinant factor VIII preparation and Monoclate showed higher values, and Hemofil M lower values. The higher values may have been due to inactivation of the clotting activity during the preparation. Our FVIII:Ag ELISA measures only the light chain of factor VIII, and possibly the batches of Hemofil M used had a relatively low content of factor VIII light chain. The results of FVIII:Ag determinations for the preparations diluted in hemophilia A plasma are noteworthy. For most of the preparations, the values were lower than those obtained with buffer as diluent. This was checked for 22 different hemophilia A plasmas. This might indicate that multitransfused hemophiliacs, despite having no demonstrable FVIII:C inhibitory activity, may have inhibitors directed against non-coagulation active epitopes of factor VIII. Fulcher et al [14], using immunoblotting techniques, also found a multitransfused individual with severe hemophilia A and no detectable inhibitor titre to have silent anti-factor VIII antibodies.

As expected, the recombinant preparation contained no vWF (Table 3). The monoclonal antibody purified preparations contained varying but small amounts of vWF; the ratios FVIII:C to vWF were 9, 7, 79 and 65 for Monoclate, Monoclate P, Hemofil M and Octonativ M, respectively. The superpure concentrates Octavi and FVIII VHP, prepared by conventional protein chemistry purification methods, contained considerable amounts of vWF and their FVIII:C to vWF ratios were 2 and 3, respectively. Corresponding values were obtained for vWF:Ag, ristocetin cofactor activity and collagen binding activity of vWF. The two high/intermediate pure concentrates tested contained large amounts of vWF, the FVIII:C to vWF ratios being 0.2 and 0.4. Figure 1 shows the multimetric pattern of vWF in the concentrates as analyzed by low resolution SDS agarose electrophoresis. Octavi and FVIII VHP manifested patterns similar to that of normal plasma, except that some of the highest molecular weight multimers were lacking. The monoclonal antibody purified concentrates differed from each other by their vWF multimeric pattern. The high/intermediate purity concentrates both lacked the high molecular weight multimers.

Specific activity, in terms of units of FVIII:C/mg protein, has been used to express the purity of factor VIII concentrates. Factor VIII itself has a specific activity of 4000 units/mg protein. The recombinant preparation and the monoclonal antibody purified concentrates are all dissolved in albumin, and the purity of the concentrates cannot be evaluated by measuring specific activity. Octavi and FVIII VHP had the highest values for specific activity, 43 and 45 units/mg, respectively (calculated using IgG as the protein standard; using albumin as the standard, the respective values were 105 and 126 units/mg); Kryobulin had the lowest value, 1.8 units/mg. The best assessment of the purity of factor VIII concentrate is obtained by determining its content of other protein contaminants. The recombinant preparation contained no fibrinogen or fibronectin, but small amounts of IgA and IgG. Fibrinogen, fibronectin or IgG could not be detected (or only in trace amounts) in Hemofil M and Octonativ M. The concentrates purified by vWF monoclonal antibodies contained small but measurable amounts, whereas the superpure concentrates prepared by conventional protein chemistry methods contained larger amounts. Huge amounts were demonstrated in the two high/intermediate purity concentrates.

In vivo studies

The single-dose pharmacokinetic data for 14 patients are given in Tables 4 and 5. Mean in vivo recovery varied between 101 and 128% for the monoclonal antibody purified concentrates, and 80 to 82% for Octavi and Profilate SD. The peak values were observed between 5 and 30 minutes after injection. The higher recovery figures obtained with the monoclonal antibody purified products, as compared with those purified conventionally, do not necessarily reflect a true biological difference. As already mentioned, in our in vitro studies we obtained higher potency values for Monoclate, Monoclate P and the recombinant preparation than those quoted by the manufactures. The findings in several other studies have also shown that the label potency of factor VIII concentrates may differ from the actual content of the vial [12,15,16]. Owing to the formula used for the calculation of in vivo recovery, a high recovery value may be due to a higher actual factor VIII content than declared by the manufacturers, and vice versa.

As discussed previously, e.g. by Messori et al [17], the calculation of in vivo recovery is subject to several other sources of error, such as the difficulty of pinpointing peak values, imprecision in indirect methods of plasma volume measurement, and the assumption that factor VIII distributes only into the plasma. Although conclusions drawn from pharmacokinetic data obtained in a small series are uncertain, our data nevertheless indicate no major difference in recovery between the products studied, especially if the actual FVIII:C content of the vials is taken into account.

Values for FVIII:C half-life were very similar for all the products tested, despite their different degrees of purity and difference in the

Table 4. In vivo recovery (%) in 14 severe hemophilia A patients (A-O) after injection of 25 IU labeled FVIII:C/kg.

	A	B	C	D	E	F	G	H	J	K	L	M	N	O	Mean
Monoclate	151	92	127	98	102	167	110	121	113						120
Monoclate P	152	104	118	107	151	171	124	120	106						128
Hemofil M		74			128										101
Octonativ M			104	97						57	120	128			112
Octavi										78			94	68	80
Profilate SD				84										80	82

Table 5. Half-life (h) of FVIII:C in 14 patients (A-O) with severe hemophilia A after injection of 25 IU labeled FVIII:C/kg.

	A	B	C	D	E	F	G	H	J	K	L	M	N	O	Mean
Monoclate	13	18	11	12	20	10	15	20	21						16
Monoclate P	15	18	11	13	17	11	12	20	16						15
Hemofil M		16			15										15
Octonativ M			11	12						15	8	11			11
Octavi										17			17	17	17
Profilate SD				12										18	15

viral inactivation procedures used (Table 5). It should be borne in mind that approximately the same half-life values were obtained in a given patient, irrespective of which concentrate had been given. Thus, for example, the half-life value was 11 hours in case C, 12 hours in case D, and 20 hours in case H. In all probability, the relatively short half-life observed for Octonativ M (mean 11 hours) is a consequence of this preparation having been given to subjects in whom low half-life values were usual. When comparing different concentrates, it is thus extremely important to use the same patients.

In previous studies we found that the values for recovery and half-life did not vary between heat-treated and non-heat-treated concentrates [18,19]. In agreement with our present results, others have also found that differences in the virus inactivation procedures applied to factor VIII concentrates, or in the degree of purity, do not affect the in vivo properties, whether determined by model dependent analysis or by model independent analysis [20-23].

If a concentrate has a normal in vivo recovery and disappearance rate of FVIII:C, it follows that it is clinically effective if given in adequate doses in connection with bleeding episodes and surgical procedures. Figure 2 shows the course in one patient with severe hemophilia A undergoing plastic surgery of the hip on two different occasions. On the first occasion, he was given intermediate purity concentrate and on the second a monoclonal antibody purified concentrate. No difference in clinical efficacy was seen. In Sweden we routinely give prophylactic treatment with factor VIII to boys with severe hemophilia A at a dosage of 25 IU FVIII:C/kg, usually three times a week. We used to give low or intermediate purity concentrates for the past, but since 1-2 years we have given monoclonal antibody purified concentrates. We have observed no difference in effect.

Concentrates containing no vWF, or only traces, can not, of course, be expected to control the hemostatic defect in vWD. We have previously shown that concentrates such as cryoprecipitate, fraction I-O and Hemate P (Behring) containing high molecular weight multimers of vWF can correct the defect in vWD [24,25]. Mazurier and coworkers [26] have shown that the concentrate from Biotransfusion, FVIII VHP, can normalize the bleeding defect in vWD. Recently pure vWF concentrates have become available.

Conclusion

The in vitro properties of one recombinant factor VIII preparation, four monoclonal antibody purified factor VIII concentrates, two superpure factor VIII concentrates prepared by conventional protein chemistry methods and two high/intermediate purity concentrates indicate that the purity of superpure factor VIII concentrates, should be evaluated by measuring other protein contaminants and not by specific activity.

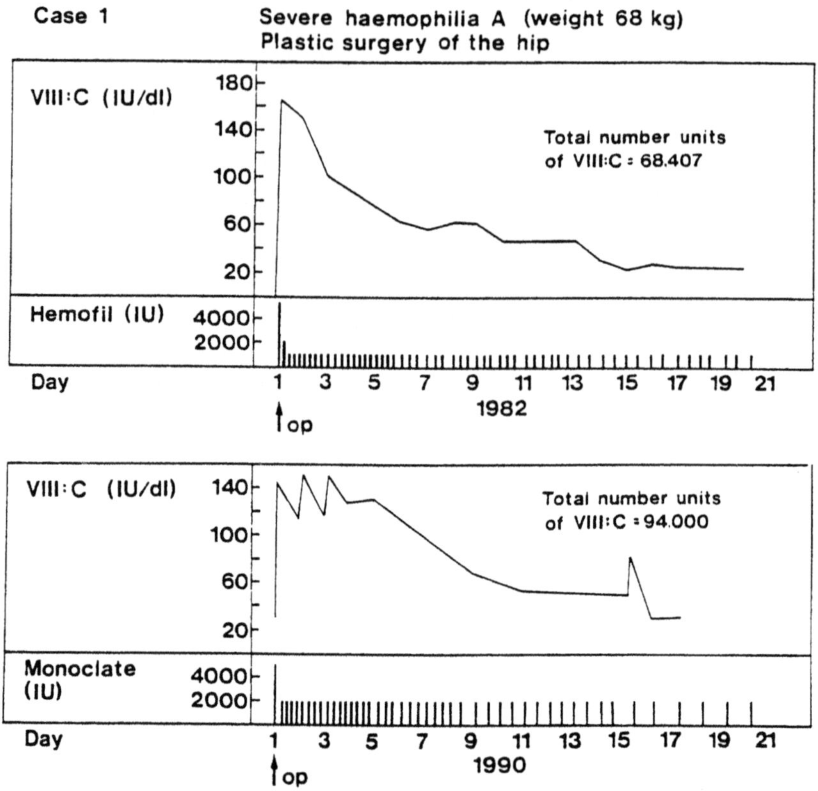

Figure 2. The course in one patient with severe hemophilia A undergoing plastic surgery of the hip on two different occasions.

Dilution in hemophilia A plasma gave the same FVIII:C values as dilution in BSA buffer except in the case of the recombinant factor VIII concentrate. Two of the monoclonal antibody purified preparations yielded higher potency values in one-stage assay than in chromogenic values were obtained with the two methods. FVIII:Ag diluted in hemophilia A plasma gave lower values than those obtained with the dilution in BSA buffer, indicating that multitransfused hemophiliacs may have inhibitors directed against non-coagulation active sites on factor VIII.

The recombinant preparation contained no vWF, fibrinogen or fibronectin but small amounts of IgA and IgG. Monoclonal antibody purified concentrates contain only trace amounts of vWF, the FVIII:C to vWF ratio varying from 7 to 79. Fibrinogen, fibronectin and IgG could not be detected, or only in trace amounts. Superpure concentrates prepared by conventional protein chemistry methods (Octavi, FVIII VHP) contain vWF of almost normal multimeric pattern, as well as fibrinogen, fibronectin, IgG and IgA. They have high specific activity. Both the high and intermediate purity concentrates contained huge amounts of vWF, fibrinogen, fibronectin, IgA and IgG.

In the in vivo studies, 14 patients with severe hemophilia A were given four different monoclonal antibody purified concentrates, one superpure concentrate prepared by conventional protein chemistry method (Octavi) and one high purity concentrate. In vivo recovery and half-life were similar for all the concentrates tested. In a given patient the half-life was the same, irrespective of which concentrate was given. No difference was seen in clinical efficacy between superpure and intermediate purity concentrates.

References

1. Nilsson IM, Kirkwood TBL, Barrowcliffe TW. In vivo recovery of factor VIII: A comparison of one-stage and two-stage assay methods. Thromb Haemostas 1979;42:1230-9.
2. Lethagen S, Östergaard H, Nilsson IM. Clinical application of the chromogenic assay of factor VIII in hemophilia A, and different variants of von Willebrand's disease. Scand J Haematol 1987;37:448-53.
3. Nilsson IM, Berntorp E, Zettervall O, Dahlbäck B. Non-coagulation inhibitory factor VIII antibodies after induction of tolerance to factor VIII in hemophilia A patients. Blood 1990;75:378-83.
4. Laurell CB. Quantitive estimation of proteins by electrophoresis in agarose gel containing antibodies. Anal Biochem 1966;15:45-52.
5. Ingerslev J. A sensitive ELISA for von Willebrand factor (vWF:Ag). Scand J Clin Lab Invest 1987;47:143-9.
6. Zuzel M, Nilsson IM, Åberg M. A method for measuring plasma ristocetin cofactor activity. Thromb Res 1978;12:745-54.
7. Lamme S, Wallmark A, Holmberg L, Nilsson IM, Sjögren HO. The use of monoclonal antibodies in measuring factor VIII/von Willebrand factor. Scand J Clin Lab Invest 1985;45:17-26.
8. Brown JE, Bosak JO. An ELISA test for the binding of von Willebrand antigen to collagen. Thromb Res 1986;43:303-11.
9. Bradford MM. A rapid sensitive method for the quantitation of microgram quantities of protein utilizing the protein dye binding. Anal Biochem 1976;72:248-54.
10. Allain JP, Verroust F, Soulier JP. In vitro and in vivo characterization of factor VIII preparations. Vox Sang 1980;38:68-80.
11. Cinotti S, Boni E, Morfini M. Factor VIII:C potency assay in two rDNA and in plasma derived concentrates. International Symposium on Biotechnology of plasma proteins: Hemostasis, thrombosis and iron proteins. Florence, Italy, April 1990:60(Abstract).
12. Dawson MJ, Kemball-Cook G, Barrowcliffe TW. Assay discrepancies with highly purified factor VIII concentrates. Haemostasis 1989;19:131-7.
13. Barrowcliffe TW, Dawson NJ, Kemball-Cook G. Activated factor VIII in concentrates prepared by monoclonal antibody and recombinant technology. Thromb Haemostas 1989;62:198(Abstract).

14. Fulcher CA, de Graaf Mahoney S, Roberts JR, Kasper CK, Zimmerman TS. Localization of human factor VIII inhibitor epitopes to two polypeptide fragments. Proc Natl Acad Sci USA 1985;82:7728-32.
15. Lusher JM. Factor VIII concentrates: Matching what you see with what you get. JAMA 1985;254:802-3.
16. Ratnoff OD. Factor VIII concentrates. JAMA 1986;255:325-6.
17. Messori A, Longo G, Matucci M, Morfini M, Rossi Ferrini PL. Clinical pharmcokinetics of factor VIII in patients with classic hemophilia. Clin Pharm 1987;13:365-80.
18. Nilsson IM. Clinical characteristics of the factor VIII concentrates. In: Smit Sibinga CTh, Das PC, Seidl S (eds). Plasma fractionation and blood transfusion. Boston, Dordrecht, Lancaster: Martinus Nijhoff Publishers, 1985: 197-209.
19. Berntorp E, Nilsson IM. Biochemical and in vivo properties of commercial virus-inactivated factor VIII concentrates. Eur J Haematol 1988;40: 205-14.
20. Matucci M, Messori A, Donati-Cori G, et al. Kinetic evaluation of four factor VIII concentrates by model-independent methods. Scand J Haematol 1985;34:22-8.
21. Longo G, Matucci M, Messori A, Morfini M, Rossi-Ferrini P. Pharmacokinetics of a new heat-treated concentrate of factor VIII estimated by model-independent methods. Thromb Res 1986;42:471-6.
22. Brettler DB, Forsberg AD, Levine PH, Petillo J, Lamon K, Sullivan JL. Factor VIII:C concentrate purified from plasma using monoclonal antibodies: Human studies. Blood 1989;73:1859-63.
23. White G, McMillan C, Courter S, Gomperts E and the Recombinate Collaborative Group. Safety and efficacy of antihemophilic factor (recombinant) in hemophilia A patients. Abstract book XIX International Congress of the World Federation of Hemophilia, Washington DC, 1990:25(Abstract 85).
24. Holmberg L, Nilsson IM. Von Willebrand disease. Clin Haematol 1985;14: 461-88.
25. Berntorp E, Nilsson IM. Use of high-purity factor VIII concentrate (Hemate P) in von Willebrand's disease. Vox Sang 1989;56:212-7.
26. Mazurier C, de Romeuf C, Parquet-Gernez A, Goudemand M. In vitro and in vivo characterization of a high-purity, solvent/detergent-treated factor VIII concentrate: Evidence for its therapeutic efficacy in von Willebrand's disease. Eur J Haematol 1989;43:7-14.

DISCUSSION

M. Mikaelsson, J. Sixma

P.C. Das (Groningen, NL): Dr. Brozovic and Mr. McShine, you have shown a very simple system which is able to detect the platelet volume change in response to EDTA. Could you utilize that for routine quality control in the production of platelets in a Blood Bank? If so, where would you put it: At the stage of whole blood collection or after you make your platelet concentrate?

R.L. McShine (Groningen, NL): I suspect the most appropriate stage to do it will be after preparation of platelet concentrate.

P.C. Das: But that presumes that you have followed a bag of blood, which has got a good platelet volume change, that was retained in the platelet concentrate stage. Have you done that kind of experiment?

B. Brozovic (London, UK): If you use the test as a rejection test for poor quality product, then you can do it at two different times during the storage period. The first one is immediately after preparation, where you can set your limits and reject anything which does not meet your specification on the basis of the test. The second time to use it, is before release. Because of simplicity, that test has a potential to be used as a release test. Units of platelets stored over a period of time, which show no change in mean platelet volume on addition of EDTA, could be discarded because they do not meet the specification.

S. Stienstra (Nijmegen, NL): Dr. Brozovic, I agree with you that during ageing platelets are shrinking. We have done measurements on flow cytometry as well and we have seen that while the platelets are shrinking they become more spherical and get some activation markers on their surface. We have heard that after filtration the platelets have lower MPV. Having the yield figures in mind when using the commercially available platelet filters, I cannot believe that this lower MPV is only a matter of selection by the filters. I think it might be the same effect but more rapid than the ageing effect. Can you give any comment on that.

B. Brozovic: First of all, I would like to make it absolutely clear that I did not say that during storage the platelets are shrinking or swelling. What I am saying is that there is a change in the mean platelet volume. What kind of changes are going to be registered, depends on the counting system which we use. When we use Technicon H1 flow cytometry counter, we are going to see the decrease in the mean platelet volume, which does not mean that the platelet volume is shrinking. When we use a Coulter counter or a Sysmex 2000 counter, we see that the mean platelet volume is increasing during storage. So, what we are registering is the change, which is dependent on the technology of the measurement. We have done this with all three machines.

S. Stienstra: With the flow cytometric technique you are looking at side scatter and we have validated this with beads. With the hematological cell counter techniques it is done by electrostatic measurements. I can imagine that more roundish platelets have a different electrostatical way of acting in the measurement chamber.

J.J. Sixma (Utrecht, NL): Dr. de Wolf, what is the safe level of platelets above which one should want to keep one's patients with leukemia. What is the level that you would recommend from your reading: Is that 20×10^9/l or can we get lower.

J.Th.M. de Wolf (Groningen, NL): It depends on what your purpose is. If you want to prevent any kind of bleeding, you have to stay above 20. Studies show that serious bleedings are more frequent when you come below 5.0×10^9/l.

J.J. Sixma: When looking at a study from 1982, one should realize that certainly in bone marrow transplantation today cytostatic treatments are more severe and certainly give more damage to the gastrointestinal tract than was usual in the early 80's. Platelet levels that might have been safe in those days might no longer be so today. On the other hand, a policy by which you keep platelets above 20×10^9/l versus one in which you keep platelets above 15×10^9/l may already mean some 30% or 40% increase in platelet concentrate use.

J.Th.M. de Wolf: Well, we are using in Groningen a level of 10×10^9/l. When platelets come below 10×10^9/l patients will be transfused. But the point I think is that there is so few literature on which you can say well that is the level. You can theorize about it. There are much more antibiotics and more chemotherapy is used. It should be logical that patients are facing bleeding problems much more easily than in the early days, but there are no studies available.

M. Harvey (Leiden, NL): I like to comment on what Dr. de Wolf said. In Leiden we try to substitute at a level of about 10×10^9/l, but it really depends on the clinical data of the patient. For instance a patient known to be a high-risk bleeder, somebody who is infected or has shown decreasing response over the last few days. I think it is wrong to transfuse on a number.

J.J. Sixma: You are talking from the laboratory side. But in a busy clinic you get all these numbers and you have to think in every case: "Is this a patient that has at this moment...". Obviously you do that, but you need a general policy, a sort of minimum figure. And that might be 10×10^9/l. When we say the patient should not have a platelet count below 10×10^9/l, the residents begin to transfuse when there is a drop from 30 to 18×10^9/l. Because they know that the next day the patient will be at 6×10^9/l and they know that their supervisor does not like that. So, they already take a higher level anticipating a further drop. That is the reality and that determines the amount of platelets transfused. For our own unit with 30 bone marrow transplantations a year, it meant a 30% increase in platelet concentrate consumption over the last year. We now set the limit at 15×10^9/l and platelets should not be given, unless there are obvious complications and unless the platelets are below that level. I do not yet know how this will work out.

M. Harvey: If I understand you correctly you have just confirmed what I said, you do not treat a number only, you treat a patient.

J.J. Sixma: We do both; obviously we treat the patient in the first place, but then we also have a lower limit below which we do not want to go.

P.C. Das: Dr. Sintnicolaas, that was an excellent presentation. My question relates to ELISA crossmatching where you have used fresh platelets versus frozen platelets indicating that frozen platelets missed some of the crossmatching problem. But a group in Charleston has shown that when crossmatching by FACS technique there are no differences at all, whether they use fresh or frozen platelets[1] I wonder since the FACS cell sorter is now quite common, have you used this in parallel and found any difference in your ELISA versus FACS?

K. Sintnicolaas (Rotterdam, NL): As you said fluorescence measurements are very common. We also use the FACScan for antibody detection, but we did not compare the donor selection by FACScan, because

1. Lazarchick J, Das PC, Jones TJ, Russell RJ, Hall SA. Utility of frozen platelets for a platelet antibody assay using flow cytometric analysis. Diag Clin Immunol 1988;5:338-43.

we are doing FACScan on platelet suspensions and it is much more time consuming than to do large series of crossmatches. However, we recently did some radiolabeling studies with the platelets in the ELISA and the first experiments indicate that following cryopreservation, we lose platelets from the bottom of the plate. It could thus very well be that the platelets retain their antigenic activity, which would be in agreement with the flow cytometric data. But in the ELISA the problem is that they are washed away from the plate. When we could improve the coating of the plates, we might solve the problem.

J.J. Sixma: Have you ever tried poly-lysine covered trays?

K. Sintnicolaas: We did try that when we developed the ELISA, but we saw the background values going up using poly-lysine.

J.J. Sixma: Dr. Pflugshaupt, you showed levels of total protein S and free protein S that were in the same range. But the free protein S was expressed as a percentage of a mean value, I mean the actual protein S that is free is about half of what there is in total, is not that so? I make this question for those who are not familiar with it.

R. Pflugshaupt (Bern, CH): That is correct.

C.Th. Smit Sibinga (Groningen, NL): Dr. Pflugshaupt, what actually is the purpose. Would there for instance be a place for looking into the average protein C levels in donors in order to find out what plasma might have an effect on factor VIII_a inactivation or the stability over the further processing in the purification. What are you going to do with it.

Dr. Pflugshaupt: That was not the idea of the study. It is just because we have an analytical laboratory for coagulation and thrombosis where we do protein C and S analyses. We were not sure on what the level is in normal individuals and what their normal range is. It has nothing to do with preparation of anything.

C.Th. Smit Sibinga: Dr. Lindhout pointed out that protein C in its activated state has an effect on the activity of factor VIII, once activated. So, one could imagine that in the present coarse and crude methodology to purify factor VIII from plasma, we might have a beneficial effect from those plasmas in which you have this “neutralizing effect” so to speak of protein C in its activated state on the activity of factor VIII. I am just postulating an idea.

J.J. Sixma: I think two years ago Dr. J. Koedam in our laboratory showed that you do not have to worry about factor VIII as it is present in plasma, because factor VIII on von Willebrand factor is protected against degradation by protein C[2]

A. Greinacher (Giessen, FRG): Dr. Sintnicolaas, we worked quite a long time on this problem storing platelets prepared for crossmatching. We had the same experiences you discussed. So, we came back to a method using platelets stored in saline, where Azide was added to. This combination worked perfectly well. So, I think this type of ELISA technique with saline stored platelets, which do not have any function at all, might be a tool for testing for crossmatch activity.

K. Sintnicolaas: Thank you for this comment.

M.K. Elias (Groningen, NL): Dr. Brozovic or Mr. McShine, how would you explain the more significant increase in mean platelet volume in products containing red cells, as you have shown us. How would the change in mean platelet volume, or the delta mean platelet volume as it says, be used as a quality control test if other factors such as a presence or absence of red cells influence this.

R.L. McShine: Because of the centrifugation process of the whole blood, you probably get separation of the platelets in different populations. The population nearest to red cell concentrate would be different to the population present in platelet rich plasma. Most of the larger platelets are lost in the red cell sediment and these seem to be more sensitive to EDTA delta MPV changes compared to smaller platelets in platelet rich plasma.

J.J. Sixma: Mr. McShine, is it possible that there are differences in pH. Most platelet rich plasmas tend to be rather alkaline, whereas the red blood cell containing blood has a lower pH. Could that influence your results?

R.L. McShine: Possibly! I did not do any pH measurements.

C.Th. Smit Sibinga: Dr. Barrowcliffe, you quite nicely showed that we run slowly into trouble now that we are dealing with much more purified material. Purified in many senses, also according to the definition of Prof. Nilsson, which I like very much. There are different contaminants, different determinants, different matrices. The problem, however, is to obtain from a centre, like yours, appropriate standards to do the assays. What is on the horizon? could you tell us whether in the

2. Koedam JA, Meijers JCM, Sixma JJ, Bouma BN. Inactivation of human factor VIII by activated protein C. Cofactor activity of protein S and protective effect of von Willebrand factor. J Clin Invest 1988;82:1236-43.

concept of WHO reference standardization there is something which first of all really meets the definition of conventional purity, and secondly whether there is something on the horizon which meets the definition of super high purity with completely different matrix.

T.W. Barrowcliffe (Potters Bar, UK): There are things on the horizon. For the conventional products we do not have too much of a problem. We can get a good agreement at least in the studies that we have organized. I am not saying that there are no problems at all. But the problems are fairly well identified and resolvable. For the very high purity products we have seen that we can reduce the variability if we pay attention to some details of the methodology. There are really two general approaches to this. One approach would be to propose "like versus like", which is predominant. So we perhaps need separate standards for the different types of products, in other words more than one factor VIII concentrate standard. We have rather resisted that approach, because it introduces a whole lot more complications. But it may be, for instance, that when the recombinant product comes on the market, we might have to have a separate recombinant standard. The other approach, which I prefer, is to try and find out what are the important things in the assays that contribute towards this variability. Because, after all, if you have a completely specific assay, the contaminants should not matter that much. The aim is to try and allow for this by specifying the details and methodology which are important like for instance the albumin concentration and the method of predilution. Perhaps one could come up with a reference method which people can follow and which can be used in a whole lot of different laboratories, not just in reference centres. So, there are two approaches; one is the possibility of establishing different standards for the different purity products and second is tightening up on the specifications of the methodology.

C.Th. Smit Sibinga: Could I then turn the question to Dr. van den Besselaar, because it immediately relates to the methodology of the testing. When we deal with these extremely pure materials as for instance we have them in our laboratory running off the column, we run into trouble with a number of the premises you need for doing a standardized assay. One of them is in the substrate plasma, which has a completely different matrix than the superpure material coming out of a monoclonal antibody bound column. Secondly the elution buffers also do disturb the system. What would you advise to do.

A.M.H.P. van den Besselaar (Leiden, NL): Well, in fact you dilute your buffers in the assay system. So, I would expect that the more you dilute them, the less effect you experience of the buffer. The buffers used in the one-stage factor VIII clotting assay are usually buffers that do not bind calcium ions. I am not sure what kind of buffers you are using to elute your columns!

K. Koops (Groningen, NL): The buffer we are using contains for instance KI and lysin; that is the main part. We found that especially KI is interfering in the assays and the albumin which is in the buffer, is interfering as well. So, we had a buffer without and with albumin. Without albumin we found normal recoveries of the factor VIII. But with the albumin in it, we found recoveries of more than 150% (calculated), which was of course not possible, otherwise we were generating factor VIII.

A.M.H.P. van den Besselaar: One possibility would be to add the same concentration of your KI to the standards. That would possibly allow to avoid the stabilization problems. According to the principle of assay "like versus like", the test and standard samples should have similar matrix and similar interference with other components. Perhaps you could add the same concentration of KI to your standard plasma.

K. Koops: So, you want to change the matrix of the standard by adding some of the buffer components. I do not know what will be the effect.

A.M.H.P. van den Besselaar: The alternative would be to eliminate the interfering components by dialysis or something.

K. Koops: We have done these experiments by gel filtrating the samples and then looked at the effects of several amounts of KI and albumin, but still there are some discrepancies in the assays.

M. Mikaelsson (Stockholm, S): What type of assay do you use: One-stage or chromogenic assay?

K. Koops: We use the chromogenic assay. However, the KI especially was interfering in the clotting assay.

A.M.H.P. van den Besselaar: Does it interfere with the chromogenic assay?

K. Koops: No, not in the chromogenic assay, but on the other hand albumin is interfering in this assay.

M. Mikaelsson: I am very surprised, because we do not see that type of discrepancy in the chromogenic assay. Do you use the same amount of albumin for your standards etc.?

K. Koops: Yes, it is the same amount as in the dilution buffers for the samples and what is used normally.

T.W. Barrowcliffe: I think one of the points is that your standard is a cryoprecipitate. You have very extreme differences in purity between your material and your standard. Whatever the detailed explanation, I think probably you need to get away from that kind of situation, probably needing a new standard.

J. Over (Amsterdam, NL): Dr. Barrowcliffe, looking at your assay for activated factor VIII, it is quite obvious that the lag phase in generation is decreasing with increasing purity of the factor VIII preparation. Can you exclude that contaminants in the preparations are inhibiting X_a generation?

T.W. Barrowcliffe: No, we cannot exclude that completely. But first of all, there are three lines of evidence which suggest that (it) is not the complete explanation. One is that in some of the intermediate purity preparations, there are quite short lag phases, almost as short as one of the monoclonal products, even though they have all the contaminants of the other intermediate purity including the high von Willebrand factor etc. Another point is the von Willebrand factor, that could be partly responsible for this because a shortening of the lag phase goes with decreasing levels of von Willebrand factor. However, we added von Willebrand factor back to one of the monoclonal products and it did not make any difference. The third point is that I think in your centre the assay of these materials was studied with chromogenic systems. By prediluting in hemophilic plasma an increase rather than a decrease in the rate of X_a generation was observed. So, in other words adding back, if you like, the impurities that are present in hemophilic assay does not depress the rate of X_a generation, at least in your assays.

J. Over: Yes, but that is a completely different system.

T.W. Barrowcliffe: It is a different system, I agree. But I am not saying that it could not be partially responsible. The question is what is activating the factor VIII in this system, because there is no thrombin. If we believe that it is necessary for activation of factor VIII to take place before you get significant X_a generation to happen, how is it that there is extremely rapid X_a generation with recombinant factor VIII in the absence of thrombin.

M. Mikaelsson: Dr. Barrowcliffe, I would like to challenge your interpretation of the activated factor VIII. We have used your assay method and we have been able to reproduce your results, but our interpretation is different. I agree that with an activated factor VIII, you can measure a short X_a generation time. But I do not agree with the interpretation that a short X_a generation time indicates an activated factor VIII. We have performed some experiments where we have added back impurities and thereby we were able to prolong the lag phase. So, I think that if you take your diagrams and add another variant of diagram, where you have on one axis the purity of the concentrate, you will also be able to show a very nice correlation.

T.W. Barrowcliffe: Can you say what impurities you find having most effect?

M. Mikaelsson: I think it is von Willebrand factor, but we have not done studies enough to be sure, yet.

C.Th. Smit Sibinga: Prof. Nilsson, I am extremely delighted with the information you have provided, that actually among the patients there is no difference between the different products used. That is a very important piece of information. The question now comes up, what would you prefer now that we find that these concentrates of different qualities in terms of manufacturing and purities are available. Which one would have your preference?

I.M. Nilsson: I would anyhow prefer to use the most high purity concentrates. First, because of safety reasons, as their virus inactivation is better. The second reason is the immunodepressive effect which contaminants can have. After all, if you have factor VIII deficiency, you need factor VIII and you do not need all the other proteins. In Sweden we now try to use only the superpure concentrates except when we are treating patients with von Willebrand's disease.

IV. CLINICAL CONSEQUENCES

PRINCIPLES IN THE TREATMENT OF BLEEDING[1]

P.M. Mannucci, A.B. Federici

Introduction

When spontaneous or postoperative bleeding is due to an established and recognized defect of the hemostatic system, congenital or acquired, the first treatment of choice should be the specific correction of the defect with blood or blood products. A typical example is replacement of the coagulation factor missing or defective in hemophilias. Frequently, however, either no apparent surgical or hematological cause for abnormal bleeding can be recognized, or recognized defects cannot be corrected. In these situations pharmacological compounds that facilitate control of bleeding by potentiating hemostasis would be a welcome therapeutic weapon. Even though a large number of drugs are marketed as "hemostatic agents" that can stop spontaneous and surgical bleeding and prevent or reduce blood losses, very few of them have been proven by adequate clinical trials to be of clinical value.

In this paper, the principles governing the replacement therapy of patients with congenital coagulation disorders will be illustrated, taking as an example the treatment of factor VIII deficiency (classical hemophilia, hemophilia A), by far the most frequent bleeding disorder of clinical importance. In the second part, we shall review the evidence that led to the demonstration that 1-deamino-8-D-arginine vasopressin (DDAVP, desmopressin) can be used as a hemostatic agent in a number of acquired bleeding disorders of clinical importance.

General principles for treatment of congenital coagulation disorders

There are a number of basic principles for the treatment of patients with congenital coagulation disorders:

1. This work was supported in part by NIH grant RO1/HL41136.

1. Replacement therapy with plasma factor concentrates is the mainstay of treatment.
2. Choosing among the therapeutic concentrates available is based on careful evaluation of such factors as their availability, cost, safety in terms of transmission of blood-borne viral infections and purity, i.e., their content in unnecessary plasma proteins other than the deficient factor.
3. The goal of replacement therapy may be either the prompt arrest of bleeding after its onset (episodic treatment) or prevention of bleeding through the regular administration of the deficient factor (prophylactic treatment).
4. The choice of the system of care delivery (episodic or prophylactic) will depend on the frequency and severity of bleeding episodes, the age of the patient and the status of his joints.
5. Supervised self-treatment is the best system of care of congenital coagulation disorders wherever hematologists are willing to set up such a program and the patients or their parents are sufficiently motivated to implement it.
6. Integration of the multidisciplinary expertise of a team of specialists is necessary for a global approach to the many clinical and psychological problems that a chronic disease such as hemophilia and allied disorders create in patients, their relatives, and in the society in which they live.

Since recently there have been spectacular developments in the availability of safer and purer factor VIII concentrates, we shall address particularly this field and the criteria that can be used to choose among different factor VIII concentrates.

Purer factor VIII concentrates

The industrial preparation of highly-purified factor VIII concentrates, which are commercially available in lyophilized forms, involves a considerable loss of factor VIII during the fractionation process (90% or more for some preparations) and recovers products that are considerably expensive. Depending on the fractionation procedures used by manufacturers, concentrates vary widely in terms of purification and content of contaminating proteins. Until recently, the specific activity of commercial concentrates (units of FVIII:C/mg protein) varied between 0.5 and 2.0, being much greater than that of cryoprecipitate (less than 0.5). In addition to factor VIII, concentrates contained large amounts of other plasma proteins, such as immunoglobulins, fibrinogen and immunocomplexes [1,2]. There is now the tendency for the commercial manufacturers to produce more purified concentrates, with specific activity ranging from 30 to as much as 2,000-3,000 IU/mg protein [3].

Basically, two methods are used to achieve this greater degree of purity. One employs immunoaffinity chromatography with monoclonal antibodies directed against factor VIII or von Willebrand factor (vWF). The other adds a chromatographic step to the production of intermediate-purity concentrates. Purer concentrates have the advantage of containing almost exclusively factor VIII, reducing the infusion of extraneous plasma proteins. The purification process also achieves another important goal, i.e., the removal of a substantial amount of blood-borne viruses which cause life-threatening complications such as the acquired immunodeficiency syndrome and hepatitis (see below). With the addition of virucidal methods, such as various forms of heating the concentrate or a solvent/detergent mixture [4,5], the concentrates now licensed can be considered substantially free from the risk of transmitting HIV and at low risk of transmitting the hepatitis viruses. It was initially demonstrated that the hepatitis viruses were frequently resistant to virucidal methods based on heating the concentrates in the lyophilized state at temperatures from 60°C and 68°C for 24 to 72 hours. Hence, virucidal methods based on "dry heating" have been abandoned (except for heating at 80°C) and replaced by methods in which heating is applied to the concentrate in solution (pasteurization), as hot vapour or in suspension in the organic solvent n-heptane. Clinical trials have now established that virucidal methods based on "wet heating" quite effectively inactivate the hepatitis non-A, non-B viruses, but the hepatitis B virus seems to be more resistant. Finally, virucidal methods other than those based on heating have been developed. The use of a solvent/detergent mixture, for instance, appears to render commercial factor VIII concentrates quite safe [4,5].

Hence, virucidal methods have tremendously increased the safety from hepatitis of large-pool concentrates, and methods are continuously improving. There are good reasons to hope that liver disease will not be a problem for hemophiliacs who are now treated with these safer concentrates from diagnosis. Large-pool concentrates are probably now safer than single-donor or small-pool cryoprecipitate, because virucidal methods cannot yet be applied succesfully to cryoprecipitate. Therefore, the viral safety of this fraction rests only on the screening of the donors, which at the moment gives only limited guarantees.

Choice of concentrates

How should the physician involved in the treatment of hemophilia choose among the multitude of high-technology products that are being offered? Are purer concentrates truly necessary, notwithstanding their higher cost due to much lower yield from source plasma? The evidence in favour of purer concentrates rests on in vitro data and on limited clinical data showing stabilization of T-helper lymphocytes in HIV-infected patients treated exclusively with a monoclonally-purified concentrate [6]. There are, in addition, several theoretical reasons for preferring high-purity concentrates, such as that there will be less bombardment of the immune system with exogenous plasma proteins and less chance that a breakthrough of viral contamination occurs, since the purification procedure per se reduces the potential burden. The tendency of all the manufacturers to switch their production towards purer concentrates is compelling, so that it can be predicted that factor VIII concentrates with specific activity lower than 100 will soon no longer be available. Therefore, while waiting for the wide spread availability of recombinant factor VIII, which impact on the therapy of hemophilia cannot be predicted at the moment, it seems inevitable that we will treat hemophiliacs with purer concentrates, which offer many theoretical advantages over the less purified concentrates available until few years ago. Whether or not it is necessary to resort to the use of concentrates of very high specific activity (2,000-3,000 IU/mg) produced by immunoaffinity chromatography using monoclonal antibodies or whether it is sufficient to use concentrates of lower specific activity (130-250 IU/mg) purified by conventional chromatographic techniques, remains to be established by long-term comparative studies of the effects of these concentrates on the immune system. At the moment, monoclonally-purified concentrates should perhaps be the treatment of choice for HIV-infected patients, on the basis of the hypothesis that their negligible content in exogenous proteins would avoid or slow activation of T-helper (CD4) lymphocytes, HIV replication and infection of previously uninfected cells. For patients not infected with HIV, concentrates with lower specific activity are probably adequate and should be preferred because their price is lower than that of monoclonally-purified concentrates.

Conclusion

There have been shadows and lights around hemophilia in the last few years. Although the infection of hemophiliacs with HIV contaminated clotting factor concentrates is still a threatening and formidable shadow, the gloomy picture brought about by the AIDS epidemic is partially lightened by spectacular improvements in therapy. An important step-forward towards the elimination of the risk of blood-borne infections transmitted by plasma products was recently made through the development of virucidal methods and their application to clotting factor concentrates. Since HIV appears more vulnerable to such methods than the hepatitis viruses, currently available concentrates can be considered substantially free from the risk of transmitting HIV infection. Even though transmission of hepatitis is much reduced but not totally abolished, virucidal methods are continuously being improved, so that it can be foreseen that concentrates will become safer and safer. Another important recent advance is the production of ultrapure factor VIII concentrates using immunoaffinity chromatographic techniques based on monoclonal antibodies. Not only these concentrates are at least as safe as less pure concentrates in terms of transmission of blood-borne viral infections, there is also a hint that the deteriorating immune system of HIV-positive hemophiliacs may be stabilized by these highly purified concentrates. Since the bombardment of lymphocytes with multiple alloantigens can activate latent HIV, the use of ultrapure factor concentrates may keep the virus latent longer, although clinical trials are needed to validate this hypothesis. Finally, factor VIII produced by recombinant DNA technology is undergoing the first clinical trials in hemophiliacs. Hopefully, it will be free from the risk of transmitting infections and will be available in sufficiently large amounts to meet the need of hemophiliacs worldwide.

DDAVP as hemostatic agent

Recently 1-deamino-8-D-arginine vasopressin (DDAVP, desmopressin), an analogue of the antidiuretic hormone vasopressin, gained the status of hemostatic agent, because not only does it stop bleeding and reduce blood losses in patients with some congenital and acquired disorders of hemostasis, it also reduces blood losses in individuals with normal hemostasis.

Unlike the parent hormone, DDAVP has little or no effect on V_1 vasopressin receptors of the smooth muscle, with the ratio of its antidiuretic activity (related to stimulation of V_2, cyclic AMP-dependent receptors) to its pressor activity (related to V_1, phosphatidylinositol-dependent receptors) approximately 3,000 to 4,000 times greater than that of vasopressin. Hence, DDAVP causes little or no vasoconstriction and does not increase blood pressure or contract the uterus or the gastrointenstinal tract, all effects resulting from stimulation of V_1 receptors. Molecular tailoring has created a derivative of vasopressin with fewer side effects than the parent hormone.

DDAVP does increase factor VIII and vWF when given intravenously to healthy volunteers and patients with mild hemophilia and von Willebrand disease (vWD)[7,8]. This property, based upon the release into plasma of the factors from endogenous stores, has been exploited to treat patients with deficiencies without using blood products, with their inherent risk of transmitting blood-borne viral infections. On the whole, more than ten years of experience have now established the place of DDAVP for management of bleeding in selected patients with hemophilia and vWD. The relationship in these disorders between the levels of the deficient factors (and of the bleeding time in vWD) obtained after DDAVP treatment and the arrest of clinical bleeding is so direct that no controlled, double-blind trial has ever been deemed necessary.

More recently DDAVP has also been used to treat bleeding disorders other than factor VIII- and vWF-deficiency states, such as those that accompany uremia, platelet function defects and liver cirrhosis. The efficacy of DDAVP in these acquired disorders led to postulate that DDAVP may be efficacious in stopping bleeding and reducing surgical blood losses whatever the reason underlying their bleeding tendency. Accordingly, there have been controlled clinical trials to see whether or not DDAVP is useful during surgical operations in which blood losses are unusually large and for which blood transfusions are often needed (with a high risk of transmitting blood-borne viruses). When given to hemostatically normal subjects before spinal fusion surgery for scoliosis, DDAVP shortened their bleeding times, even though they were previously normal for all subjects [9]. In addition, the average operative blood losses were reduced by about one third in the group given DDAVP. This is especially important because many of the patients undergoing this operation are children. DDAVP or placebo were also given to patients undergoing cardiac surgery requiring cardiopulmonary bypass (not uncomplicated coronary artery grafts) [10]. In those patients, postoperative bleeding adds significantly to the morbidity and the cost of the surgery. There are probably many pathophysiological factors in the hemorrhagic tendency. One of the major ones is acquired platelet dysfunction, causing a prolongation of the postoperative bleeding time out of proportion to the degree of thrombocytopenia. DDAVP reduced operative and early (12 hours) postoperative blood loss and transfusion requirements by about one third [10]. On the other hand, in another controlled trial of patients undergoing cardiopulmonary bypass surgery there were no significant differences in either total blood loss or in red cell transfusion requirements after DDAVP and placebo, although intraoperative blood loss was reduced by DDAVP [11].

On the whole, these studies indicate that DDAVP is effective for reducing blood losses and transfusion requirements in both patients with defective hemostatic systems (such as those on cardiopulmonary bypass) and hemostatically normal individuals (such as those undergoing spinal fusion). More general use of DDAVP to reduce blood losses and transfusion requirements in other surgical operations remains to be explored in clinical trials. It is obvious that such trials are urgently needed because the acquired immunodeficiency syndrome and post-transfusion hepatitis are so threatening to those who require blood transfusions.

References

1. Berntorp E, Nilsson IM. Biochemical and in vivo properties of commercial virus-inactivated factor VIII concentrates. Eur J Haematol 1988;40:205-14.

2. Morfini M, Rafanelli D, Filimberti E, et al. Protein content and factor VIII complex in untreated, treated and monoclonal factor VIII concentrates. Thromb Res 1989;56:169-78.
3. Brettler DB, Levine PH. Factor concentrates for treatment of hemophilia: Which one to choose? Blood 1989;73:2067-71.
4. Mannucci PM, Colombo M. Virucidal treatment of clotting factor concentrates. Lancet 1988;ii:782-5.
5. Pierce GF, Lusher JM, Brownstein AP, Goldsmith SC, Kessler CM. The use of purified clotting factor concentrates in hemophilia. JAMA 1989;261: 3434-7.
6. Brettler DB, Forsberg AD, Levine PH, Petillo J, Lamon K, Sullivan SL. Factor VIII:C concentrate purified from plasma using monoclonal antibodies: Human studies. Blood 1989;73:1859-63.
7. Mannucci PM, Aberg M, Nilsson IM, Robertson B. Mechanism of plasminogen activator and factor VIII increase after vasoactive drugs. Br J Haematol 1975;30:81-93.
8. Mannucci PM, Pareti FI, Holmberg L, Ruggeri ZM, Nilsson IM. Studies on the prolonged bleeding time in von Willebrand disease. J Lab Clin Med 1976;88:662-9.
9. Kobrinsky NL, Letts RP, Patel RL, et al. DDAVP shortens the bleeding time and decreases blood loss in hemostatically normal subjects undergoing spinal fusion surgery. Ann Intern Med 1987;107:446-50.
10. Salzman EW, Weinstein MJ, Weitraub RM, et al. Treatment with desmopressin acetate to reduce blood loss after cardiac surgery. N Engl J Med 1986;314:1402-6.
11. Rocha E, Llorens R, Paramo JA, et al. Does desmopressin acetate reduce blood loss after surgery in patients on cardiopulmonary bypass? Circulation 1988;77:1319-23.

THE EFFECT OF CHRONIC EXPOSURE TO CLOTTING FACTOR CONCENTRATES ON THE IMMUNE SYSTEM[1]

C.R.M. Hay

Introduction

Abnormalities of immune function occur in hemophilic patients independently of HIV infection [1-3]. These abnormalities arise as a result of the treatment, since untreated hemophiliacs are unaffected. These defects develop during childhood and adolescence [4,5] but remain stable over long periods in adult life. Although abnormalities of almost every aspect of immune function have been described in treated hemophiliacs, they are milder than the immune defects observed in AIDS and are not associated with opportunist infection.

The abnormalities observed in these patients include decreased T-helper cell and increased T-suppressor cell numbers [1-3], defective [6], and impaired cell-mediated immunity as reflected by cutaneous anergy [7]. B-cell abnormalities including an increased incidence of autoantibodies [8] and increased concentrations of B-cell growth and differentiation factors [9] have also been described. Monocytes from patients with hemophilia show impaired phagocytosis and antigen presentation [10,11], decreased Fc receptor expression and decreased oxygen radicle production [12].

Causes of immune dysfunction in hemophilia

Why does immune dysfunction develop in hemophilia? Although links with NANB hepatitis or CMV have been suggested immune dysfunction is also observed in CMV-seronegative patients and patients without active liver disease. In any case, phagocytosis is subnormal within two hours of factor VIII infusion [10,11], and lymphocyte dysfunction is induced by incubation with factor VIII concentrate [3], arguing against a viral etiology. Others point to the importance of chronic ex-

1. This work was supported by the Haemophilia Society, grant no. 431932, and the University of Liverpool grant no. RD5267.

posure to alloantigens. Levine calculates that a typical patient exposed to factor VIII concentrate 40-60 times a year may be exposed to blood from between 1 to 2,000,000 people annually. This represents parenteral contact with multiple alloantigens and viruses without parallel in medicine. Most authorities attribute immune dysfunction to some contaminant or contaminants in the concentrate although the culprit contaminant remains to be identified, and its mode of action is still speculative.

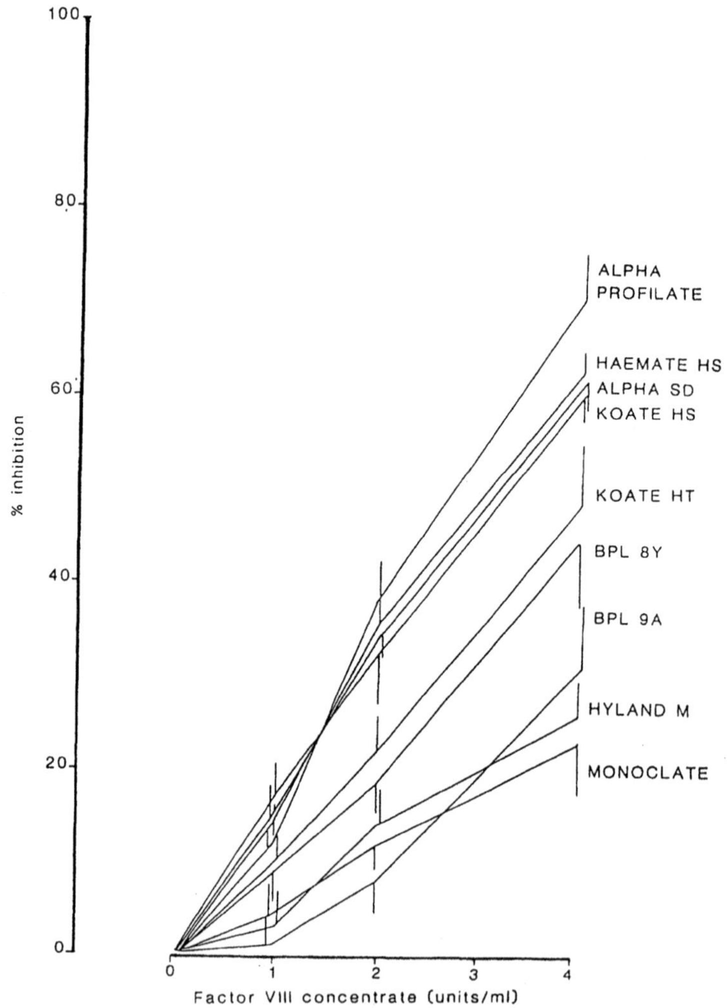

Figure 1. The variable inhibitory effect of diverse clotting factor concentrates on lymphocyte transformation with PHA expressed as percentage inhibition relative to the control (taken as zero).

Eible and Mannhalter have suggested that monocyte dysfunction in hemophilia is caused by immune complexes and immunoglobulin aggregates [10,12]. These are present in very small amounts in all concentrates and are thought to cause Fc-receptor blockade. This concept is supported by the work of Pasi et al who found that concentrates varied in their capacity to inhibit monocyte phagocytic activity in vitro [11]. They found that the degree of inhibition of monocyte phagocytic activity correlated loosely with the presence of immune complexes and with purity, the purest immunopurified concentrate having only a minimal effect on monocyte function. Eible suggestes that even the nanomolar concentrations of murine antibodies present in immunopurified concentrates may cause some impairement of monocyte function. If true, this would almost certainly also complicate treatment with recombinant factor VIII concentrate.

The contaminant responsible for lymphocyte dysfunction in hemophilia has not been identified. Various groups have attempted to identify the culprit by comparing concentrates prepared by various processes. Concentrates vary considerably in their capacity to impair immune function, both in vivo and in vitro. The effect of various factor VIII concentrates, in several concentrations, on lymphocyte transformation to PHA expressed as percentage inhibition relative to a control value is shown in Figure1. Similar results are obtained with other lectins, phorbol esters and in the mixed lymphocyte reaction. We can see that BPL factor IX and high purity immunopurified factor VIII cause little inhibition of lymphocyte transformation whereas "intermediate-purity" concentrates cause a variable but far greater degree of inhibition. Similar results have been obtained by a number several investigators, and they correspond with the limited data available on the effects of these products in vivo.

Such experiments have given rise to a plethora of reports, many appearing in abstract form only, in which the degree of inhibition of lymphocyte function has been said to correlate with the concentration of one contaminant or another. The possible culprits include total protein, immunoglobulin, immune complexes, factor VIII:C, VIIIRA, high molecular weight von Willebrand multimers, fibrinogen, factor XIII, fibronectin, citrate, and decreased ionized calcium. None of these apparent associations has survived closer examination, however. Whenever the effects of a larger number of brands is tested, the association between the contaminant and degree of immune modulation always disappears.

Mechanisms underlying lymphocyte dysfunction in hemophilia

Although the cause of these abnormalities of lymphocyte function is unknown, the underlying mechanisms are perhaps a little less obscure. The effect of factor VIII concentrate on lymphocyte IL-2 secretion has been particularly intensively investigated since proliferation of lymphocytes is largely IL-2 driven. Several groups have shown that concentrates cause profound, dose-dependent, reduction in IL-2 secretion [13-15]. Madhok et al have also shown that hemophilic patients have subnormal IL-2 secretion indicating that this is not merely a test-tube phenomenon [14]. Thorpe et al have shown that concentrates vary in their effect on lymphocyte IL-2 secretion, intermediate purity being far more inhibitory than high purity concentrates [15]. These investigators suggest that suppression of IL-2 secretion is the principal cause of lymphocyte dysfunction in hemophilia.

Lymphocyte transformation also requires up-regulation of the IL-2 receptor, since optimal IL-2 secretion is dependent upon this in a classical positive feedback loop [16]. Concentrate may therefore in-

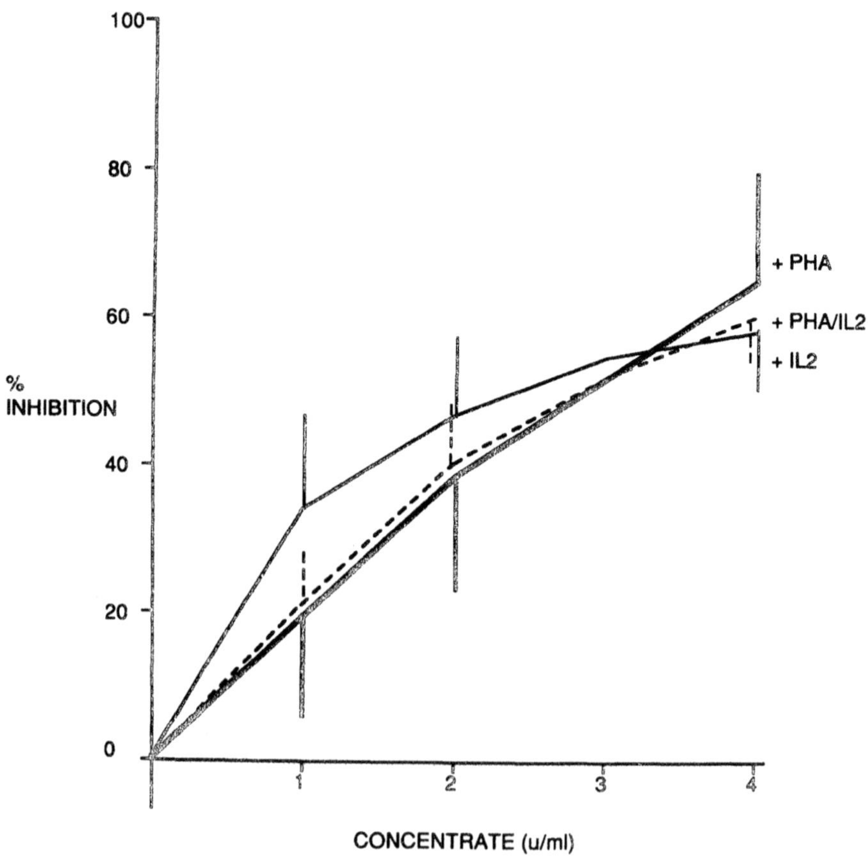

Figure 2. The percentage inhibition (mean +/– SEM) of lymphocyte transformation by factor VIII concentrate using PHA, PHA and IL-2, and IL-2 alone as stimulators.

hibit lymphocyte function not only by reducing IL-2 secretion but by inhibiting IL-2-receptor expression.

We investigated the effect of concentrate on lymphocyte IL-2 secretion by attempting to correct the inhibitory effect of factor VIII concentrate on lymphocytes stimulated with PHA, and incubated with factor VIII concentrate, by adding an excess of IL-2 [17]. The percentage inhibition caused by the concentrate was unaffected by this, and remained unchanged whether PHA alone, IL-2 alone, or both IL-2 and PHA were used as stimulators (Figure2). Although concentrates do inhibit IL-2 secretion, this cannot be the sole cause of lymphocyte dysfunction in hemophilia, since optimal concentrations of IL-2 do not correct the defect.

We investigated the effect of concentrate on IL-2-receptor expression using mononuclear cells stimulated with PHA and incubated in the presence or absence of factor VIII concentrate [17]. The effect of concentrate on the expression of several cell-surface receptors was analysed in a flow-cytometer using a dual-staining technique.

The presence of factor VIII concentrate caused a marked 7-fold reduction in the percentage of CD4 and CD8 cells expressing the IL-2 receptor with far lesser reductions in HLA-DR and CD71 expression (Figure3). A substantial 50% reduction in the number of IL-2 receptors expressed per cell was also observed, CD4 and CD8 lymphocytes being equally affected. This suggests that inhibition of lymphocyte function by pooled blood products is largely mediated by inhibition of IL-2 receptor expression. This may account for the failure of exogenous IL-2 to correct the defect, and may also account for the reduced IL-2 production observed by other authors since up-regulation of the IL-2 receptor is required for optimal IL-2 secretion.

Clinical significance of immune dysfunction in hemophilia

Is immune dysfunction in HIV-seronegative hemophilic patients clinically significant? This is the $64,000 question. Certainly the evidence that these immune defects cause clinical problems is not immediately obvious. HIV-negative hemophilic patients do not suffer opportunist infections, but do they have an increased susceptibility to standard pathogens or an increased incidence of malignancy?

An association between the mild immunosuppressive effects of clotting factor concentrates and an increased incidence of malignancy might be expected since similar immune defects occurring secondary to blood transfusion have been associated by some authors with an increased risk of metastases and decreased survival following cancer surgery [18]. Indeed, some authorities report that this association is found with the transfusion of whole blood but not packed cells, thus implicating the plasma component [19]. This contrasts with enhanced

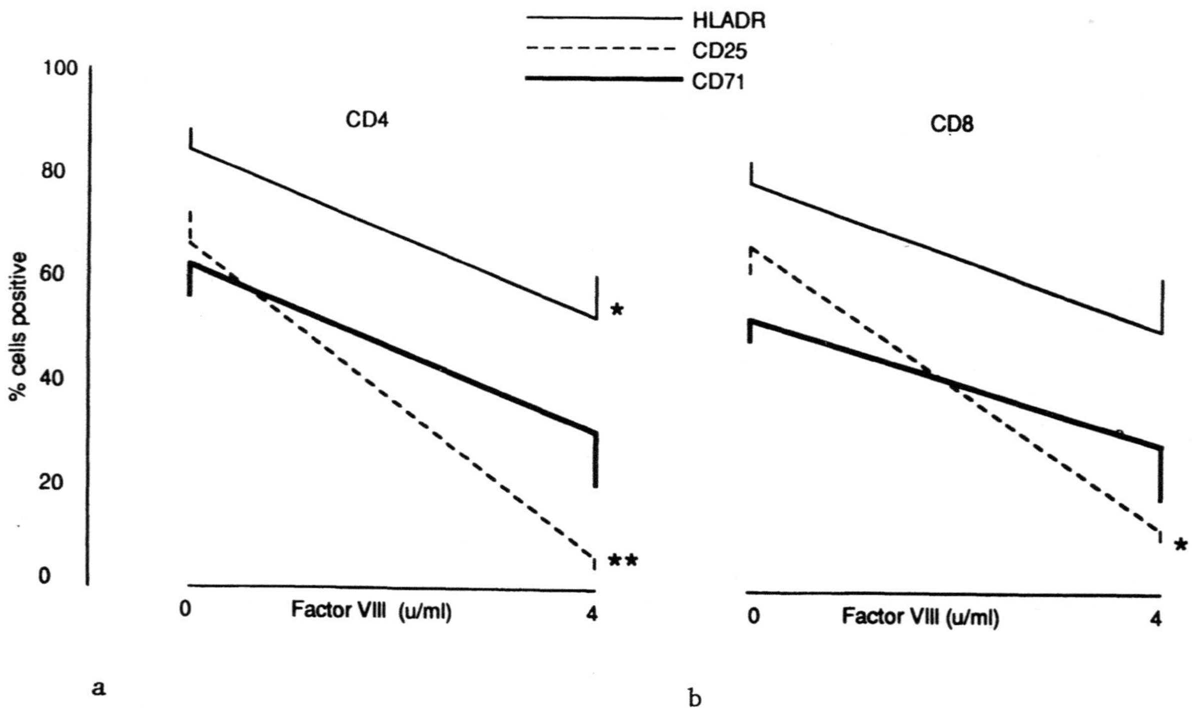

Figure 3. The effect of factor VIII concentrate on the percentage of CD4 and CD8 lymphocytes expressing HLA-DR, CD71 and CD25 following incubation with PHA (mean +/– SEM, * P<0.01, ** P<0.001).

renal graft survival observed following multiple blood transfusion, an effect usually attributed to transfused leukocytes [20].

Reports of the cause of death in hemophiliacs dying in the pre-HIV era suggest that immune dysfunction may be significant, but can be difficult to interpret. Aronson reported an increased mortality from pneumonia in 949 US hemophilic patients dying before 1979 [21]. Rizza et al observed a similar excess of pneumonia when reviewing the cause of death of 89 UK hemophiliacs who died between 1976 and 1980 [22]. Aronson also noted a high incidence of carcinoma of the lung, but was unable to assess whether the age adjusted mortality from malignancy was increased, even though the median age at death of his patients was only 44 years [21]. Rosendaal et al observed a 2.5-fold age-adjusted excess incidence of carcinoma, mainly carcinoma of the lung, but decreased mortality from ischemic heart disease amongst 43 Dutch hemophiliacs who died between 1973 and 1986 [23]. These authors did not observe increased mortality from pneumonia. Although other explanations are possible, the immunosuppressive effects of clotting factor concentrates may be responsible for this increased risk of carcinoma and pneumonia.

It is interesting that none of these surveys show an increased prevalence of lymphoma. Isolated reports of lymphoma occurring in HIV-seronegative patients have appeared [24]. These lymphomas have sometimes been extranodal and small clusters have been described, although it is not clear whether they are more frequent than expected by chance. Ludlam in Edingburgh is currently conducting a survey of UK hemophiliacs to determine whether the prevalence of lymphoma in HIV-seronegative hemophiliacs is increased. If hemophilic patients do suffer an excess incidence of malignancy secondary to immune dysfunction this may only become apparent after a latent period. Pooled blood products have only been widely available over the past fifteen years, and so an increased risk of malignancy may only now be becoming apparent as the population ages.

Evidence that hemophilic patients may be unusually susceptible to non-fatal infections is, by its very nature, difficult to come by, particularly since meaningful statistics on the prevalence of such infections in age-matched normal males are often unavailable.

Blood transfusion has been reported to interfere with macrophage function, and to be an independent risk factor for post-operative infection in non-hemophilic patients [25,26]. Hemophilic patients might also be expected to have an increased risk of post-operative infection in much the same way. HIV-seronegative hemophilic patients subjected to joint arthroplasty have a 2% incidence of late joint infection compared with 0.5% in non-hemophilic patients and 10% in HIV-seropositive hemophilic patients [27]. Staphylococci, pneumococci, or Hemophilus influenzae are the commonests isolates. The increased risk of infection has been attributed to an increased risk of hematogenous spread relating to hemarthroses. Joint replacement is usually accompanied by a dramatic reduction in the frequency of hemarthroses. It could be equally well argued that immunosuppression by blood products may be responsible for this increased susceptibility to infection.

Beddall et al reported an outbreak of tuberculosis occurring on a hematology ward in 1981 [28,29]. The index case was a parent subsequently discovered to have open tuberculosis who visited the ward over a three week period. Of the 15 boys with severe hemophilia admitted to the ward during this time eight developed a positive Mantoux test, and six developed primary tuberculosis. This rate of infection was similar to that found in the inpatients with hematological malignancy, some of whome developed miliary tuberculosis, and far greater than that found in the general pediatric patients on the ward [29]. This suggests that although they dealt with the infection normally, hemophilic boys may be more susceptible to tuberculosis, possibly because of faulty monocyte antigen presentation.

Scanty evidence is also available that immune dysfunction in hemophilia may result in abnormal susceptibility and handling of virus infections. Ludlam et al, reporting an outbreak of HIV-infection relating to a single contaminated batch of concentrate in a previous HIV-negative population, was able to show that those patients with the lowest T4-helper cell counts prior to exposure to HIV were most likely to become infected with the virus [30]. Hemophilic patients may also deal with hepatitis viruses abnormally. More than 80% of hemophilic patients treated with unheated concentrates have chronic liver disease [31,32]. This is a greater proportion than can be accounted for by the main known pathogens, hepatitis C and hepatitis B, usually associated with chronic liver disease in 50% [33] and 10% [34] of infected patients, respectively. Although this very high prevalence of liver disease may be accounted for by exposure to multiple hepatotropic viruses [35] including viruses not yet characterized, it may also result from clinically significant immunosuppresion by blood products.

There is thus a large, if not overwhelming, body of evidence to suggest that intermediate-purity clotting factor concentrates cause defective immunity, and that this is probably associated with a moderately increased susceptibility to standard pathogens and possibly an increased prevalence of malignancy. There are alternative explanations for many of the observations. Carefully conducted prospective monitoring is necessary to establish the clinical significance of immune dysfunction in HIV-seronegative hemophiliacs.

Clinical trials: "Is purer better?"

Will high-purity concentrates, either recombinant or immunoaffinity purified, be any better than the more traditional products? Certainly previously untreated patients (PUPS) treated only with immunoaffinity purified factor VIII over a period of at least four years develop no abnormalities of immune function. Whether previously treated patients with established immune dysfunction will benefit from treatment with high-purity concentrates is a more difficult question to answer.

Following the suggestion of Margolick et al [36], several groups, most notably that of Levine, have investigated the effect of high-purity factor VIII concentrate on HIV disease progression, since activation of the immune system may increase the rate of viral replication. It is hoped that the T4-helper cell counts of patients using only high-purity concentrates might stabilize or at least decline more slowly than in patients using intermediate purity concentrate. The inconclusive results of Levine's pilot study will be familiar [37]. The interim results of their current study, reported in June 1990 are shown here. In this study 34 HIV-seropositive hemophiliacs have been randomized to continue treatment with intermediate purity factor VIII concentrate, and 35 randomized to treatment with immunoaffinity purified Monoclate. The Monoclate group had a lower mean age, and slightly higher T4s at the outset. Although these differences did not achieve statistical significance, both may influence disease progression. After between 20 and 24 months the mean T4-count in the Monoclate group had risen from 0.41 to 0.49, whereas it had fallen from 0.32 to 0.25 in the intermediate purity group. This trend does not achieve statistical significance, but suggests that patients on high-purity will do better, and it is planned to continue the trial for a further twelve months.

The two groups in this trial were arguably not ideally matched at the outset. Rocino et al from Napels adopted a slightly different approach taking two groups of ten HIV-positive patients, carefully matched for age and T4-helper cell count, and allocated one group of Haemophil M whilst the other group continued treatment with intermediate purity concentrate [38]. The T4 count remained stable in the Monoclate group whereas it declined to such an extent in the intermediate purity group that the trial was discontinued after twelve months on ethical grounds. By this time the difference between the two groups had achieved statistical significance with a p-value of less than 0.0007. This is a small study but again suggests that HIV-positive patients may benefit from high-purity concentrate.

As the natural history of HIV unfolds such trials become progressively more difficult to conduct and confounding variables more difficult to deal with. Such trials may never provide a definitive answer to the question "is purer better"? Similar trials have started in seronegative individuals and when the results become available in a couple of years, they should be a little easier to interpret.

How pure is pure factor VIII concentrate? All recombinant and immunoaffinity purified concentrates are stabilized with plasma-derived, pasteurized albumin. This is presumed inoccuous although there is no long-term experience of repeated administration of albumin and despite the fact that it is not pure, as the list of impurities demonstrates. Since Parvovirus has been shown to be resistant to pasteurization, human albumin cannot be regarded as totally safe from the virological point of view. Although Monoclate and Haemophil M have a lower final specific activity after the albumin stabilizer is added than some of the newer chromatographically purified concentrates, they inhibit immune function far less in vitro, suggesting that the albumin is much less likely to cause immune dysfunction than the impurities in the chromatographically purified concentrate. Ideally, however, some other stabilizer should be found.

Immunosuppression by blood products may not always by harmful, and may have a favourable influence on factor VIII inhibitor development. PUP studies of rVIII:C and Monoclate certainly show a very high 28% and 15% incidence of FVIII:C inhibitors, the latter study after a startingly short mean follow-up period of only nine months. The Haemophil M study with its low incidence of inhibitors, is not directly comparable since it was conducted in a far older population. The true prevalence of inhibitors in newly treated patients is probably unknown, however, since testing is not usually done on such a regular basis. It has been argued that these studies show no more than the expected prevalence of inhibitors although most authorities would expect inhibitors in only 10-12% of patients. The mild immunosuppression caused by intermediate-purity concentrates may reduce or at least defer inhibitor development but larger studies and longer follow up will be required before these arguments can be resolved.

Conclusions

To return to the important question, is immune dysfunction harmful to HIV negative hemophilic patients? It may be years before we can be sure. Is purer better? This is unknown. If and when the answer becomes known it may not be a straight choice especially if the prevalence of inhibitors is increased. Indeed, will this question ever be answered? The large prospective study required to provide the answer is becoming increasingly difficult to conduct and many clinicians are already turning to the newer products. Even though Levines' laws 87a through 87c do not constitute a scientific argument they strike a cord with clinicians who cautiously waited until liver disease and HIV were proved to be genuine problems before adopting heat treated concentrates and now want to give the patient the benefit of the doubt. No-one wants another sad legacy in five or ten years. As one hemophilia centre director said to me "which concentrate would you give yourself"? If the answer is high purity, is it reasonable to use another product merely because of cost. Thus, despite their high cost, and the lack of irrefutable scientific evidence in their favour high purity concentrates account for a growing market share, and may well be the way forward.

References

1. Carr R, Edmond E, Prescott RJ, et al. Abnormalities of circulating lymphocyte subsets in haemophiliacs in an AIDS-free population. Lancet 1984;i: 1431-4.
2. Madhok R, Gracie A, Lowe GDO. Impaired cell mediated immunity in haemophilia in the absence of infection with human immunodeficiency virus. BrMedJ 1986;293:978-80.
3. Menitove JE, Aster RH, Casper JT, et al. T-lymphocyte subpopulations in patients with classical haemophilia treated with cryoprecipitate and lyophylised concentrates. NEngl JMed 1983;308:83-6.
4. Kessler CM, Schulof RS, Alibaster O, et al. Inverse correlation between age related abnormalities of T-cell immunity and circulating thymosin alpha-1 levels in haemophilia A. BrJ Haematol 1984;58:325-36.
5. Shannon BT, Roach J, Cheek-Luten M, Orosz C, Ruymann FB. Progressive change in lymphocyte distribution and degree of hypergammaglobulinaemia with age in children with hemophilia. JClin Immunol 1986;6: 121-9.
6. Froebel KS, Madhok R, Forbes CD, Lennie SE, Lowe GDO, Sturrock RD. Immunological abnormalities in haemophilia: Are they caused by American factor VIII concentrate? BrMedJ 1983;287:1091-3.
7. Brettler DB, Forsberg AD, Brewster F, Sullivan JL, Levine PH. Delayed cutaneous hypersensitivity reactions in hemophilic subjected treated with factor concentrate. AmJ Med 1986;81:607-11.
8. David J. Immune response mechanisms. In: Rubenstein E, Federman DD (eds). Scientific American Medicine. New York, NY: Scientific American Inc, 1987;111:1-15.
9. Matheson DS, Green BJ, Fritzler MJ, Poon MC, Bowen TJ, Hoar DI. Humoral immune response in patients with haemophilia. Clin Immunol Immunopathol 1987;4:41-50.
10. Mannhalter JW, Zlabinger GJ, Ahmad R, Zielinski CC, Schramm W, Eible MM. A functional defect in the early phase of the immune response observed in patients with haemophilia A. Clin Immunol Immunopathol 1986; 38:390-7.
11. Pasi KJ, Hill FGH. In vitro and in vivo inhibition of monocyte phagocytic function by factor VIII concentrates: Correlation with concentrate purity. BrJ Haematol 1990;76:88-93.
12. Eible MM, Ahmad R, Wolf HM, Linnau Y, Gotz E, Mannhalter JW. Acomponent of factor VIII preparations which can be separated from factor VIII activity down modulates human monocyte functions. Blood 1987;69:1153-60.

13. Lederman MM, Saunders C, Toosi Z, Lemon N, Everson B, Ratnoff OD. Antihaemophilic factor preparations inhibit lymphocyte proliferation and production of interleukin 2. JLab Clin Med 1986;107:471-8.
14. Madhok R, Gracie JA, Smith J, Lowe GDO, Forbes CD. Capacity to produce interleukin 2 is impaired in haemophilia in the absence and presence of HIV 1 infection. BrJ Haematol 1990;76:70-4.
15. Thorpe R, Dilger P, Dawson NJ, Barrowcliffe TW. Inhibition of interleukin-2 secretion by factor VIII concentrates: A possible cause of immunosuppression in haemophiliacs. BrJ Haematol 1989;71:387-91.
16. Smith KA. Interleukin 2. Annual Reviews of Immunology 1984;2:319-33.
17. Hay CRM, McEvoy P, Duggan-Keen M. Inhibition of lymphocyte IL2-receptor expression by factor VIII concentrate: A possible cause of immunosuppression in haemophiliacs. BrJ Haematol 1990;75:278-81.
18. Burrows L, Tartter P. Effect of blood transfusion on colonic malignancy recurrence rate. Lancet 1982;ii:662-5.
19. Blumberg N, Heal JM, Murphy P. Association between transfusion of whole blood and recurrence of cancer. Br MedJ 1986;293:530-3.
20. Proud G, Shenton BK, Smith BM. Blood transfusion and renal transplantation. Br J Surgery 1979;66:678-82.
21. Aronson DL. Cause of death in haemophilia A patients in the United States from 1968 to 1979. AmJ Haematol 1988;27:7-12.
22. Rizza C, Spooner RJD. Treatment of haemophilia and related disorders in Britain and Northern Ireland during 1976-80: Report on behalf of the directors of haemophilia centres in the Untied Kingdom. Br MedJ 1983;286: 829-33.
23. Rosendaal FR, Varekamp I, Smit C, et al. Mortality and causes of death in Dutch haemophiliacs, 1973-86. BrJ Haematol 1989;71:71-6.
24. Madhok R, Lowe GDO, Forbes CD, Stewart CJR. Extranodal lymphoma in a haemophiliac negative for antibody to HIV-1. Br MedJ 1987;294:679-80.
25. Tartter PI, Quintero S, Barron DM. Perioperative blood transfusion associated with infectious complications after colorectal cancer operations. AM J Surgery 1986;152:479-82.
26. Dawes LG, Aprahamian C, Condoin RE, Malangoni MA. The risk of infection after colon injury. Surgery 1986;100:796-803.
27. Green WB, DeGnore LT, White GC. Orthopaedic procedures and prognosis in hemophilic patients who are seropositive for human immunodeficiency virus. JBone Joint Surg 1990;72:2-11.
28. Beddal AC, Hill FGH, George RH, Williams MD, Al-Rubei K. Unusually high incidence of tuberculosis among boys with haemophilia during an outbreak of the disease in hospital. JClin Path 1985;38:1163-5.
29. Hill JD, Stevenson JK. Tuberculosis in unvaccinated children, adolescents and young adults: A city epidemic. Br MedJ 1983;286:1471-3.
30. Ludlam CA, Tucker J, Steel CM, et al. Human T-lymphocyte virus typeIII (HTLV-III) infection in seronegative haemophiliacs after transfusion of factor VIII. Lancet 1985;ii:233-6.
31. Hay CRM, Preston FE, Triger DR, Underwood JCE. Progressive liver disease in haemophilia: An understated problem? Lancet 1985;i:1495-8.
32. Spero JA, Lewis JH, van Thiel DH, Hasiba U, Rabin BS. Asymptomatic structural liver disease in haemophiliacs. NEngl JMed 1978;31:779-83.

33. Koretz RL, Stone D, Gitnick GL. The long-term course of non-A, non-B hepatitis. Gastroenterology 1980;79:893-8.
34. Wright R, Millward-Sadler GH. Chornic hepatitis. In: Wright R, Millward-Sadler GH, Alberti KGMM, Karran S (eds). Liver and biliary disease: Pathophysiology, diagnosis and management. Baillière Tindall: Saunders Corp 1985:769-820.
35. Lee CA, Kernoff PBA, Karayiannis P, Farci P, Thomas HC. Interactions between hepatotropic viruses in patients with haemophilia. JHepatology 1985;1: 379-84.
36. Margolick JB, Volkman DJ, Folks TM, Fauci AS. Amplification of HTLV-III/LAV infection by antigen-induced activation of T cells and direct suppression by virus of lymphocyte blastogenic responses. J Immunol 1987; 138:1719-23.
37. Brettler DB, Forsberg AD, Levine PH, Petillo J, Lamon K, Sullivan JL. Factor VIII:C concentrate purified from plasma using monoclonal antibodies: Human studies. Blood 1989;73:1859-63.
38. Rocino A, Miraglia E, Mastrullo L, Quirino AA, Ziello L, De Biasi R. Prospective controlled trial of an ultra-pure factor VIII concentrate to evaluate the effects on immune status of HIV antibody-positive hemophilia patients (preliminary results). Estratto da: "Acta Toxicologica et Therapeutica" 1990;XI:(1):49-58.

LIVER TRANSPLANTATION AND BLOOD USAGE

R.A.F. Krom, S.R. Rettke, H.F. Taswell, K.R. Williamson, R.H. Wiesner

Liver transplantation and blood usage

During the last 20 years, liver transplantation has been characterized as a long procedure, technically difficult for surgeons and anesthesiologists, and a nightmare for the blood bank. Blood loss, the common denominator in the problems, is found to be directly related to survival after liver transplantation [1] and creates an enormous challenge for the blood bank in order to support the sometimes excessive need for blood products during the operative procedure.

Per operative blood loss can be caused by:

1. surgical complications, leading to a major blood loss;
2. a poor quality of the graft, possibly caused by unfavorable donor circumstances or by preservation factors, leading to severe coagulopathy and blood loss;
3. the poor clinical condition of the patient with end-stage liver disease and its related abnormal coagulation.

Surgical technical complications are often caused by the sequelae of previous abdominal surgery like bile duct operations and porto-systemic shunts. Previous abdominal surgery leads often to an above-average blood loss [2] but with the exception of a protocaval shunt does not influence patient survival [3].

Poor early graft function is related to factors in the organ donor, like prolonged hypotension and sepsis, and to preservation like its total duration and the period of warm ischemia. Immediately after recirculation of the donor liver, activation of fibrinolysis and subsequent destruction of factor VIII, factor V and factor I have been demonstrated [4]. This is thought to be caused by release of tissue plasminogen activator from vascular endothelium or inhibition of the tissue plasminogen activator by activated protein C. The worse the quality of the donor liver, the more severe is this fibrinolytic process. Moreover, the lack of production of clotting factors due to poor synthetic function will lead to severe shortage of these factors and increased coagulopathy and bleeding. Although some of these risk factors for diminished graft function can be identified prior to the actual transplant procedure, most of this information comes too late to let the blood bank prepare for an excessive demand for blood products.

Patient related factors, like the type and severity of liver disease and the history of previous abdominal surgery, are known prior to transplantation and therefore can provide an indication about the risk of the patient for excessive blood loss. Pre-operative risk factors that have been analyzed are: the type of liver disease, age of the patient, coagulation profile (prothrombin time, activated partial thromboplastin time (APTT), thrombotest, fibrinogen, platelet count, antithrombin III, and euglobulinlysis time) and history of previous surgery [1-3,5,6]. The type of liver disease, age, and pre-operative serum creatinine level [7] are also considered important risk factors for diminished survival. However, these risk factors are generated by different transplant programs, using different definitions and approaches. Therefore, this information is inconsistent and sometimes contradictory, often due to a relatively small number of patients involved in the analysis.

The blood bank, in order to prepare an adequate stock supply for the individual patient, needs a reliable indication for the expected blood loss based on consistent data. An analysis of a sufficient sample size of patients in one liver transplant program may provide a set of reliable risk factors for blood usage in the individual patient.

Therefore, pre-operative data of 210 patients in whom a liver transplantation was performed were analyzed in relation to per-operative data (Table1).

The 210 patients were transplanted for the following diagnoses: chronic active hepatitis (CAH, n=58), primary biliary cirrhosis (PBC, n=56), primary sclerosing cholangitis (PSC, n=51), acute fulminant hepatitis (AH, n=15) and a rest group of various diagnoses (other, n=30).

For the 210 patients the median usage of RBCs was 15.1 units (range 1-130 units) and of platelets 12 units (range 0-76 units). The difference between the various diagnositic groups was only significant for the

Table 1. Pre- and per-operative data used in the analysis.

Pre-operative data	**Per-operative data**
Diagnosis	Red blood cell usage (units)
Age (years)	Platelet usage (units)
Serum creatinine (mg/dl)	Operating time (min)
Child-Pugh's classification	Preservation time (min)
Childscore 0-16	
Prothrombin time (sec)	
Activated partial thromboplastin time (sec)	
Platelet count × 1000/ml	

Table 2. Diagnosis and the usage of RBCs and platelets.

Diagnosis	n	Usage (units) RBC	(range)	platelets	(range)
CAH	58	19.6	(3-97)	18*	(0-70)
PBC	56	11.6	(1-73)	6*	(0-37)
PSC	51	15.2	(4-130)	12	(0-67)
AH	15	12.8	(6-119)	24	(0-40)
Other	30	17.8	(2-79)	12	(0-37)

* Newman-Keuls test $p<0.05$.

usage of platelets, (the groups CAH versus PBC). No statistical difference was found in the usage of RBCs between the diagnostic groups (Table2).

The wide range of requirements of RBCs and platelets within the various groups suggest that other pre-operative factors than the primary diagnosis of the patient are of more importance. One hundred sixty two of the total of 165 patients with chronic liver disease in the groups (AH, PCB, and PSC) could be stratified according to the child Pugh's criteria (Table3). Independent from the primary diagnosis, the usage of RBCs and platelets increases with the severity of the liver disease (Table4). The blood product requirement in the group Child C is significantly worse than in that of the groups A and B. As the length

Table 3. Child-Pugh's classification.

	Points 1	2	3
Encephalopathy (stage)	0	1-2	3-4
Ascites	0	mild	mod-sev
Bilirubin * mg/dl	<2	2-3	>3.0
Albumen g/dl	>3.5	3.5-2.8	<2.8
Prothrombin time (sec)	<15	15-17	>17
PBC: bilirubin	<4	4-10	>10.0

Table 4. Child-Pugh's classification and the usage of RBCs and platelets.

Child classification	n	Usage (units) RBC		platelets	
A	19	8.5[1]	(3--46)	6	(0-42)
B	97	12.8[1,2]	(1-97)	12[2]	(0-76)
C	46	24.7[2]	(5-130)	19[2]	(0-64)

1. A vs B $p=0.056$
2. B vs C $p<0.001$ Wilcoxon test

Table 5. Pretransplant risk factors in correlation with the usage of RBCs and platelets.

Univariate regression analysis RBC usage		platelet usage	
Childscore	r= 0.30	platelet count	r= –0.30
Prothrombin time	r= 0.31	childscore	r= 0.29
Age	r= 0.29	Prothrombin time	r= 0.20
APTT	r= 0.24	APTT	r= 0.15
Creatinine	r= 0.21	creatinine	r= 0.09
Platelet count	r= –0.14	age	r= 0.06

of the operation (425-440 min) and the duration of preservation (446-458 min) were the same for the three Child classes, these factors did not have an effect on the difference in the usage of blood products.

When the impact of the six factors: Childscore, prothrombin time, APTT, platelet count, age, and creatinine were analyzed, each of these factors had a different impact on the usage of RBCs and platelets. The RBC requirement (Table5) is strongly related to the Childscore, prothrombin time and age of the patient; the APTT and serum creatinine have less impact, while the pre-operative platelet count has no important effect. The platelet requirement is strongly related to the pre-operative platelet count and the Childscore, while the other four factors appear to have less effect. When the quantitative effect of each of these factors was determined, it appeared that a childscore above 9, prothrombin time above 15 seconds, age above 50 years, APTT above 50 seconds, a serum creatinine level above 1.2 mg/dl, and a platelet count less than 100 ? 109/l results in an above medium usage of RBCs and platelets (respectively, 15 and 12 units).

The results from this analysis can be summarized as follows: The type of liver disease itself has hardly any predictive value on the pre-operative requirement of blood products. However, the severity of the disease, Child C class, or Childscore above nine predict strongly the chance of increased usage of RBCs and platelets. Not surprisingly, as the prothrombin time is one of the variables in the Child-Pugh's classification, a prothrombin time above 15 seconds is an important risk factor for increased requirements of blood products. An age above 50 years and, less clearly, an impaired renal function (creatinine above 1.2 mg/dl) lead to increased usage of RBCs, while a platelet count below 100 ? 109/l increases the need for platelet transfusions.

References

1. Bontempo FA, Lewis JH, van Thiel DH, et al. The relation of preoperative coagulation findings to diagnosis, blood usage, and survival in adult liver transplantation. Transplantation 1985;39:532-6.

2. Brems JJ, Hiatt JR, Colonna JO II, et al. Variables influencing the outcome following orthotopic liver transplantation. Arch Surg 1987;122:1109-11.
3. Motschman TL, Taswell HF, Brecher ME, et al. Intraoperative blood loss and patient and graft survival in orthotopic liver transplanation: their relationship to clinical and laboratory data. Mayo Clin Proc 1989;64:346-55.
4. Lewis JH, Bontempo FA, Awad SA, et al. Liver transplantation: Intraoperative changes in coagulation factors in 100 first transplants. Hepatology 1989;9:710-4.
5. Butler P, Israel L, Nusbacher J, Jenkins DE Jr, Starzl TE. Blood transfusion in liver transplantation. Transfusion 1985;25:120-3.
6. Ritter DM, Owen CA, Bowie EJ, et al. Evaluation of preoperative hematology-coagulation screening in liver transplantation. Mayo Clin Proc 1989; 64:216-23.
7. Cuervas-Mons V, Millan I, Gavaler JS, Starzl TE, van Thiel DH. Prognostic value of preoperatively obtained clinical and laboratory data in predicting survival following orthotopic liver transplantation. Hepatology 1986; 6:922-7.

THE USE OF APROTININ IN CARDIOPULMONARY BYPASS AND THE IMPACT ON HEMOSTASIS AND BLOOD TRANSFUSION[1]

W. van Oeveren, Ch.R.H. Wildevuur

Cardiopulmonary bypass (CPB) during open-heart surgery causes massive activation of blood, resulting in an inflammatory reaction. One of the consequences of this activation process is impairment of the per-operative hemostasis. Invariably "oozing" of the wound area is observed, which requires drainage of the thoracic cavity until the first or second postoperative day and most often blood substitution. Oozing is a feature of capillary bleeding, primarily due to an impaired platelet function. Therefore improvement of the CPB circuit has been mainly directed to reduction of platelet damage. These efforts have resulted in the construction of a membrane oxygenator so to replace the bubble oxygenator. Although the platelet aggregatory function could be preserved by using a membrane oxygenator, the postoperative bleeding tendency was still considerable.

A recent approach to inhibit part of the inflammatory reaction by aprotinin appears to be more succesful to preserve hemostasis.

Aprotinin is known as inhibitor of plasmin, kallikrein, trypsin, and to a lesser extent also of other serine proteases. Due to this broad spectrum inhibitory capacity of aprotinin the inflammatory reaction, including complement activation, was thought to be reduced. However, the only apparent favourable effect of aprotinin was seen on hemostasis [1]. Although this effect could have been due to inhibition of fibrinolysis, there were indications that aprotinin preserved platelet function during CPB. First, the capillary bleeding (oozing) from the wound area during cardiac surgery, known to occur by a defect of platelet adhesive function or by a von Willebrand deficiency, appeared to be reduced by aprotinin treatment, despite full heparinization of the patient. Second, a markedly reduce thromboxane release in aprotinin treated patients was measured compared to untreated patients.

1. This work was supported by grants from the Netherlands Heart Foundation and from Bayer AG.

In successive studies we have tried to elucidate the effects of aprotinin on platelets and hemostasis.

First, we could reproduce the observation of the initial small, randomized study on reduced blood loss and blood transfusion by the use of aprotinin in a placebo controlled double blind trial on 80 patients [2]. Interestingly, the largest reduction of blood loss by aprotinin was achieved during surgery. The absolute amount of blood loss in gauzes and the suction system during surgery appeared to be two third of total. Therefore the clear benefit by aprotinin was obtained by reduction of the intraoperative next to the most often studied postoperative bleeding.

We observed furthermore that the platelet release reactions and platelet receptor alterations occurred immediately after the start of CPB [3]. Therefore we compared patients receiving aprotinin only in the prime of the heart-lung machine (2 million KIU) with patients who received in previous studies a high dose aprotinin (6 million units in total) to maintain a continuous high plasma concentration of aprotinin, from the start of anesthesia until the end of CPB. A similar benefit of preserved hemostasis was observed in both groups and most importantly the same protective effect against platelet damage was observed [4,5]. Although commonly the high dose aprotinin is used, directed by the initial observations, we advocate the low dose in the prime, not only for economic reasons, but most of all for safety reasons.

These safety reasons concern a possible hypercoagulability by inhibition of the fibrinolytic system as result of the use of aprotinin. In addition, our in vitro studies show that in the presence of aprotinin thrombin is less effectively inhibited by heparin/ATIII and activated protein C. These findings indicate that during situations of reduced anticoagulation, existing before and after CPB, high concentrations of aprotinin might promote clotting. This could occur particularly when the extrinsic pathway is activated. In contrast the intrinsic clotting system is inhibited by aprotinin already at low heparin concentrations, as shown by the high ACT values [6]. Next to these effects of aprotinin on the clotting system, the effects on platelets might potentially reduce the vein graft patency. However, our results indicate that platelet aggregation, responsible for thrombus formation, is reduced rather than promoted by aprotinin. This effect might be related to the inhibition of thromboxane release by platelets during aprotinin treatment. Furthermore, we found that the combined use of aprotinin and aspirin during CPB inhibits platelet aggregation, while the preservation of platelet adhesive function remains [7]. Aspirin specifically reduces arachidonic acid and collagen induced aggregation and decreases the mean number of GPIIb/IIIa antigen by 50% independent of aprotinin treatment during CPB. However, the protective effect of aprotinin on the platelet adhesive function was not affected by aspirin and blood loss was similarly reduced by aprotinin in aspirin as in non-aspirin treated patients.

Although the mechanism of an improvement of hemostasis by aprotinin is still not fully clarified, we could demonstrate that the platelet GP-Ib receptors are affected by the first pass blood activation which is protected by aprotinin. Since aprotinin is known as an inhibitor of plasmin, which can affect the platelet GPIb receptor, the improved hemostasis could be explained as a secondary effect of plasmin impairment of platelets.

Conclusions

The use of aprotinin in open-heart surgery marks a major step in the reduction of blood loss and consequently blood transfusions. At the same time we have demonstrated that the concept about the main cause of platelet dysfunction during CPB has to be reconsidered. It appears that impairment of the platelet aggregatory function is only of minor importance for the blood loss during and after CPB, whereas the platelet adhesive function is pivotal.

In routine CPB procedures with use of a membrane oxygenator the platelet aggregatory function appeared to remain fully intact, as determined by different methods. This might be in contrast with studies performed in the past in which a bubble oxygenator was used.

It is important to note that aprotinin appeared to improve hemostasis despite the use of aspirin before operation. Since aspirin treatment should preferably start before CPB to optimalize the patency of the vein grafts for coronary bypass, the combination of aspirin and aprotinin can be advocated to meet both criteria of reduced blood loss and improved graft patency rate.

The increased use of aprotinin will decrease blood transfusions after open-heart surgery, because 70% of patients for routine coronary artery bypass surgery could leave the hsopital without transfusion of any blood or blood products. Because the reduction of blood transfusions is most striking in complicated operations, such as reoperations and endocarditis, which usually needs large amounts of blood products, the contribution of aprotinin for blood salvage in CPB is quite considerable and contributes to the safety of cardiac surgery.

Acknowledgements

The work of this review has been accomplished by all authors and co-authors mentioned in the references. Dr. P.H. Mook and J. de Haan are acknowledged for their critical review. Especially we are grateful to the cooperation we obtained in the OLVG, Amsterdam, The Netherlands.

References

1. Van Oeveren W, Jansen NJG, Bidstrup BP, et al. Effects of aprotinin on hemostatic mechanisms during cardiopulmonary bypass. Ann Thorac Surg 1987;44:640-5.
2. Harder MP, van Oeveren W, Roozendaal KJ, Eijsman L, Wildevuur ChRH. Aprotinin reduces intra- and postoperative blood loss in cardiopulmonary bypass, a placebo controlled double blind trial. Ann Thorac Surg 1991;(in press).
3. Van Oeveren W, Eijsman L, Roozendaal KJ, Wildevuur ChRH. Platelet preservation by aprotinin during cardiopulmonary bypass. Lancet 1988;i: 644.
4. Wildevuur ChRH, Eijsman L, Roozendaal KJ, Harder MP, Chang M, Van Oeveren W. Platelet preservation during cardiopulmonary bypass with aprotinin. Eur J Cardio Thorac Surg 1989;3:533-8.
5. Van Oeveren W, Harder MP, Roozendaal KJ, Eijsman L, Wildevuur ChRH. Aprotinin protects platelets against the initial effect of cardiopulmonary bypass. J Thorac Cardiovasc Surg 1990;99:788-97.
6. De Smet AAEA, Chang MNJ, van Oeveren W, et al. Increased anticoagulation during cardiopulmonary bypass by aprotinin. J Thorac Cardiovasc Surg 1990;100:520-7.
7. Tabuchi N, van Oeveren W, Eijsman L, Roozendaal KJ, Gu YJ, Wildevuur ChRH. Preserved hemostasis during the combined use of aprotinin and aspirin in CABG operations. In: Blood use in cardiac surgery, Publ. Symposium Berlin, 1991;(in press).

DISCUSSION

P.M. Mannucci, J.Th.M. de Wolf

J.Ph.H.B. Sybesma (Dordrecht, NL): Prof. Mannucci, are you giving DDAVP in patients to reduce blood loss in big operations, in the same dose as is given in hemophilia or von Willebrand's disease or is it a different dosage?

P.M. Mannucci (Milan, I): The dosage of DDAVP given to patients undergoing surgery to reduce blood loss is the same as is being used in hemophiliacs: 0.3 mg/kg of bodyweight.

J.Th.M. de Wolf (Groningen, NL): May I ask, how many days can you use desmopressin?

P.M. Mannucci: In that specific case I mentioned, desmopressin was given in only one dose before surgery to reduce intraoperative blood loss, which is of course the main period of blood loss. So, I think one dose was justified. In more general terms, if you want to know how many days it can be given, it depends on the clincial situation. We are doing now a study in patients with hemophilia and von Willebrand's disease to see what really are most frequent problems, but we have not yet the answer. Certainly, it can be given to patients that respond, but side-effects have to be considered. Some patients do not respond after two or three infusions.

P. Haeyaert (Destelbergen, B): Prof. Mannucci, in the beginning period the use of DDAVP in von Willebrand and hemophilia A patients was always accompanied by the use of anti-fibrinolytic agents, because of that small fibrinolytic response to DDAVP, which has already been used I think as a test for fibrinolytic response. Is it beneficial to use anti-fibrinolytic agents in combination with DDAVP in hemophilia A and von Willebrand patients?

P.M. Mannucci: The answer for me is a clear cut no. The evidence stems from the study that I presented. These patients undergoing spinal fusion were treated with DDAVP without anti-fibrinolytic agent and yet, the net effect was in favour of hemostasis. So, I think for me that is quite convincing. Additionally I can tell you that we have never used anti-fibrinolytic agents except at the very beginning of our experience with DDAVP. We have carried out many surgical operations in patients with von Willebrand's disease and hemophilia without any anti-fibrinolytic agent. Nevertheless, some people may wish to still use it. This brief effect on fibrinolysis is probably relevant from the point of view of hemostasis.

M. Harvey (Leiden, NL): Dr. Hay, there is increasing evidence that the immunomodulatory effect in some cancers, like in colon cancer, may be related to the presence of mismatches in the DR and the class II HLA complex on cells. Have you ever looked for HLA antigens in concentrate?

C.R.M. Hay (Liverpool, UK): I have not, but Christine Lee and Dr. Kernoff at the Royal Free have.[1] They were able to correlate the degree of immunosuppression in vitro and in vivo with the concentration of β-2 microglobulin which correlates with HLA antigens in the concentrates. So, they probably do circulate to some extent.

T.W. Barrowcliffe (Potters Bar, UK): Dr. Hay, you mentioned some results from our laboratory. It is certainly true that we found that in vitro inhibition of IL-2 secretion was less or non-existent with high purity concentrates. But one of the unexpected findings was also that amongst the intermediate purity concentrates there were quite a lot of differences. There were some concentrates which had relatively little inhibitory activity. What I am wondering is, do you think that it could be one specific or perhaps more than one specific contaminant which could be eliminated or is it simply a question of protein load.

C.R.M. Hay: I increasingly despair of finding one and I really do not know whether it is a single contaminant that is responsible or whether it is just protein load. When all said and done, most studies have only been able to correlate the inhibitory activity with purity, whatever that is and not with anything more specific.

1. Lee CA, Kernoff PBA, Karayiannis P, Waters J, Thomas HC. Abnormal T-lymphocyte subsets in hemophilia: Relation to HLA proteins in plasma products. N Engl J Med 1984;310:1058.

C.Th. Smit Sibinga (Groningen, NL): Prof. Mannucci, in surgical cases at what point in time would you preferably administer desmopressin. Would you do it prophylactically, or would you wait for what is happening at the operation room.

P.M. Mannucci: I think it depends on the situation. If you have an operation like spinal fusion, where because of the nature of the operation, you do expect a lot of blood loss, I would give it prophylactically; that is immediately before surgery starts. But if in a given operation blood loss is expected to be normal, not dangerous, then I would not give it prophylactically and I would give it only if the patient starts to bleed too much. Of course, I want to maintain doing all the screening coagulation tests that are necessary and I would like to be sure that there is no cause left that could be eliminated in the circumstance.

C.Th. Smit Sibinga: It is not really the platform here to discuss that in full length, but a point which for quite obvious reasons you did not mention is the surgeon himself. I think that the need for more meticulous and careful surgery and surgical hemostasis also needs attention. Taking more professional skill and time in comprehending hemostasis actually should be in the training courses of surgeons.

Dr. Hay, Peter Levine showed in his initial studies and mentioned this summer in Washington again, that there is also an obvious defect in hemophilia A patients on a number of immune functions including the skin test as a monitor. When changing the therapeutic regimen to superhigh purity concentrates, these disturbed functions tend to normalize. Could you comment on that. Is there also an effect on the alteration of the B-cell population in converting to the production of the immunoglobulins notable when patients are challenged on a long-term receiving more crude type of products.

C.R.M. Hay: Well, to answer the second question first, because I do not actually know very much about it, there is a great deal of doubt in the literature about the B-cell defect and I have not looked into it, so, I do not know the answer to your question.

Certainly, in all of Dr. Levine's studies he has also shown some improvement in cutaneous anergy in groups of patients treated with superhigh purity factor VIII concentrate, which I did not refer to just through lack of time. In some respect the changes in cutaneous anergy have been statistically a little bit more impressive than the T4's. But on the other hand, even using a standard test, cutaneous anergy is really a rather semiquantitative test, a rather soft endpoint. So, you have to interpret such results with a good deal of caution I think.

C.Th. Smit Sibinga: Yet, on the B-cell side I think one could speculate, on what might occur. When one sees what happens to the T-cells, as you have shown in a number of monitoring systems, the effect on the cytokine production signalling to the B-cell population might therefore certainly lead on the long term to some effects.

L.W. Hoyer (Rockville, MD, USA): First a comment and that is simply to indicate for fairness sake that there is a study, that is been going on with, although small numbers, of HIV-negative hemophilia patients. There was a random assignment either to the more highly purified or the conventional concentrates. My understanding from Joan Gill[2] is that these patient groups in Milwaukee have not shown any significant difference over the first year of study. In fact if anything looked slightly better, it was for the patients receiving the conventional concentrates. So, I think it is a plea for caution here as we look at small numbers. We must not make decisions based on small trends, but we should wait for a really definitive study which is going to be important.

C.R.M. Hay: That is true, there are lots of studies with such a protocol and one cannot refer to them all. Lots of studies, most of them in HIV-positive patients, are mostly quite small. I understand that someone in the Unites States is planning to do a meta-analysis of these studies, [Dr. L. Aledort], so, that they can achieve adequate numbers.

L.W. Hoyer: I would think this is going to be very useful, but we feel we probably are going to get much more important information from the HIV-negative patients. That is even more important.

C.R.M. Hay: I am inclined to agree with you, because there are far fewer variables in the HIV negatives. But, one further reservation I have about these studies is that they may have little hope of showing a change. Ludlam for example has shown that by the time you reach adulthood the abnormalities of T4 numbers are stable.[3] At that point there is no relationship between the degree of reduction of T4's and the treatment intensity. If that is the case, will changing these people with an established abnormality of their immune system to a high purity product make any difference? It may not.

L.W. Hoyer: Of course you need to start as early as possible in the treatment period.

A question to you or the others on the panel: Are you aware of any animal model studies? Perhaps we will really only get the answer to

2. Personal comment.
3. Cuthbert RL, Ludlam CA, Tucker J, et al. 5 Year prospective study of HIV infection in the Edinburgh cohort. Br Med J 1990;301:956-61.

this if we start looking at some animal model in which the comparable proteins of the intermediate concentrates are given and the immunologic parameters are monitored very carefully.

C.R.M. Hay: I do not know of any animal studies.

C. Smit (Amsterdam, NL): Dr. Hay, is there a relation between the immune function in HIV-positive people and the use of drugs for the treatment of full blown AIDS or the early intervention therapy on HIV-positive people with AZT.

C.R.M. Hay: Well, a lot of the early studies showed some probably transient increase in T4's after starting AZT, although that probably depends on how low the T4's are to start with. In most of my patients on AZT, I have not noticed any particular change in T4's, which seem to continue to go down. That is a problem for trials of the sort that I discussed. One of the reasons that they are becoming more and more difficult to conduct is because more and more variables emerge, patient's HIV infection progresses and they need to go on the specific treatment which may have some effect on the endpoint.

S. Elödi (Budapest, H): Dr. Krom you were talking about the red blood cell and platelet requirements of liver transplantation. Would you tell me something about the other blood components, like fibrinogen, because our surgeon insists having prothrombin complex concentrate, fresh frozen plasma, fibrinogen or anything else we have.

R.A.F. Krom (Rochester, MN, USA): Our anesthesiologists are monitoring clotting during the liver transplant with the thromboelastograph. If on the thromboelastogram the R or R plus K is prolonged, then fresh frozen plasma is their choice of treatment. If the maximum amplitude is small first platelets are being given to improve the thromboelastogram. If no effect is noted cryoprecipitate is added. These are basically the three products, of course, that every anesthesiologist uses to manipulate clotting and to restore the thromboelastogram. But, I cannot tell you how much is used in what specific case and actually I believe it is the individual preference of the anesthesiologist. The platelets and the cryoprecipitate are not being transfused when the patient is on the veno-bypass; it is used after recirculation when hemostasis is really wanted. Prior to recirculation usually only FFP is used to maintain adequate coagulation. In general the number of units of RBCs matches the number of units of FFP.

J.A. van der Does ('s-Gravenhage, NL): Dr. Krom, you mentioned that for each patient there has to be a separate stock of blood components. I wonder why.

R.A.F. Krom: Well, I can imagine that the blood bank does want to have some stock in case something happens. If you have an indication that the patient is a low risk for per-operative bleeding the blood bank probably can have less blood in stock than for a patient who is expected to be a high risk. Moreover, some patients have blood group antibodies which might be important to know. Also, a stock of blood products becomes important if one wants to respond to CMV matches. So, yes it is probably very important for the blood bank to know if they need to have to stock a large or a smaller batch for this particular patient.

J.A. van der Does: But then it is only for CMV negative or special request, not for the group as a whole.

R.A.F. Krom: Well again, for a high risk patient our blood bank will stock twice as much as for a low risk patient. If you do not do that, you might be in trouble with a considerable amount of patients especially when other high risk surgery is performed on the same day. The unpredictability of the moment of donor availability and the needed amount of blood products makes it desirable to have more blood products in stock for high risk patients.

C.Th. Smit Sibinga: Actually here in Groningen, as a transplant centre with ten years' experience in liver transplantation, the blood bank is a member of the liver transplant team. As such we are provided weekly and even sometimes more frequently with a total list of potential candidates, those patients who need to be transplanted in a very short period of time. The information includes whether these patients are supposed to be high risk bleeders or not, their ages, whether they are CMV negative and what their blood group is. That means that we could set aside in the specific blood groups what is anticipated to be transfused. It does not matter then whether patients' group is A or B for as long as you have the stock in these blood groups available, because there is only one transplantation done at the time. There may be a second one the next day, but there is only one at the time at the operation table. In principle the stock is rotating. So, that is the way it is really handled.

Dr. Krom, you very nicely showed the relationship to the different criteria. I think that is a most important and valuable piece of information which you did on the analysis since the Mayo Clinics started the liver transplant program. What I noticed, however, separate from the question of the correction of the defect before you start the operation, is that the total consumption of blood, even if I take the range, is half of what we in general still use here in Groningen. Elaborating on your figures, it means that, if we would introduce in a similar fashion the criteria in our centre, there could be reduction of 50% and a saving, specifically on the red cell side, and probably also platelets, at least in the lower risk patients. What is issued now for each transplantation, irrespective of the risk, as a basic amount of red cells is the highest amount you have shown in these regular groups of patients. I am not talking about the disasters, which may come up. I think, that a continuation of the program in the way we do it is not justified. Are there other centres for instance in Pittsburgh or others in the US that apply a similar approach in predicting, by and large, the anticipated blood loss and therefore the transfusion need and what is their experience?

R.A.F. Krom: I do not know by what methods other centres are anticipating per-operative blood loss. In the literature a number of individual risk factors are analyzed, for example, creatinine and age. However, there is a substantial centre specificity in the absolute numbers of required blood products. Patient selection, individual approach by anesthesiologists in handling clotting abnormalities, and surgical teams are three important factors that make a difference from one centre to another. Despite these differences, every centre can analyze the degree of abnormality of various per-operative factors related to the median blood loss in that specific centre. These centre's specific data can direct the supporting blood bank to anticipate the need of blood products for each patient.

C.Th. Smit Sibinga: The second point acutally is: Might there be also a useful additive effect in trying to support these patients also with desmopressin. Probably Prof. Mannucci could add to that.

R.A.F. Krom: We have never used it and we are looking, of course, with curiosity to the effect of aprotinin. It is something that is being considered. Unfortunately, aprotinin is not yet approved by the FDA. But it is obvious that, if aprotinin works as being presented by Dr. van Oeveren, it might be very useful during and after the bypass procedure when we see most of the coagulation problems.

A.M.H.P. van den Besselaar (Leiden, NL): Dr. Krom, you have developed criteria for the prothrombin time and the APTT and you have reported those criteria as clotting time in seconds. Now, that is probably all right within your institute, but you are probably aware that the prothrombin time and the APTT are very much dependent on the reagent and also the instrument that is used for its assessment. While your criteria are all right within your institute, they probably are different in other institutes or hospitals. So, I would advise that you report the prothrombin time and the APTT as a ratio, representing the patient time divided by the mean of your healthy population. That is the first step towards standardization of these overall clotting tests which I would recommend.

R.A.F. Krom: I apologize that I am not aware of the use of ratios for prothrombin time and APTT. I agree that this would give a better standardization of clotting tests. Definitely I should have given the normal values of our institution.

A.M.H.P. van den Besselaar: But for scientific reasons I think it is very important to report the ratio as well, together with the brand names of reagents and instruments.

R.A.F. Krom: I should have put it on the slides.

P.M. Mannucci: The point that is being made is that as Dr. van den Besselaar said this is valid only in you clinic and no general information can be drawn by presenting the data in the way you did, because my prothrombin time could be different from yours. So unfortunately by giving the time in seconds you do not really get the general message. Also within your clinic, it probably would be better to express the resulting ratio, because even if your normal prothrombin time is 11 and even if the reagents are very standardized, there might be one day in which your normal is not 11, but 12. In that day the system functions slightly different and then also the results of the patients are going to be affected. The message should be conveyed to the laboratory.

I wanted to comment on the story of the thromboelastogram. This is a test, rightly or wrongly not being used by the so-called clotters. Even though the test gives overall information on the clotting, platelet and fibrolysis system, the test is not very sensitive. I know that the Pittsburgh group is using it. I think this stands for the fact, that originally they were not in contact with the clotting group. So they had this system that worked very simple and automatically in the operation theatre. They are still using it, and I am puzzled, I do not understand why. I noticed that you also use other screening tests of hemostasis such as the prothrombin time, the APTT and the platelet count. I understand the rationale of using one test that gives a comprehensive information. But then I do not understand why you also use other tests that, put together, would give the same information. So, I am a little bit puzzled by this situation.

R.A.F. Krom: The reason is, I think, very simple. First of all the prothrombin times that I mentioned here are pretransplant values, so it is done on elective situation. The laboratory turn-around time of the prothrombin time and the APTT is about 20 minutes and takes more time than a glance of the anesthesiologist on the piece of paper in the back of the OR. The anesthesiologists have three or four TEG machines running simultaneously providing an almost ongoing view on how the clotting situation evolves. They can respond to that immediately. Probably the main reason why the anesthesiologists like to work with the thromboelastogram is that they have immediate feedback. They can monitor continuously and respond to it immediately.

P.M. Mannucci: Yes, I think you are probably right, that is the reason.

B. Brozovic (London, UK): Dr. Krom, if I may just make a comment. You presented absolutely brilliant results on the use of blood and blood products in US surgery and predictive values of great importance to the providers of blood and blood products. However, that needs a word of caution, based on our experiences in supporting a team which carried out 49 liver transplants. When ever we have a request for liver transplantation, we take into account to provide the maximum possible need and not the median need based on predictions. Because there is no risk factor as far as I know, which can predict or give you an idea whether you are going to deal with a catastrophe. So, in spite of all the predictors we are asked to provide quite large volumes of blood and blood products. If we have not got them in stock and readily available, we either stop the surgery or we take measures to get supply from other centres.

R.A.F. Krom: Of course, one should not prepare for median need of blood products and that is not what my message was. The parameters related to the median need for blood products may help to define patients as low or high risk for per-operative bleeding and if the parameters of a particular patient point to a high-risk situation, the blood bank can prepare itself better for that particular patient. Besides these preoperative parameters one has to deal with unknown donor factors and per-operative situations that lead to increased blood loss like poor graft function and a surgical complication. But when a blood bank is low on blood products for a particular recipient, it might be an advantage to know if this patient can be considered low risk as the decision to go ahead with the procedure might be made more easily. While on the contrary if the patient is high risk, the procedure might be cancelled.

B. Brozovic: Your are absolutely right.

A.C.J.M. Holdrinet (Breda, NL): Dr. van Oeveren, the ultimate question is the patency rate in the patients who are treated with the hemostatic agent you mentioned. Are there controlled studies done?

W. van Oeveren (Groningen, NL): We have not done this study in the most proper way, that is making angiography. Studies are going on in the United States, because it is also connected to the FDA approval required in the States. In the Cleveland Clinic they can handle, I think, 50 patients a week and then it might be feasible in a few years to get results out of such a study, because the most difficult point is that the differences might be so small that you need thousands of patients to get an answer whether the graft patency is affected or not. The less precise studies sofar do not show an increase of clotting tendency, no differences in products generated as a result of occluded grafts. So, the rough screening does not show differences.

C.Th. Smit Sibinga: Dr. van Oeveren, could I congratulate you with this beautiful presentation. I am very pleased that you came back to the issue which we discussed on the platelet vessel wall interaction, a most important aspect which we tend to overlook from the blood banking point of view. What would you recommend in using aprotinin in this specific indication, as they are used more in the surgical field. At what point would you give the dosage and how long would you proceed. I understand that you did the study on two dosages 2 and 6×10^6 units of aprotinin, and came to the conclusion that 2×10^6 was sufficient actually. Is that a single dosage or are you giving it repeatedly, could you tell something about that?

W. van Oeveren: You must realize that the studies are conducted in routine cases, which all have a bypass time of about one to two hours. We do not have experience in very long bypass times. We found that the single dose, one bolus in the pump prime, was sufficient to have the same hemostatic effect as the continuous dose which extends until the end of the operation. As I also showed, at the end of bypass the levels of aprotinin in the single dose might be insufficient to protect and yet these patients do not bleed. So, we think that really the first bypass of blood is doing most harm.

C.Th. Smit Sibinga: I quite agree on that point, because that has been proven also by Wildevuur's department. For instance de Jong and others have shown that the very initital contact of the blood in the extracorporeal circuit causes a tremendous activation and a sharp drop in initial platelet count as well as in the function.[4] If you could prevent that you would be much better off, I quite agree on that. So, you do it already in the prime, that is well understood.

W. van Oeveren: Yes, the prime is prepared in advance. In terms of feasibility it is a great advantage. There is no need of a continuous infusion, or infusion during the anesthetic procedure. In the Netherlands this method is used now in most clinics. You asked whether it would be of advantage to give aprotinin at another timepoint, perhaps later on or a second time. I think there is a danger to give aprotinin at the end

4. De Jong JCF. Cardiopulmonary by-pass. The effect on blood elements in dogs. Academical Thesis University of Groningen. Speciaaldrukkerij Europrint bv Veendam 1983.

of the operation, because whilst one neutralizes heparin, the clotting system is functional again. When fibrinolytic system is strongly inhibitied, I think that could cause problems.

P.M. Mannucci: Yes, but you did show that the drug has an anticoagulant effect!

W. van Oeveren: Yes, we are looking at these effects now. The anticoagulant effect seems to be only on the intrinsic clotting system, not on the extrinsic clotting system. Especially the introduction of catheters in the patient might induce extrinsic clotting and therefore we do not recommend to use aprotinin after the operation.

P.M. Mannucci: Because the drug has been also proposed as an anticoagulant I would suggest you to see what happens. Not only on fragments produced by plasmin, but also on fibrinopeptide A and prothrombin, because I think the effect on the activated coagulation time is very impressive. I think it gives some evidence that it acts as an anticoagulant.

W. van Oeveren: We studied all these fragments, and fibrinopeptide A (FPA) levels for instance are lower in aprotinin treated patients, also thrombin-antithrombin III (TAT) levels are lower. So, there is indeed a suppression of the clotting system. I think the intrinsic clotting is a major activator during these procedures, but we cannot discriminate intrinsic from extrinsic as far as these products are concerned.

R.A.F. Krom: Dr. van Oeveren, you mentioned that even the bypass surgery is being done without any transfusion. But in the liver transplantation, despite the use of aprotinin, we will still have quite a need for transfusion of blood products. Therefore, my first question is, is it essential to treat every batch of platelets with aprotinin? My second question is, when in liver transplantation the graft is damaged or has damaged endothelium, is it worthwhile to put aprotinin in the preservation fluid?

W. van Oeveren: Difficult questions! We have done a cooperative study here in the blood bank to see if we could improve the function of stored platelets by adding aprotinin even during the collection of blood. It did not work; the platelets had the same function during storage as non-treated units. We think in these cases most damage to the platelets was caused by centrifugation and the aggregation that occurs in the pellet of platelets. If you do not protect that, the adhesive function does not play a role. Also the main cause of platelet damage in the cardiac surgery procedure might be fibrinolytic activity on platelets, because the GP-Ib is very sensitive to plasmin degradation. In the patients we have tissue plasminogen activator (tPA) which generates plasmin, which is not in a bloodbag, of course. tPA is generated in liver transplantation. I think the function of platelets should be studied in these patients, but you can as well give the patients aprotinin with the stored platelets. As to the second question on the graft preservation, I think I cannot say a reasonable word about it.

P.M. Mannucci: You studied glycoprotein Ib because of the possibility of bleeding due to action by plasmin and that is probably the rationale as you did explain. But glycoprotein Ib is important in platelet vessel wall interaction, but also IIb-IIIa complex is important. Are you planning to study that as well?

W. van Oeveren: We studied that and we did not see a difference on IIb-IIIa complex during the bypass procedure. Also not on fibrinogen binding to platelets. Therefore, we think that aggregation is of less importance in this hemostatic mechanism.

INDEX

α_1-antitrypsin, 11
α_2-macroglobulin, 11
a-granula, 83
acquired immunodeficiency syndrome (AIDS), 221, 227
activated partial thromboplastin time (APTT), 165, 172, 242
adhesive molecules, 85
affinity chromatography, 99, 103
albumin, 95, 106, 182, 236
albumin monomer, 94
albumin polymers, 94
alloantigen, 227
alloimmunization, 152, 162
aluminium hydroxide gel, 99
analysis of variance, 169
anti-factor VIII monoclonal antibodies, 120
anticoagulant exchange reagent, 50
antithrombin III (ATIII), 10, 11, 47, 98, 178, 179, 180, 242
apheresis machines, 70
aprotinin, 247
artificial medium, 143

B-cell, 227
b-TG release, 69
basement membrane, 85
beta-propiolactone, 98
bio-assay, 165
blood usage, 241, 242
buffy coat (BC), 68

C3a, 70
C4b-binding protein, 187
calcium, 3, 18, 29, 49, 67, 83, 86, 229
cancer, 231
cardiac surgery, 224
cardiopulmonary bypass (CPB), 224, 247
cell-mediated immunity, 227
chaotropic reagent, 95
Child-Pugh's criteria, 243
chromogenic assay, 194
chromogenic method, 172, 182
chromogenic substrate assays, 166
chromogenic substrates, 173
chronic liver disease, 234
citrate, 29, 138
CMV, 141, 227
coagulation factor assays, 165
coagulation proteins, 17
collagen, 85
collagen type I, 86
collagen type III, 86
collagen type VI, 86
collagen type VII, 86
collagen type VIII, 86
complement activation, 70, 247
concentrate standard, 176, 177
conformational transition, 31

corrected count increment (CCI), 159, 160
cryoprecipitate, 34, 49, 96, 107, 193, 220
cryoprecipitation, 39, 96
cryopreservation, 157
cutaneous anergy, 227
cyclic-AMP, 90
cyclic-GMP, 90
cytoadhesins, 87

1-deamino-8-D-arginine vasopressin (DDAVP, desmopressin), 219, 223
dense granula, 83
disappearance rate, 203
double-stage apheresis systems, 71

EBV, 141
EDTA, 138
ELISA crossmatch, 151
endothelial cell derived relaxing factor (EDRF), 89
endotoxin, 89
extrinsic pathway, 3

factor I, 241
factor II, 98
factor IX, 8, 17, 18, 31, 97, 119, 177, 229
factor V, 4, 6, 18, 22, 29
factor VII, 5, 18, 172
factor VII-tissue thromboplastin complex, 31
factor VIII (FVIII), 6, 17, 29, 49, 68, 93, 119, 175, 177, 220, 227, 241
factor VIII coagulant antigen (FVIII:Ag), 177, 195
factor VIII coagulation activity (FVIII:C), 165
factor VIII concentrates, 193
factor VIII deficiency, 219
factor VIII inhibitor, 236
factor VIII/von Willebrand factor, 33
factor X, 18, 31, 98
factor XI, 8, 100
factor XI deficiency, 100
factor XII, 8
factor XIII, 31, 100, 229
factor XIII deficiency, 100
Fc receptor, 227
fibrin adhesive, 99
fibrinogen, 4, 17, 40, 83, 94, 106, 195, 220, 229, 242
fibrinolysis, 187, 241, 247
fibrinopeptides A (FPA), 40, 50
fibronectin, 83, 106, 195, 229
frameshift mutations, 19
FVIII/vWF complex, 103
FVIII:C, 177
FVIII:C half-life, 201

gas permeability, 68
gelfiltration, 109
Gla domain, 31
glycoprotein Ia-IIa, 87
glycoprotein Ibab-IX, 88
glycoprotein Ic-IIa, 87
glycoprotein Icé-IIa, 87
glycoprotein IIb-IIIa (GPIIb-IIIa), 83, 139, 248
glycoprotein IV, 88
GP-Ib, 88, 139
GP-Ib receptors, 249
half-life, 199
half-strength citrate, 34
haptoglobin, 95
HBV, 93, 221
HCV, 93
hemoglobin, 89
hemopexin, 95
hemophilia, 84, 227
hemophilia A, 17, 49, 122, 193, 219
hemophilia B, 17, 122
hemophilic plasma, 183, 199
hemostatic plug, 83
heparin, 7, 32, 49, 98
heparin cofactor II (HCII), 12
hepatitis B, 234

hepatitis C, 234
hepatitis non-A, non-B virus, 221
high molecular weight von Willebrand multimers, 229
HIV, 67, 221, 227
HIV-1, 93
HLA, 141
HLA-matching, 151
HMW multimers, 97
HTLV-I, 141
hypercoagulability, 248
hypotonic shock response, 73

IgA, 195
IgG, 94, 195
IL-2 secretion, 229
IL-2-receptor, 230
immune complexes, 220, 229
immune defects, 227
immune dysfunction, 227
immune function, 227
immune modulation, 93, 229
immuno affinity chromatography (IAC), 99, 103, 221
immuno-affinity purification, 97, 103
immuno-affinity reagent, 95
immunodepleted plasma, 183, 199
immunoglobulin aggregates, 229
immunoglobulins, 220
immunopurification, 120
immunosuppression, 236
in vivo recovery, 196, 197, 198, 199
integrins, 87
inter-a-trypsin inhibitor, 98
interleukin-1, 89
international standard, 176
intrinsic pathway, 3
irradiation, 71
ischemic heart disease, 233

Josso loop, 8
Josso pathway, 31

kallikrein, 10, 247

laminin, 86
Leucams, 87
leukocyte depletion filters, 71
liver cirrhosis, 224
liver transplantation, 241
lymphocyte dysfunction, 227
lymphoma, 233
macrophage function, 233
magnesium, 86
mean platelet volume (MPV), 144, 145
membrane oxygenator, 247
metal-chelate chromatography, 97
MGP140, 139
missense mutations, 19
modified tissue thromboplastin time, 165
molecular defects, 19
monoclonal antibodies (MAbs), 26, 95, 103
monoclonal antibody purification, 180
monocyte dysfunction, 229
monocytes, 227
murine antibodies, 229

n-heptane, 221
NANB hepatitis, 227
neoantigenicity, 122
nidogen, 86
nitric oxide, 89
nonsense mutations, 19

one-stage assay, 181, 194
opportunist infection, 227
osteonectin, 86
oxygen radicle production, 227

parallel line assay, 166
Parvovirus, 236
pasteurization, 96, 221
Pentosan polysulphate, 7
perfusion chambers, 85
phagocytosis, 227
phorbol myristate acetate (PMA), 89

phospholipid interface, 5
photochemicals, 71
plasma standard, 176, 177
plasma volume, 196, 197, 198, 199
plasma-free synthetic medium, 74
plasmapheresis, 34
plasmin, 247
plasminogen activator-inhibitor (PAI), 187
platelet additive solution, 69
platelet adhesion, 88
platelet aggregation, 141
platelet apheresis, 152
platelet concentrates (PC), 67
platelet factor 4 (PF4), 7, 50
platelet function defects, 224
platelet increments, 159
platelet recovery, 159
platelet refractoriness, 67
platelet storage, 90
platelet storage lesion, 138
platelet surface glycoproteins, 70
platelet survival, 159
platelet viability, 67
platelet-rich plasma (PRP), 68
platelet"flip-flop" reaction, 8
pneumonia, 233
point mutations, 24
polymerase chain reactions (PCR), 25
post-operative infection, 233
post-tranfusion platelet recovery, 153
post-transfusion hepatitis, 224
potency ratio (R), 166
pre-dilution, 180
procoagulant activity, 29
prostacyclin, 89
protein C, 10, 18, 31, 98, 178, 187, 241, 248
protein S, 11, 18, 98, 187
proteoglycans, 86
proteolysis, 4
prothrombin, 4, 18
prothrombin complex, 94, 177
prothrombin Metz, 7
prothrombin time, 175, 242
prothrombinase, 31

recombinant DNA (rDNA), 180, 223
recombinant factor IX, 98
recombinant factor VIII (rVIII), 96, 119, 193, 199, 222, 229
recombinant FVIII variants, 120
recombinant human FIX, 119
reference standard, 175
refractoriness, 162
renal graft survival, 232, 233
replacement therapy, 219
ristocetin cofactor activity (vWF:Rcof), 97, 195

scoliosis, 224
Scotts syndrome, 8
serine protease, 31, 247
serotonin, 83
shape change, 72
shear rate, 30, 84
site-directed mutagenesis, 26
slope ratio assay, 166
solvent-detergent, 96
solvent/detergent mixture, 221
SPARC, 86
specific activity, 200, 201, 220, 236
spinal fusion surgery, 224
standardization, 175
sterile docking device, 69
storage pool deficiency, 7
subendothelium, 30
supervised self-treatment, 220
T-cell mitogen responses, 227
T-helper cell, 227
T-helper lymphocytes, 221
T-suppressor cell, 227
temporal drift, 168, 194

tenase, 31
thrombin, 3, 23, 40, 76, 83, 99, 120, 248
thrombin activation, 120
thrombocytopenia, 67, 160, 224
thrombomodulin, 11
thromboplastin, 3, 172
thromboplastin-factor VII complex, 172
thrombosis, 84, 94, 98
thrombospondin, 86
thrombotest, 242
thromboxane release, 247
thrombus, 84
tissue plasminogen activator, 241
trans-hepatomas, 122
transgenic mice, 121
transimmortalization, 121
trypsin, 247
tuberculosis, 234
tumor necrosis factor, 89
two-stage assay, 181
ultraviolet (UV) irradiation, 71
uremia, 224
vasopressin, 223
vessel wall, 83
viral replication, 235
virucidal methods, 221
virus inactivation, 93, 106, 193
virus safety, 93
vitamin K-dependent enzymes, 31
vitamin K-dependent factor, 98
vitamin K-dependent proteins, 17
vitronectin, 83, 86
VLA-2, 87
VLA-5, 87
VLA-6, 87
VLA-proteins, 87
von Willebrand deficiency, 247
von Willebrand disease (vWD), 86, 97, 104, 193, 223, 268
von Willebrand factor (vWF), 22, 30, 83, 94, 97, 104, 105, 120, 177, 193, 221
von Willebrand factor antigen (vWF:Ag), 195

zymogen, 31

DEVELOPMENTS IN HEMATOLOGY AND IMMUNOLOGY

1. H.R. Lijnen, D. Collen and M. Verstraete (eds.): *Synthetic Substrates in Clinical Blood Coagulation Assays.* 1980 ISBN 90-247-2409-0
2. C.Th. Smit Sibinga, P.C. Das and J.O. Forfar (eds.): *Paediatrics and Blood Transfusion.* Proceedings of the 5th Annual Symposium on Blood Transfusion, organized by the Red Cross Bloodbank Groningen-Drenthe, The Netherlands (1980). 1982 ISBN 90-247-2619-0
3. N. Fabris (ed.): *Immunology and Ageing.* 1982 ISBN 90-247-2640-9
4. G. Hornstra: *Dietary Fats, Prostanoids and Arterial Thrombosis.* With an Introductory Chapter by A. Bleakley Chandler. 1982 ISBN 90-247-2667-0
5. C.Th. Smit Sibinga, P.C. Das and J.J. van Loghem (eds.): *Blood Transfusion and Problems of Bleeding.* Proceedings of the 6th Annual Symposium on Blood Transfusion, organized by the Red Cross Bloodbank Groningen-Drenthe (1981). 1982 ISBN 90-247-3058-9
6. J. Dormandy (ed.): *Red Cell Deformability and Filterability.* 1983 ISBN 0-89838-578-4
7. C.Th. Smit Sibinga, P.C. Das and H.F. Taswell (eds.): *Quality Assurance in Blood Banking and Its Clinical Impact.* Proceedings of the 7th Annual Symposium on Blood Transfusion, organized by the Red Cross Bloodbank Groningen-Drenthe (1982). 1984 ISBN 0-89838-618-7
8. A.M.H.P. van den Besselaar, H.R. Gralnick and S.M. Lewis (eds.): *Thromboplastin Calibration and Oral Anticoagulant Control.* 1984 ISBN 0-89838-637-3
9. P. Fondu and O. Thijs (eds.): *Haemostatic Failure in Liver Disease.* 1984 ISBN 0-89838-640-3
10. C.Th. Smit Sibinga, P.C. Das and G. Opelz (eds.): *Transplantation and Blood Transfusion.* Proceedings of the 8th Annual Symposium on Blood Transfusion, organized by the Red Cross Bloodbank Groningen-Drenthe (1983). 1984 ISBN 0-89838-686-1
11. H. Schmid-Schönbein, L.J. Wurzinger and R.E. Zimmerman (eds.): *Enzyme Activation in Blood-perfused Artificial Organs.* 1985 ISBN 0-89838-704-3
12. J. Dormandy (ed.): *Blood Filtration and Blood Cell Deformability.* 1985 ISBN 0-89838-714-0
13. C.Th. Smit Sibinga, P.C. Das and E. Seidl (eds.): *Plasma Fractionation and Blood Transfusion.* Proceedings of the 9th Annual Symposium on Blood Transfusion, organized by the Red Cross Bloodbank Groningen-Drenthe (1984). 1985 ISBN 0-89838-761-2
14. S. Dawids and A. Bantjes (eds.): *Blood Compatible Materials and their Testing.* 1986 ISBN 0-89838-813-9
15. C.Th. Smit Sibinga, P.C. Das and T.J. Greenwalt (eds.): *Future Developments in Blood Banking.* Proceedings of the 10th Annual Symposium on Blood Transfusion, organized by the Red Cross Bloodbank Groningen-Drenthe (1985). 1986 ISBN 0-89838-824-4
16. A. Berlin, J. Dean, M.H. Draper, E.M.B. Smith and F. Spreafico (eds.): *Immunotoxicology.* Proceedings of the International Seminar on the Immunological System as a Target for Toxic Damage – Present Status, Open Problems and Future Perspectives, in collaboration with the UNEP-ILO-WHO IPCS and the Commission of the European Communities. 1987 ISBN 0-89838-843-0

DEVELOPMENTS IN HEMATOLOGY AND IMMUNOLOGY

17. T. Ottenhoff and R. de Vries: *Recognition of M. leprae Antigens*. 1987
ISBN 0-89838-887-2
18. J.-L. Touraine, R.P. Gale and V. Kochupillai (eds.): *Fetal Liver Transplantation*. 1987
ISBN 0-89838-975-5
19. C.Th. Smit Sibinga P.C. Das and C.P. Engelfriet (eds.): *White Cells and Platelets in Blood Transfusion*. Proceedings of the 11th Annual Symposium on Blood Transfusion, organized by the Red Cross Bloodbank Groningen-Drenthe (1986). 1987
ISBN 0-89838-976-3
20. C.F.M. Hendriksen: *Laboratory Animals in Vaccine Production and Control*. 1988
ISBN 0-89838-398-6
21. C.Th. Smit Sibinga, P.C. Das and L.R. Overby (eds.): *Biotechnology in Blood Transfusion*. Proceedings of the 12th Annual Symposium on Blood Transfusion, organized by the Red Cross Bloodbank Groningen-Drenthe (1987). 1988
ISBN 0-89838-404-4
22. C.Th. Smit Sibinga, P.C. Das and C.F. Högman (eds.): *Automation in Blood Transfusion*. Proceedings of the 13th Annual Symposium on Blood Transfusion, organized by the Red Cross Bloodbank Groningen-Drenthe (1988). 1989
ISBN 0-7923-0488-8
23. S. Dawids (ed.): *Polymers: Their Properties and Blood Compatibility*. 1989
ISBN 0-7923-0491-8
24. C.Th. Smit Sibinga, P.C. Das and H.T. Meryman (eds.): *Cryopreservation and Low Temperature Biology in Blood Transfusion*. Proceedings of the 14th Annual Symposium on Blood Transfusion, organized by the Red Cross Bloodbank Groningen-Drenthe (1989). 1990 ISBN 0-7923-0908-1
25. C.Th. Smit Sibinga and L. Kater (eds.): *Advances in Haemapheresis*. Proceedings of the 3rd International Congress of the World Apheresis Association. April 9–12, 1990, Amsterdam, The Netherlands. ISBN 0-7923-1312-7
26. C.Th. Smit Sibinga, P.C. Das and P.M. Mannucci (eds.): *Coagulation and Blood Transfusion*. Proceedings of the Fifteenth Annual Symposium on Blood Transfusion, organized by the Red Cross Bloodbank, Groningen-Drenthe (1990). 1991
ISBN 0-7923-1331-3

KLUWER ACADEMIC PUBLISHERS – DORDRECHT / BOSTON / LONDON

GPSR Compliance

The European Union's (EU) General Product Safety Regulation (GPSR) is a set of rules that requires consumer products to be safe and our obligations to ensure this.

If you have any concerns about our products, you can contact us on ProductSafety@springernature.com

In case Publisher is established outside the EU, the EU authorized representative is:

Springer Nature Customer Service Center GmbH
Europaplatz 3
69115 Heidelberg, Germany

Batch number: 10682323

Printed by Printforce, the Netherlands